Side Effects

With epidemics, the timing is everything.[1]

Laurie Garrett, 2000
BETRAYAL OF TRUST

Side Effects
The story of AIDS in South Africa

Lesley Lawson

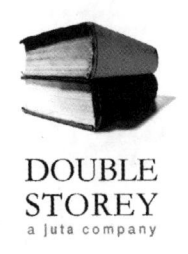

DOUBLE
STOREY
a juta company

First published 2008 by Double Storey Books,
a division of Juta & Co Ltd,
Mercury Crescent, Wetton, Cape Town

© 2008 Lesley Lawson

Editor: Gail Jennings
Cover Designer: John Blignaut, Pulling Rabbits
Typesetter: Ashley Richardson

ISBN: 978-1-77013-067-8

All rights reserved. No part of this publication may be reproduced or transmitted in any form or by any means, electronic or mechanical, including photocopying, recording, or any information storage or retrieval system, without permission in writing from the publisher.

The authors and the publisher have made every effort to obtain permission for and to acknowledge the use of copyright material. Should any infringement of copyright have occurred, please contact the publisher, and every effort will be made to rectify omissions or errors in the event of a reprint or new edition.

Opinions expressed in this book do not necessarily reflect those of the publisher.

Printed by Creda Communications

The story of politics, people and the AIDS epidemic is ultimately a tale of courage as well as cowardice, compassion as well as bigotry, inspiration as well as venality and redemption, as well as despair.

It is a tale that bears telling, so that it will never happen again, to any people, anywhere. [2]

Randy Shilts, 1987
AND THE BAND PLAYED ON

Contents

A note on terminology	8
PROLOGUE:	
1996, *Mashayabhuqe* – AIDS kills everything	9
PART ONE: FERTILE GROUND 1982 TO 1994	**19**
Peter	20
Chapter One: FROM 'GAY PLAGUE' TO 'AFRICAN AIDS'	21
Lucky	34
Chapter Two: THE VIRUS UNDERGROUND	35
Toni	48
Chapter Three: SEX IN THE CITY	49
Shaun	64
Chapter Four: BAD BEHAVIOUR	65
PART TWO: FAULT LINES 1994 TO 1998	**81**
Mercy	82
Chapter Five: FREE AT LAST!	83
Florence	93
Chapter Six: A SONG AND DANCE	94
Mercy	108
Chapter Seven: OF HEARTS AND MINDS	109
Themba	120
Chapter Eight: DRUG WARS	121
Nonhlanhla	134
Chapter Nine: POISONED BARBS	135
Mercy	148
Chapter Ten: 'PILLS COST PENNIES'	149
Nkosi	159
Chapter Eleven: A STATE OF DENIAL	160

Part three: Reason on trial 1998 to 2003 — 175
  Lucky — 176
  Chapter Twelve: Positive lives — 177
  Busi — 190
  Chapter Thirteen: Securing the future — 191
  Lucky — 201
  Chapter Fourteen: Where the truth lies — 202
  Mercy — 218
  Chapter Fifteen: Behold a pale horse — 219
  Busi — 237
  Chapter Sixteen: In the court of public opinion — 238
  Lucky — 252
  Chapter Seventeen: Little white crosses — 253
  Florence — 264
  Chapter Eighteen: The moral economy — 265
Epilogue:
  2005, and the band played on — 277

  Endnotes and References — 283
  Timeline — 324
  Annual Antenatal Survey Results — 330
  Dramatis Personae — 331
  Glossary And Abbreviations — 334
  Sources — 336
  Acknowledgements — 338
  Index — 339

About this book

Today HIV and AIDS affect the lives of all South Africans. The virus has infected over five million people causing an estimated 1 000 deaths a day. But the epidemic has also invaded the body politic, creating new polarities in a society so wounded by the divisions of the past.

This book tells the story of how and why this happened.

Part One, Fertile Ground, investigates the socio-economic and political context that enabled the virus to enter the country, and spread so rapidly in the late 1980s. It also describes the initial strategies that failed to combat the growing epidemic. Part Two, Fault Lines, shows how the response to the disease became so entangled in the politics of political transformation that it put the new liberation government on a collision course with the pharmaceutical industry and civil society organisations. Part Three, Reason on Trial, follows these conflicts to their conclusion in the highest courts of the land. The government's belated commitment to provide antiretroviral drugs in the public sector represents a climax in this narrative, and it is for this reason that the book ends in November 2003. The dénouement — the full story of the rollout of the treatment plan — is a story has been told and retold in the mass media and popular accounts of the day.

Readers will notice that this book favours the now-unpopular term AIDS. In the early days of the epidemic, before HIV was identified, the acronym AIDS was used to describe a range of HIV- and AIDS-related conditions. Later it became more common to use the term HIV/AIDS in order to confirm that these were two separate phenomena: HIV as infection with a virus; and AIDS as the disease syndrome that eventually resulted from this infection. In early 2000 the formulation 'HIV and AIDS' became common usage. While this may be scientifically preferable, used often it makes for uncomfortable reading. For this reason I have chosen to use the term 'AIDS' to describe the epidemic in a generic way. When specifically referring to the virus, I have used the term 'HIV'.

Prologue

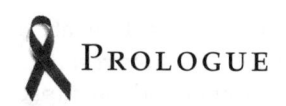

1996, *Mashayabhuqe* – AIDS kills everything

The round room is almost bare. Sizakele sits upright on a narrow bed, a sleeping child upon her lap. Her elderly mother is seated on a mat on the floor, her legs stretched out in the traditional manner. She is also cradling a baby in her arms, and two more toddlers drowse against her side. As Siza tells her story she gently slaps the hand of the sleeping child against her own, as if for emphasis.[3]

'I started losing strength and energy,' she says, 'and I went to the hospital in town, but I was discharged. Then I came back home and attended another hospital. They gave me X-rays, but they said there was nothing wrong. Then they took my blood and they told me I have this disease.'

Her story is punctuated by a cough that tears through her spare frame. Despite her illness she is still quite beautiful. In the background, cows are lowing and birds call above the shouts of distant conversations. In the round room the children snore. Siza's mother sighs. 'It breaks my heart to see my daughter in this condition, and now there is nobody in this family who is working.'

It seems that Siza used to support all the children with her meagre wage. Although her sisters are doing 'piece work' in the towns they seldom send any money home. Now the family must rely on the kindness of neighbours for the occasional dish of food.

The grandmother looks down at the baby and wipes a hand across her face. She knows what is to come. Soon, very soon, she will be the sole carer of all these children.

It is by chance that I am here, in the early summer of 1996, in this hell of hidden death. I am working for a small television company that has been commissioned to make a film about AIDS. The film is to be used to forewarn non-governmental organisations (NGOs) about the coming epidemic and the impact it is likely to have on their beneficiaries, on communities, on civil society at large.

The visit to Siza has been one of our first, and the crew and I are sobered by it: people's lives are already too difficult, and now there is AIDS. It particularly affects our young assistant, who has grown up in the relative privilege of Soweto. Before we leave the homestead he empties his pockets into Siza's hands.

Here, in the rural hinterland of the post-apartheid state, tragedy is layered upon injustice. A century of labour migration has disrupted traditional patterns of life and notions of kith and kin. There are few men in evidence and even fewer young people of working age. Before, these migrants would send money from the factories, the mines and the suburban kitchens to the wives and elderly parents at the rural homestead. But now there is a steady stream of young people returning ill and in need of care themselves. Instead of cash, they bring orphans.

By 1996, this area of KwaZulu-Natal has the highest HIV prevalence in the country, with nearly one-fifth of adults infected. But the epidemic is yet young, and most are unaware of their status. Fewer still are visibly ill.

The country is yet to face the enormity of the coming crisis. So far there have been a few 'AIDS scares', and one major scandal in which the new democratic government was found to have spent a large chunk of the annual AIDS budget on a play with dubious educational messages. The mass media are unconcerned about the mounting epidemic. Indeed, recently *The Star*, one of the country's largest circulation broadsheets, had seen fit to dismiss the whole subject in an editorial concluding that the AIDS epidemic was not going to be as serious as we thought. Instead, it opined, we should direct our energy and resources at clear and present health dangers, like malaria and TB. At the time I had found this an interesting observation — for ten years now a small clique of AIDS experts had been warning that the plague was upon us, but so far it was nowhere to be seen. We had been told that AIDS would hit South Africa with such severity that the hospitals would be unable to cope, and a novel system of home-based care would have to be devised. This was the common talk of the day, and we braced ourselves for the crisis: the people huddled in blankets, dying on street corners. But so far, it had not happened.

My path to Siza's hut had been arduous, involving intensive research and painful soul-searching. One of the first people I had seen was Mary Crewe, the director of the Community AIDS Centre in inner-city Johannesburg. To her I had voiced my doubts about the real extent of the epidemic. In response Mary reached into a file and produced a chart of five years of antenatal HIV survey results. It was the first time I had heard of it. I could see that from the beginning of the survey in 1990, national HIV prevalence had soared from under 1 per cent to over 10 per cent. I was stunned.

'But where is the evidence, the dying people?' I asked.

Crewe responded by saying that the predictions had been based on uncertainty about how long Africans could live with HIV. It was now apparent, she said, that the average person, in Africa as in the north, had six to ten years of healthy life. It's the people infected in 1990 — the under 1 per cent — who are beginning to die at this time.

Turns out the good news is also the bad news. Ten healthy years also means ten years of being able to transmit the virus without realising it. Thus each year the numbers grow in an almost exponential curve.

In time our film team acquires a consultant. Peter Busse has been HIV-positive for eleven years, and open about his status for the last four years. Peter presides over our induction into this secret world with kindliness and patience. He emphasises the importance of distinguishing between HIV and AIDS. Young people who are diagnosed must not be allowed to think that HIV is a death sentence, when they have many healthy years ahead.

In a workshop Peter goes through all the basics, some of which, to my shame, I do not know. For example, when I hear that HIV is present in saliva I wince at the memory of an HIV-positive toddler chewing on my pen, and my mind wanders.

(What happened to that pen? Oh, but I must be OK. I had that HIV test when I bought my house, remember. I never did get the lab results, but I got the insurance, so I must be OK. Slight guilt at this memory... at the time, I knew the corollary was that HIV-positive people could not get insurance, could not buy houses; but I went along with it, without protest. I did, though, challenge the nurse to provide me with pre-test counselling, which was my right by law. She responded aggressively: what do you want that for? The test is routine for anyone buying a house. You haven't got it, you are a decent person, she said.)

In my mental meanderings I miss the next important bit of Peter's spiel where he explained that casual transmission, ie other than via direct exchange of body fluids, has not been proven to occur.

In Peter's workshop we all have stories to tell. It turns out that none of us are as innocent as we would like to have thought.

We may not know the statistics, but the epidemic has been hovering just outside our field of vision for so many years and we have turned our heads away. 'Close your eyes,' says Peter, 'think of the person you hold most dear. Can you see his face, can you hear her laugh? Now I want you to imagine that that person has HIV. How do you feel?'

As part of the film research, I make contact with a range of organisations and support groups for people living with HIV and AIDS in Johannesburg. They are not easy to find — no names advertising their presence in office blocks, no signs on the doors. It is like the underground world of the apartheid years — informal groups working for a common cause, virtually unfunded. And in secret.

At *Friends for Life*, which runs a buddy scheme for 60 HIV-positive people in the city, I learn why this is so. I hear stories of sick people thrown out of parental homes, women beaten by their husbands (who had infected them in the first place), people being made to eat off separate plates in separate rooms, mothers parted from their children. The immense stigma and vengeful discrimination has already set up a vicious circle of secrecy and ignorance that seems impossible to break.

The time of my appointment at *Friends* has been very carefully arranged so that I will not meet any of its members. Chris and Mark, the two men who run the project, tell me that every film they have ever seen about AIDS has insulted and offended them with images of wasting, dementia and open sores. That is not the reality of HIV and it is counterproductive, they say. People think: 'I am not like that, therefore I am not infected, and neither is anyone else I know.'

'I call HIV/AIDS "the other people's disease",' says Chris. 'It's time to tell the truth. HIV-positive people are just like everyone else.'

It's a hard one. I put it to them that a film that portrays people living positively with HIV is unlikely to shake us up. Why should we change our behaviour if being HIV-positive seems OK? This is so clearly not the right thing to say, but Mark and Chris tolerate my comments and we chew through this dialectic until it's time for me to go. The biggest problem with filming here is that few of the members are open about their HIV status. Confidentiality, in the context of film, means an absence of all evidence.

This was to be an ongoing problem for the film research. Across the country I meet dozens of people living with HIV, but the vast majority of them have very good reasons to keep their identities secret. Many had not even disclosed to their families, friends and employers out of fear of losing the love and support they would need to survive.

Back home I spend my spare time reading mounds of literature. It is the World Bank projections that make me cry. All our hard-won gains are to be washed away in this tidal wave of distress. When I broach the subject with friends and acquaintances in the NGO sector and government jobs I am rebuffed. They resent me for disturbing their peace of mind. They shock me with their determination not to hear the truth. Why are you always going on about AIDS, they ask? Why don't you talk about TB, or malnutrition, or any number of other diseases? We haven't managed to beat poverty yet, they say, and here you are presenting us with another intractable problem.

Most often they remind me that they are engaged in the reconstruction of the country, in righting apartheid's wrongs, in redressing inequality, in fighting racism, providing for basic needs. How can they be asked to dilute their energies with a hypothetical problem?

I take to carrying around the HIV prevalence graph for them to see what lies ahead, but they are not convinced. This whole period recalls the early 1970s when, as a young adult, I tried to talk to my mother's friends about apartheid. Like then, I feel as if I am in a parallel universe.

I am particularly disturbed by one comment from a friend that links 'this new obsession' of mine with my unhappy childhood. Yet, I have to concede that there is some truth in it. My father died a painful and protracted death in full view of the family, without the 'C word' being said aloud. Though I was only

11 years old at the time I have always felt implicated. Perhaps my whole political life has been one of infinite reparation.

In the end I resist what I feel is a reductionist view. Back in the 1970s my mother's friends, no doubt, felt the same about my abnormal concern for human rights. If it is only the damaged and the doubtful who can take these things to heart, then what hope for humanity?

Inevitably my research leads me to the battered office door of paediatrician Dr Neil McKerrow, at Edendale Hospital in KwaZulu-Natal province. I have been here before. While writing a story about adoption I had stumbled upon the amazing story of Pietermaritzburg's abandoned babies. The aftermath of the bloody civil war between the Inkatha Freedom Party and the African National Congress seemed somehow to have created great swathes of abandoned babies and children in the area. This was a new phenomenon, as in African culture the extended family has always cared for orphans. *Ubuntu*, the humanistic culture of Africa, tells us that to be human is to be part of a community. In this culture, all children are the children of all adults; and all adults are the parents of all children.

McKerrow and his colleagues had done their research and discovered that, far from this tradition breaking down, communities surrounding Pietermaritzburg were almost saturated with 'surplus' children. Nearly one-third of families were hosting children not their own — children of parents who had fled the hit squads, been killed in the fighting, or simply disappeared. When families and neighbours could absorb no more, the children found themselves on the street. At the time of my first visit to this hospital in 1995, there were at least a dozen children living permanently in the wards.

Though the root cause was the political conflict, a new problem was worming its way into this crisis. HIV.

One year on, the situation has deteriorated further. Not only are there increasing numbers of orphaned and abandoned babies, but McKerrow's wards are filling up with dying children for whom there is no cure. Their immature immune systems mean that they are the first in the family to show the symptoms of AIDS. One stick-thin girl of about seven years of age is stretched out motionless, tubes in her nose. McKerrow comments that they are just trying to stabilise her condition so that they can send her home to die.

It is clear that children are on the frontline of the epidemic, both in terms of the illness and its social consequences. McKerrow talks about a home he visits in the valley where a 12-year-old cares tenderly for his dying father, scratching his father's inflamed skin to ease the agonising itch. From McKerrow's perspective, as a paediatrician of long standing, the fact that AIDS targets adults of child-bearing age makes it the most serious illness that he has ever encountered.

Various organisations in the city are desperately trying to place children in homes in the local community, and when that fails, in white adoptive homes. Child Welfare is one of these. Social workers in their inner-city offices exude an air of burnout, hysteria even.

'I look out the window and I watch the women passing,' one social worker says. 'I know that one in five is infected with HIV, and if we can't even deal with the orphans today, how is it going to be in ten years' time?' He is still reeling from an earlier encounter with an HIV-positive mother who had come to see him, simply to ask: Will you look after my baby when I die?

His despair is common among those who work with young people for whom there is no hope. One counsellor I meet simply calls it 'the sadness'.

Though the child protection agencies in Pietermaritzburg are in turmoil, other NGOs are seemingly oblivious. Just across the road I visit an organisation providing educational support to out-of-school learners, whose staff will be part of the audience for this film. No, they haven't encountered HIV or AIDS. Nobody in their programme is affected. It is not a priority.

The squatter camps in the green rolling hills of the Midlands tell a more nuanced tale. Here ordinary people are slowly coming to acknowledge and understand this new threat.

'My husband comes in late every night,' says one plump, ageing wife. 'He is drunk and I know he has been round and about with many women. Then he wants to have sex with me. What can I do?'

This is countered by the men. We all know who the culprits are, they say — those women who drink and force us to have sex without a condom.

Everybody laughs. But one youth is not so amused. As the discussion about AIDS continues, he becomes increasingly agitated. 'You mean to tell me there are no signs of this virus? I could have this disease without knowing it?'

Everybody in the room knows somebody who has died. Though they may say it's from TB or pneumonia, it is young people who are dying and this is something new.

'It is going to kill us all,' says one old woman. Another nods. 'Like the death squads. We use the same name for this disease as we used for them — *mashayabhuqe*'.

Across the land, in this year of 1996, communities are in varying stages of adjustment to the new crisis. There is denial and anger; depression, despair and the grief of acceptance. The five stages of accommodation to dying, described by psychologist Elisabeth Kübler Ross, come readily to mind.

On the dusty road that leads away from Sizakele's house, our assistant realises we have left something behind, and so we return. Hearing our van pull up, Siza runs out of her hut, looking frantic. She is still clutching the crumpled notes he had given her. She thinks he's changed his mind, and wants the money back. It is less than R20.

We continue our journey through the Valley of a Thousand Hills to the village of Ndwedwe. Here we hope to meet a group of women that has been adopting Pietermaritzburg's abandoned babies. By now there are at least a dozen people in the van. Two women who live in Ndwedwe are in the front, directing — 'left', 'right', 'left', they point the way. There are no signs, and the crevassed, dirt road seems to wind impossibly around every single one of those thousand hills. The shadows are lengthening and there are voices in my head saying that this is all folly.

We are brought to a sudden halt on the brow of a steep hill. Way up top there is a row of mud houses, clinging precariously to the red earth. We extract ourselves from the van in time to be greeted by a line of ululating Zulu women dancing down the narrow path. They are momentarily dismayed when the guide explains our mission, but soon recover their pleasure in the occasion. It seems that, at first, they had thought we had brought a whole vanload of fresh babies for their care.

We meet three women from the Nzama family — all apparently married to the same man who is a migrant worker on the mines. Surprisingly, all three wives discovered in their youth that they were infertile. But now great joy has come into their lives in the form of these much-adored foundlings from the city.

'If I could show with my body how happy I am, I would be huge,' says Gertrude Nzama. 'My heart is filled with pure joy because of this child of mine.'[4]

The women are motivated by compassion, as much as their own need. 'Even if you have a mother and you lose her, it is sad,' says Ntombizakhona Nzama. 'But it is too sad to be an orphan before you have even had a chance to say "ma".'

Only one of these children is HIV positive; though at her young age this may just be a measure of her birth mother's HIV status. This child has been allotted to the eldest wife. As Pendulike Nzama cradles her baby, she tells us: 'Women shouldn't be afraid to adopt a child with HIV, because there are so many diseases on earth. Any child may be born with a disease from the mother that may or may not be cured. So you shouldn't just take the child who is well and leave the sick one. You should take care of it.'

In the years that follow, during which I try to grapple with an understanding my country's crisis, I return again and again to the memory of the good women of Ndwedwe and their message of *ubuntu*. For, if there is any solution for this tragedy, it is they, and people like them, who will lead the way.

PART ONE

FERTILE GROUND
1982 TO 1994

Nobody can be quite sure when, or where, the story of AIDS in South Africa began.

Some would date it from the highly publicised diagnosis of two local airline stewards in mid 1982. Others might say that the key narrative began some years later, with the emergence of HIV on the mines and in the black townships.

Yet others argue that the story began way back, long before the virus even skipped the species barrier into humankind. They would want to trace the forces that shaped and moulded this land and its people to be uniquely receptive to the new disease.

Peter

It is an evening in late 1985 and Peter Busse is driving alone through the Transvaal lowveld. He can't stop thinking about his recent appointment with the doctor, replaying it over and over in his mind. He keeps seeing the lines of the graph his doctor had drawn to illustrate his condition: his prognosis, a thick black line that just keeps on going down...

Peter was one of the first people in Swaziland to take an HIV test. Earlier in the year a doctor friend had offered to try out this new test on him, and out of curiosity he had agreed. The result was negative. Then something changed at home, something almost intangible, but it made him uneasy about his relationship with his partner, John. Six months later he took the test again. This time it was positive.

'It threw my doctor into a tizzy,' he says, 'because it was a completely new disease. She said, "I think you better... go to the South African Institute for Medical Research to get the disease explained." So it was a matter of getting in the car and driving across to South Africa.'

Until these events, Peter, like most of his friends, had felt invulnerable to the new disease. AIDS was for Americans, he thought, or for promiscuous people. And he was neither. 'What does promiscuous mean anyway?' he asks. 'Very few of us would use that label for ourselves. It's only for people who have more sex than you.'

But now he was returning home with a positive diagnosis. 'This was very new. This was a disease you were reading about in Time *magazine, and now you had it. You felt as if you were the only one. And it was so grand and mysterious that you had to drive from one country to the next to find out about it.'*

Beneath his confusion lurked a deeper pain. 'It was very problematic. On the one hand it was this medical thing, and on the other it was so tied in with John's relationship with me and having evidence of him being unfaithful. I can remember driving from Swaziland thinking: this is a physical illness, but it's so much to do with trust, communication, relationships, social issues... you know at that point I realised fully and clearly that this disease will never be managed by doctors alone. There's too much other stuff in it.'

During the long journey that evening nothing seemed quite real... the beautiful colours in the long grass, being alone with his thoughts in the car, thinking about John, about deception and betrayal. 'I had a lot of issues about abandonment...' he says, 'in my fantasy I always ended up dying in a Yeoville gutter with nobody around.'[5]

CHAPTER ONE

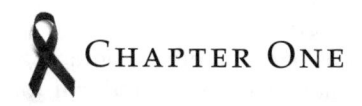

From 'gay plague' to 'African AIDS'

ISOLATED CASES

In early 1983 the first known South African deaths from AIDS made the headlines. Variously known as 'GRID' (gay-related immunodeficiency disease), the 'gay cancer' or the 'gay plague', AIDS had arrived, and it was here to stay.

The National Party government of the day reassured its people that the general population was not in danger. Senior officials in the Department of Health implied that the virus could only be transmitted sexually between homosexuals, or via the needles of drug users. They suggested that the first two gay South Africans who had died may just have been 'isolated cases'.

But their optimism was ill-founded. By the end of 1983 there had been another four cases of AIDS.[6] Doctors treating these men realised that the disease threatened to decimate South Africa's gay community, just as it was doing in the United States, where nearly half of those diagnosed had already died. It was just two years since the disease had been identified in the northern hemisphere, but aided by close friendship networks in the gay community and ease of international air travel, the new disease had found its way across the world.[7]

In South Africa, as in the United States, the response to the disease was initially left up to gay men to organise. Dr Denis Sifris was a member of a Johannesburg group that tried to set up a prevention programme in those early days. He recalls how they put together a budget of R20 000 and approached the Department of Health with a detailed proposal. An official listened patiently, and when they were done he replied, 'AIDS is not a problem in this country. TB is a problem in this country.'

The attitude of Sifris's peers was hardly more encouraging. When he visited gay clubs to promote prevention and call for volunteers for his programme, he was met with deep suspicion. 'You would have thought I was giving everybody AIDS,' he says, 'because people just spread away from me. They were scared and there was denialism: "We don't want to know about condoms... We don't want to know about safer sex... You are spoiling the party."'

The root of the government's reluctance to fund prevention programmes was revealed when the director-general of health, Coen Slabber, reportedly told the press: 'Homosexuality is not accepted by the majority of the population and certainly not by the Afrikaans-speaking population. To advocate that homosexuals use the condom is therefore very difficult.'[8]

He confirmed that the government was not planning to provide any assistance to those affected, as it was the homosexual community's 'own affair'.

'Own affairs' was the term used at the time by the apartheid government to describe policies specific to racially delineated population groups. Thus, by sleight of hand, the government had not only dismissed HIV and AIDS as unimportant, but had created a new ethnicity, the gay man, with its own speciality disease.

In 1980s South Africa, gay men lived in the shadow of the law.[9] Male-to-male sex was included in the catalogue of sexual acts that transgressed the social boundaries of that time and place, although men who had sex with men were seldom prosecuted. The Sexual Offences Act (Act 23 of 1957) even went so far as to criminalise any act designed to 'stimulate sexual passion' between men. Over the years this had been subjected to varying interpretations, including the suggestion that one could break the law by winking across a crowded room. Even during the dying days of apartheid, when the prohibitions against cross-race sex were lifted, gay sex remained outlawed. A government commission in the late 1980s classed homosexuality as a 'serious social deviation', and one of a range of evils that preyed on South Africa's youth.

In the general population, growing fear about AIDS was intimately bound up with homophobic sentiments. The numbers tell it all: one survey found that nearly three-quarters of Cape Town residents thought that homosexuality was morally wrong;

another survey showed that eight out of ten black university students believed that most gay men and women had AIDS.[10]

Even before the era of AIDS, being black and gay was a major challenge. Gay political activist Simon Nkoli wrote movingly about his experience when his mother took him to a string of sangomas to have the 'sickness' spirited out of him. She only relented after his lover's mother paid to send them both to a psychologist — who also turned out to be gay. Nkoli commented: 'My mother said "Then I have failed. If that educated man is gay, it seems like everybody is gay!"'[11]

Later, when Nkoli was one of 22 people accused of high treason against the apartheid state, he had to fight a long battle to win acceptance for his gender orientation. Initially some of his comrades even demanded a separate trial, saying they would not 'stand accused with a homosexual man'.

Signing the death certificates

In an environment hostile to both human rights and public health, the virus flourished. Sifris and his peers lobbied for a dedicated clinic to treat the growing numbers of sick and frightened gay men. Eventually this was okayed by the head of medicine at the Johannesburg General Hospital. Sifris was charged with setting it up, although he was only a general practitioner at the time. Later he was joined by other concerned doctors, including immunologist Dr Reuben Sher, who was based at the South African Institute for Medical Research (SAIMR). Together they interviewed and examined about 200 gay men and took their blood. Two years later, when the first HIV test became available, they went back and tested the samples. They found that 11 per cent were already HIV positive. But without medication there was little that could be done.

'In those days,' says Sher, 'doctors were just signers of death certificates.'

All the doctors who worked in the AIDS clinic at the Johannesburg General Hospital were volunteers (a situation that continued until 2002), and they had very little support from the hospital. Dr Clive Evian, who has worked at the clinic since 1989, says 'Even to this day it has never attained the status of a specialised clinic where you have a professor in charge. Most people who work there are community doctors, junior doctors.

There is rarely anyone specialised around.'

Despite their reluctance to engage with the issue, the government set up a technical advisory group on HIV and AIDS. Sher was asked to serve on it, but Sifris was excluded, although he was the director of the only AIDS clinic in the country.

When Sifris asked to join, he was told it would create problems, because then they would have to have a representative from every special-interest group. 'They would have to have a prostitute, and God forbid, a black person,' says Sifris. 'I said, "Look I'll bring my own coffee cups and things if you are worried," but I wasn't allowed, because I was gay.'

By the end of 1985, Sher, Sifris and others had also established an AIDS Testing and Information Centre at the SAIMR. It was housed in a faded Herbert Baker building on the edge of the inner-city Johannesburg suburb of Hillbrow. Although there were no medication, no counselling to speak of, no educational materials and no support group structure, the centre did provide a haven of sorts for the newly diagnosed.

It was here that Peter Busse came for information and support after his diagnosis in 1985. 'The key thing for me was the smallness of it,' says Busse. 'It was the only place in the country that was dealing with HIV, and it was one little room. It was incredibly isolated and you felt very scared.'

In those early days homophobia and fear of AIDS were prevalent in the medical system. In Durban the blood transfusion services put up a sign that read: 'If you are a *moffie* or have had sex with a *moffie* we don't want your blood.' When people objected, the authorities refused to change it, saying, 'That's the only language people understand.'

On Christmas Eve in 1986, 21-year-old Shaun Mellors experienced these attitudes first-hand after he collapsed at work and was rushed to the casualty department at the Johannesburg General Hospital. The attending doctor felt for swollen glands and asked if he was gay.

'I thought it was my opportunity to give a forceful, empowering "Yes",' says Mellors, 'and she looked a bit shocked. She came back a few minutes later and said, "Young man I am sorry to tell you, but you have AIDS and you have six months to live".

'I still remember… the clock on the other side of the wall — it had just gone ten past four in the afternoon.'

Mellors was admitted into an isolation ward that had biohazard stickers on the door. Everybody who entered, including his parents, was dressed in full body protection, and everything that went out — the used linen, cutlery, etc — was sealed in plastic bags. Ten days later he was discharged and sent to the SAIMR for a confirmatory blood test.

At the time, full barrier nursing was the global norm. Sifris and his group had long argued against it. Not only was it frightening for the patients and unnecessary for the medical personnel, but it threatened confidentiality. They would go into the wards and take off their masks, gowns and gloves, then hug and feed their ill and dying friends.

While this scary new disease stalked the hospital wards, outside the townships were burning. Although AIDS seemed remote from the turmoil of township uprisings and police brutality, AIDS-phobia percolated quietly through the political terrain. In a peculiarly South African mix, homophobic sentiments and AIDS were principal ingredients in a savage state campaign against South Africa's first gay conscientious objector. Dr Ivan Toms had been involved in AIDS education in his community since early 1983. He was also a medical doctor, working at a clinic in Crossroads squatter camp in Cape Town. After witnessing the actions of the police in the township, Toms's Christian conscience was roused and he decided not to complete his army service. Instead, he became an active member of the End Conscription Campaign.

The dirty tricks began after he participated in a three-week fast in Cape Town's Anglican Cathedral to protest against the presence of troops in the townships. Posters appeared all over Cape Town declaring 'Toms is a fairy', 'Toms — AIDS test positive'. His car was spray-painted with the words 'Moffie Pig' and graffiti appeared on the wall saying 'SACLA gives AIDS'. (SACLA was the acronym for the name of the clinic where Toms worked.)

'African AIDS'

Although it was predominantly gay men in affluent societies across the world who were dying, it soon became clear that there was another distinctive pattern to the disease.[12]

In the early 1980s, African men and women with symptoms of

HIV infection began appearing in the medical wards of European hospitals. Many were students and immigrants from countries in Central and East Africa. At the same time, African doctors working in hospitals in Uganda, Zaire and other countries in the region were discovering patients with symptoms remarkably similar to those described by North American AIDS researchers. The fact that there were women as well as men with the disease suggested that it was being heterosexually transmitted.

Dr David Serwadda was one of the African doctors who first identified the virus in Uganda. A young research fellow at the Uganda Cancer Research Institute in 1983, he read the description of AIDS given by US doctors and realised that two of his patients had many of the same symptoms. On his next ward round he examined them carefully, and felt even more certain. The big question was — was it something new?

Serwadda went to the library to examine the historical records, poring over hundreds of entries. He even read the early case notes of medical missionary doctor Albert Cook, but found nothing describing what he had seen. It was definitely a new phenomenon.

Over the months, the number of likely cases increased, but there was no way to be certain. In April 1984, while he was eating his lunch in a restaurant, Serwadda was flicking through *Newsweek*. He came across an article that described the new test for the virus. It gave him an idea. He sent 23 of his samples to a colleague at Porton Down, a military facility in England. Months later, he received a letter to confirm that four of them had tested HIV positive. 'I was so excited,' he says, 'though in retrospect, I should have mourned.'

Around the same time a team from the US Centers for Disease Control (CDC) went to Uganda to conduct their own research, and a team of Belgian virologists visited Zaire. They identified dozens of cases.

It was official: from Kinshasa to Kampala, HIV was spreading across Africa and it seemed certain that it could be heterosexually transmitted. Until now, it had been thought that it was mainly gay men and injecting drug users who were at risk, but now the picture was drastically altered.

The prospect of a heterosexual epidemic created panic in the rich countries of the northern hemisphere. Now that everyone was at risk, the AIDS issue emerged from the 'gay ghetto' to take the headlines of international print and broadcast media.

Sensational reporting painted a dramatic picture of 'AIDS victims' in 'darkest Africa'. In a typical piece, over images of funerals and dying people, the New York-based ABC Nightline[13] presenter's voice rang out: 'There is an epidemic of AIDS in Africa and it will have a direct effect on us...'.

But along with the threatening news of heterosexual transmission, there was also a growing sense that AIDS was somehow intrinsically linked with Africa, and 'African-ness'. Reporters wondered aloud if the source of AIDS was not one and the same as the source of the Nile. Comments and speculation about the nature of African sexual mores were common, both in the international media and the scientific community.

The growing epidemic in Africa was a hot topic at the first international AIDS conference that was held in Atlanta, US, in 1985. Because of the similarity of HIV to viruses commonly found in African primates, scientists had proposed that HIV had originated in these animals and skipped the species barrier to humankind.[14] Although elements of this theory were incorrect, the primate origins of HIV have now been confirmed by exhaustive research.[15] Today it is thought that HIV skipped the species barrier when the wounds of a hunter were infected with blood from a primate with the animal form of the virus.

But in 1985, the animal origin of HIV was just a hypothesis, a hypothesis which was seriously misunderstood by many parties. Because HIV was known as a sexually transmitted disease, many thought that it was being implied that it had been sexually transmitted from animals to humans. Journalists at the conference approached African doctors with the question: 'Do Africans have sex with monkeys?'[16] Other bizarre explanations were advanced for how the animal virus may have entered the human body, including the idea that parents gave dead monkeys to their children to play with[17], or that lovers injected monkey blood into the groin, for added stimulation. These theories were understandably offensive to Africans and other clear-thinking individuals.

Even serious broadsheets gave the African epidemic unusual treatment. One example is this lead paragraph of the English *Guardian*'s first major story on AIDS in Africa[18], which compared African women to beasts of the savannah, preying on innocent white flesh:

'The best time to observe the Nairobi hooker is at dusk when the tropical sun dips beneath the Rift Valley and silhouettes the thorn trees against the African skyline. It is then that the hooker preens itself and emerges to stalk its prey: The *wazungu* (white person). The hookers head for the city's hotels, bars and nightclubs where they know they will find herds of *wazungu* — white men looking for fun and with money to burn.'

Just one year after the virus had been named and identified, the discourse around HIV and AIDS had become infused with the prejudices of the day. The notion that ordinary people could be at risk by doing the ordinary things that ordinary people do, was far from the public mind. People living with HIV have long objected that the media portrays them as guilty, deserving victims. In the words of epidemiologist Charles Rosenberg, 'affliction implies prior transgression'.[19] This tendency in the response to epidemic diseases throughout history was much amplified with AIDS, a disease associating sex and death.

First gay men, and now Africans — already isolated by their 'otherness' — were blamed for the new disease. And in the process, the disease acquired a greater stigma. Scientists and the mass media alike began to speak as if HIV, when heterosexually transmitted, was a separate disease. 'African AIDS' was born.

Racism and denial

By the late 1980s it was clear that there were growing epidemics of HIV among heterosexuals in many African countries, but elsewhere the virus was largely confined to the gay community and injecting drug users. In many quarters, uneasiness about the disease was mounting: Africanists were suspicious of the affinity between the virus and 'Africanness'. They felt that journalists had regressed to racialised descriptions of illness and poverty that would have been at home in the Victorian era. In their influential 1987 book, *AIDS, Africa and Racism*, Richard and Rosalind Chirimuuta drew the inevitable conclusion:

'The depth to which racist ideology has penetrated the Western psyche remains profound. The association of black people with dirt, disease, ignorance and an animal-like sexual promiscuity has in no sense been eradicated. When a new and deadly sexually transmitted disease... emerged in the United States this decade, it was almost inevitable that black people would be associated with its origin and transmission.'

The origin of the virus in Africa became a particularly

inflamed topic. Critics asked why a disease that had first been noted in America was being attributed to Africa. Their suspicions were that it was racism rather than scientific evidence that explained the passage of the virus from the south to north.

Members of the African medical community also reacted with indignation. After the first symposium on AIDS in Africa in 1986 [20], representatives of 15 African countries issued their own communiqué distancing themselves from the accepted version of African origins. They said that there was no conclusive evidence for the theory, and called instead for measures to improve blood safety and the reliability of the HIV test.

Indignation turned to disbelief when early reports suggested that the new disease had already engulfed the entire subcontinent, and one-fifth of adults in many African cities were infected. Later improvements in the reliability of HIV-testing technology showed that many of these early estimates had been wildly inaccurate — false positives and over-diagnosis had been the order of the day.[21]

But it was more than just an ideological battleground. Northern countries began introducing mandatory testing for African immigrants. The scaremongering also affected tourism, damaging the economies of African countries. In response, African governments began clamping down on information about HIV, and some even rejected help from the World Health Organisation's new AIDS prevention programme.[22]

'People from the South were in denial,' says Serwadda. 'Mentally they felt it was a white, male, homosexual disease. They felt this disease could not be in Africa so soon. To exacerbate this, in Uganda the AIDS researchers were all young and the older consultants were sceptical of them.'[23]

The outraged response of African commentators to what they saw as rank racism was to have lasting and tragic consequences. Instead of reforming the discourse and science around HIV, anger and defensiveness led to rejection of the very idea that AIDS was a new disease, or that HIV caused it. AIDS denialism [24] was born.

African denialists, or dissidents, as they preferred to be known, reserved their greatest scorn for the theory that HIV might have crossed the species barrier from primates to humans in Africa. To them this theory, which advances in genetics have now confirmed, was the product of racial thinking. The nature of the reporting and the distorted understanding of sexual transmission must have contributed a great deal to these suspicions. However, it is worth noting that since then several new infectious diseases (such as SARS and avian flu) have been attributed to animal origins without controversy.

If the international response to the early AIDS epidemic could be so distorted by racialised thinking, the prospects for a South African heterosexual epidemic were chilling. For a country where race determined identity and life itself, the portent could hardly have been worse.

Alongside, and reinforcing African denialism, a group of American and European scientists and writers began to espouse an alternative AIDS paradigm. They rejected orthodox theories that AIDS was caused by the virus HIV, and contested the idea that AIDS was a novel disease in both character and scale. Some argued that the disease and death witnessed among gay Americans was caused by their libertine sexual and drug habits. In Africa, they said, immune deficiency was a result of diseases of poverty like tuberculosis and parasite infestation.

The denialist position was given credibility by eminent scientists, such as internationally renowned retrovirologist Professor Peter Duesberg and Nobel chemistry prize-winner Professor Kary Mullis.[25] In March 1987 Duesberg published a paper in a medical journal arguing that HIV was a harmless passenger virus, and the drugs that were currently being used to treat the symptoms of AIDS were, in fact, its major cause.[26] An Australian group argued that the virus had never been isolated, and there was no scientific proof of its existence.

In the early days, when little was known about HIV and AIDS, challenging voices were to be expected, and even nurtured. However, AIDS denialism attracted mavericks and conspiracy theorists whose ideas were seldom amenable to scientific analysis or rational debate.

Several activist groups, including ACTUP San Francisco, espoused the denialist theories about AIDS. By 1993 denialists had formed themselves into the Group for the Scientific Reappraisal of the HIV/AIDS Hypothesis, and called for a major audit of the current status of the science.[27] Their views were taken seriously enough for the US National Institute for Allergies and Infectious Diseases to publish a lengthy document collating the evidence that HIV leads to AIDS in 1994.[28]

The denialists' critique was seemingly compatible with the debunking mission of contemporary journalism, and several influential publications espoused their point of view.

During the 1980s the news magazine, *New African*, became a firm proponent of AIDS denialism,[29] and used every opportunity to cast doubt on the AIDS orthodoxy that had as its fundamental tenet that a virus called HIV is the cause of AIDS. In various articles over the years the magazine, widely read by South Africans at home and in exile abroad, suggested that the HIV test was not accurate for those with malaria antibodies in their blood; that Africa had been the site of US experiments to test new viruses for biological warfare; and even that HIV had been invented by the former Rhodesian and/or South African security forces in their struggle to maintain white supremacy.

African mass media were not alone in their interrogation of the AIDS orthodoxy. For several years Britain's Channel 4 television station gave prominence to the views of denialist Joan Shenton, broadcasting several of her films on their authoritative current affairs programme *Dispatches*, between 1987 and 1993. The London *Sunday Times* also published more than 20 articles by denialist journalist Neville Hodgkinson between 1992 and 1994.

During the late 1980s, South African exile Dr Sam Mhlongo became involved in this debate whilst working as a family practitioner in London.[30] When Mhlongo was asked to confirm the HIV status of 11 Ugandan couples who had been diagnosed HIV positive in their homeland, he re-tested them and found that they were all negative.[31]

This experience led Mhlongo to the denialists' door. Like many others, he became sceptical about the credentials of the new virus, concluding that AIDS itself could be caused by dozens of diseases, infections and conditions that weakened the immune system. After his return to South Africa many years later, Mhlongo was to become a leading denialist spokesperson, and was influential in shaping the controversial stance of South African President Thabo Mbeki's on HIV and AIDS.

THE VIRUS CONTINUED...

From its Central African beginnings, HIV spread slowly southwards. By 1986 it was clear that there was a serious and growing problem in Zambia, Zimbabwe and other southern

African countries. For example, a 1987 survey in three urban areas of Malawi showed that HIV prevalence among pregnant women was between three and 8 per cent.[32] People from all walks of life were affected: Zambian president Kenneth Kaunda was the first African leader to reveal HIV in his family, when his son died of AIDS in 1987.

But the virus's slow African land journey seemed to end at the northern borders of South Africa. In 1986, virologists began routine HIV monitoring at key sites in South Africa to identify the extent of the epidemic among heterosexuals.[33] They found that levels of sexually transmitted infections such as gonorrhoea were high, but by the end of March 1987 there was still no sign of HIV or of AIDS in the local heterosexual population. This was explained in part by the fact that South Africa was so isolated from the rest of the subcontinent: electric fences separated the country from Mozambique to the east, and patrols and border guards sealed off the northern borders. This strategy was designed to keep political insurgents at bay and to prevent black South Africans from being infected by the spirit of liberation in the north. However, until the late 1980s, this *cordon sanitaire* had been remarkably effective in keeping the virus out.

But the gay epidemic continued to grow, and by March 1987 there had been 64 reported cases of AIDS. By now the AIDS Training and Information Centre at the SAIMR had expanded to meet the need. Soon they were offering a professional counselling service and were recruiting volunteer counsellors for training. Busse, now resident in Johannesburg, jumped at the offer. 'I was still fine and healthy,' he says, 'but I decided that I didn't want anybody to have the same experience as me — being diagnosed with a terminal disease with nobody to talk to…'

The counsellor training course was the first course of its kind in South Africa, and most of the counsellors were white and gay. For Busse it was a life saver. 'Doing the counselling was very good for me, being altruistic and realising that other people have the same issues'.

Simon Nkoli was also becoming active in AIDS prevention. After his acquittal in the Delmas Treason Trial he had founded the Gay and Lesbian Organisation (GLOW). And then, when he realised he was HIV positive, he added AIDS to his portfolio of activism. Together, Nkoli and Busse established the first AIDS-prevention organisation in the black townships. Initially the

Township AIDS Project had a special mandate to reach gays and lesbians in Soweto. Busse found people's reactions interesting. 'Even people working in AIDS were saying, "What on earth are you going to the townships for? What a waste of time. There are so many gay men and now you are going off to do this work in Soweto."'

'At that time, it was said that homosexuality was a foreign thing in the black community, that you won't find African homosexuals,' says Busse. 'But I can remember going with Simon and running safer sex workshops with enormous numbers of gay people in Soweto.'

Lucky

It was not until Lucky Mazibuko was in his final year of high school that he heard about AIDS. He and his classmates referred to it as 'American Ideas to Discourage Sex'. The year was 1988.

'You must remember,' says Lucky, 'there was political turmoil and everyone was talking about Madiba being released from prison, and everybody was saying "No man, these white people, they are coming with some kind of trick so that we are not prepared for the war…" One of the ways of preparing for the war was to make as many babies as you can.'

It was several years later, while driving a taxi in his father's business, that Lucky had his first date with HIV; or at least the first one he was aware of. One drizzly summer evening in 1991, a stunningly beautiful young woman climbed into the back seat of the vehicle. Although Lucky's working day was almost over, he readily agreed to take her to an address in Soweto.

She was going to a party, she said, but when they arrived at the place it was in darkness. Lucky and his best friend, who was the only remaining passenger, sat and waited while she investigated. Then she came back to the vehicle saying that the party had been cancelled and she had nowhere to go.

He took her to one of the most popular shebeens in the township and they had a couple of beers. Then they went to his grandmother's house.

Some years later, when Lucky became the manager of his father's business, he decided to apply for life insurance. For that, he had to have an HIV test. The insurance cover was declined and instead, Lucky was called in to speak to the doctor. He guessed the reason. 'I knew what the problem was, because my sexual lifestyle suggested it.' Lucky didn't turn up for his appointment with the doctor — nor did he tell anyone about it. But this indirect diagnosis was a turning point in his life. 'I lost interest in sex and in women, and tended to spend a lot more time alone.'

For three years he sat on it, until he forced himself to go for an HIV test. The result confirmed all his fears.

How did he know the source of his HIV? In 1999, when Lucky became a public advocate for positive people, a woman called the national newspaper where he worked. Weeping, she told him the whole story, how on discovering her HIV-positive status she had become bitter and angry and had set out deliberately to take revenge on men. 'She told me that she had met me as a taxi driver and she felt very bad that she had infected a good man,' says Lucky. 'She was now very ill, and I begged her to give me her contact details but she refused. Up to this day I do not know what happened to her.'

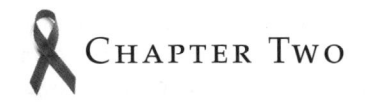

Chapter Two
The virus underground

The breach in the cordon

By 1987 the African AIDS epidemic had become a major international news story, with reports of depopulated villages and huge numbers of people dying without help or hope. So far, South Africa's isolation from its northern neighbours had afforded some measure of protection from the growing crisis: the virus had not yet been found in routine HIV monitoring outside of the gay community.

But many feared that this was just a temporary respite. The country's mining industry bosses were among the most concerned. By now, South Africa's mines were employing nearly three quarters of a million migrant workers. They were drawn from the country's impoverished rural areas, as well as from neighbouring Lesotho, Swaziland, Mozambique and Malawi. Under the apartheid system of influx control, migrant workers' contracts lasted for one year [34], during which time the men lived in dormitory accommodation near the mines. Those who lived a distance away seldom saw their wives, and many began second families in the towns, with whom they could not legally reside.

Depending as it did on recruits from northern neighbours with a growing epidemic, this system had the potential of breaching the apartheid government's *cordon sanitaire*. It was also an obvious catalyst for an explosive epidemic, because the living and working conditions of mineworkers made them particularly vulnerable to HIV. By day, the men performed dangerous and taxing work underground, and by night they were barracked in single-sex hostels. Many found their only pleasure and relaxation in the crowded shebeens, in liaisons with township girls or cash transactions with local sex workers.

The propensity for the migrant system to spread disease, particularly sexually transmitted infections (STIs), had been well known since the 1940s, when South African epidemiologist Sydney Kark investigated what he called the 'social pathology of syphilis'.

Kark found that men contracting syphilis on the mines brought it home to their partners in remote rural areas.[35] This had the effect of creating mini-epidemics in areas where such diseases were previously unknown.

The mining houses were well aware that some of their employees from high-prevalence countries were likely to have the virus in their blood, but they wanted to be sure. In May 1986 the Chamber of Mines[36] contracted a team at the South African Institute for Medical Research (SAIMR) to test mineworkers for HIV.

It was a huge undertaking. Drs Reuben Sher and Denis Sifris were the key investigators.

'We bled thousands of miners. We had a whole factory, fridges full of serum,' says Sher. 300 000 samples were taken, and of these nearly 30 000 samples were tested. The results showed that 3,76 per cent of Malawian miners were HIV positive.[37] Prevalence among South Africans was just 0,02 per cent — four men out of nearly 20 000.[38]

'We were then faced with what to do about this,' says Dr Brian Brink, medical senior vice president of the Anglo American Group of mining companies. 'Clearly it was "prevention", but how were we going to prevent this epidemic from taking hold? We had seen what had happened in East and Central Africa and it was pretty damn clear that unless we could prevent it, the same thing would happen here. Close to 4 per cent infection in Malawi was seen as a crisis.'

By now the international community was on high alert about the AIDS pandemic. In 1987 it became the first disease ever to be debated on the floor of the United Nations General Assembly. Under the dynamic leadership of a young American doctor, Jonathan Mann, the World Health Organisation had established the Global Programme on AIDS[39], which aimed to help government leaders across the world design programmes to prevent the spread of the new disease. But the white minority government of South Africa was not a welcome guest at the UN table.

At home, news of the discovery of HIV among miners was greeted with dismay by the white right wing. Arrie Paulus,

Conservative Party spokesman and former white trade union boss, demanded that the Chamber of Mines send HIV-positive miners packing. Housewives who lived near the mines complained that their domestic workers were fraternising with infected miners. They feared the import of the virus into their safe suburban homes.

By October 1987 the government had introduced new legislation requiring compulsory HIV testing for all foreign workers. The regulations [40], which also provided for quarantining, made AIDS a notifiable disease and those with HIV were deemed prohibited immigrants. The Malawian government objected to these provisions and refused testing for their workers. As a result, between 1988 and 1992, all 213 000 Malawian mineworkers were repatriated.

Brink, Sher and members of the government's AIDS advisory board consistently argued for a more progressive strategy. 'We said that it had to be based on awareness and education,' says Brink. 'We were saying you have to get involved and start working very hard. But our advice was ignored.'

This was a tragic mistake. Despite the effort to exclude the infected, levels of HIV on the mines continued to rise. In April 1988 the Chamber of Mines released figures showing that 2 000 Malawian miners were infected, along with 40 South African miners. HIV prevalence on the mines had more than doubled within one year.

Men alone

The implications of these statistics reverberated through academic and left-wing circles. In 1988, researchers from the Sociology of Work Unit at the University of the Witwatersrand, led by Professor Eddie Webster, decided to investigate the HIV-risk behaviour of migrant miners.[41] They already had a well-established working relationship with the National Union of Mineworkers (NUM), the radical grouping that represented the black mine workforce. The two parties had previously collaborated on a piece of research on health and safety on the mines, and had jointly presented it to the Chamber of Mines in an effort to improve working conditions. This new project was intended to perform a similar function. Some even hoped it would provide ammunition for the long-held union demand for the abolition of single-sex housing.

A research team that included former mineworker Monyaola Mothibele, post-graduate student Karen Jochelson and senior researcher Dr Jean Leger went off in search of evidence for mineworkers' risk and vulnerability to HIV.

Mothibele and Jochelson hung out in the neighbourhoods of working mines, drinking beer and talking to men and women about their lives and loves. The local branch of the mineworkers' union had offered help, but when the moment came, they did not seem too eager to arrange the interviews. Perhaps they found it strange, offensive even: a white girl, young enough to be their daughter, asking about their sex lives. But many knew Mothibele from his working years, so there were always a few ready companions.

The women who lived around the mines were more cooperative. Mothibele and Jochelson found a group that had set up an encampment of sorts on nearby white-owned farmland. When they were not otherwise engaged, the women slept in a disused pigsty, for which they were paying rent to the farmer, a well-known right wing political leader in the area. Many of the inhabitants of this settlement were women who had come from rural areas to find their husbands on the mines. Most were abandoned, unemployed and alone. Servicing men on the mines was one way of making do.

The women compared the act of harnessing men's desires to that of spanning donkeys or oxen, and for them it was the only route to survival.

'I worked for six months and saw that it's better to "span". I could send home money for my children to get something to eat,' said one woman. 'Just think what it is like if you have no place, no money, no husband…' said another.

For their part, the men complained about the hellish life in the hostel. 'We are locked in, like cattle in a cattle post,' they said. Many only saw their families once a month, and separation was a constant source of anxiety.

'I drink. Most of the time I think about my wife, I want to be next to her,' said one miner. 'I ask, "Is she using the money I sent her in the right way?" I think about the children.'

Most men had several sexual relationships going at a time. On paydays men and women would meet outside the hostel gate at the 'waiting place'. Some women took up to ten clients on paydays. At one hostel, the pick-up point was an open field they had nicknamed the airport: 'You produce the money, have sex and go away immediately. Then the next man follows.'

Few had heard of HIV, and of those that had, even fewer knew how it was transmitted. Although condoms were promoted by the mine management, they were not in great demand. 'I did not believe management's pamphlets,' said one miner, 'because he has locked us up in a hostel away from our wives. If these pamphlets were true, they would give us at least four days every month to be with our wives.'

The researchers concluded that the migrant labour system had 'institutionalised a geographical network of relationships' for spreading sexually transmitted disease. 'Once HIV enters the heterosexual mining community,' they wrote, 'it will spread to the immediate urban area, to surrounding urban areas, from urban to rural areas, within rural areas and across national boundaries.'

Prophetic words maybe, but in 1989 the union was having none of it. The day after the paper had been presented, Webster received a phone call from NUM's secretary-general Cyril Ramaphosa.

'Cyril was saying, no way can you publish this report — it's objectionable because it's exposing the private lives of our members,' says Webster. Ramaphosa was furious. He complained that the paper was racist, because it was just looking at black people. Maybe it should describe the sex practices of mine owners, he suggested.

For Webster's group this attitude came as a shock. 'Our argument was that it's not about black mineworkers being promiscuous, but about the fact that migrant labour takes men away from their partners and therefore creates conditions for them to develop multiple relationships,' says Webster.'It's commoditised sex, it's disrupted families, and the only answer is to allow men to settle with their families next to the mine.'

More importantly, the researchers felt something had to be done before HIV really took a hold. And the union was best placed to talk to mineworkers.

A protracted negotiation ensued. The researchers argued from a position of academic freedom, that their work should be published. The union demurred, from the perspective of the rights and dignity of their members. Finally they reached a compromise, in which the researchers agreed to moderate the language of the article and to ensure the piece would only be published abroad, and never in a local journal.

Today Webster admits that he had not fully understood the cultural dynamics of sexuality in the context of apartheid. 'A white man with NGO support driving this kind of agenda is a complete non-starter,' he says, 'because of the history of pathologising black sexuality in colonial discourse, where the black man is portrayed as diseased and promiscuous. I was aware of that in a more general way, but it became clearer to me when I began to read and reflect on President Mbeki's response to AIDS.'

THE MANY FACES OF DENIAL

When the research paper was presented to the Chamber of Mines, some months later, they also rejected it on the same grounds as the unions had.

'I call it the "celibate miner" thesis', says Webster. 'Miners were totally faithful to their wives and would not dream of having unprotected sex; and we were just a bunch of shit-stirrers trying to upset the industry.'[42]

Both parties wanted the lid on it. Today Brink agrees that the industry's response was defensive. 'Migrant labour was the way the industry had worked for decades and decades. You can imagine what changing that would mean.'[43]

In a short space of time the Chamber went on to publish its own research which concluded that '80 per cent of employees are not, as commonly believed, promiscuous and therefore not likely to spread the infection... with the proper housing and feeding and the generally responsible behaviour of the vast majority of mineworkers we believe that the industry and its employees plays a very minor role in the spread of HIV in South Africa.'

It is reasonably safe to assume that the Chamber would have a strong interest in denying the links between migration, single-sex hostels and AIDS. For one thing, if HIV was deemed to be an occupational hazard the unions might think of suing the industry and the price tag would be enormous.

But the union's denialism was a more complex matter. Like many moments in the AIDS epidemic, this one was tangled in a complex web in which sensitivities about race and sexuality were just one thread. It is worth noting that the late 1980s was the time of the big 'fear' campaigns around AIDS. Shock tactics, such as AIDS education posters depicting coffins and skulls and crossbones, were having a counterproductive effect, driving people away from the issue. On top of all of this, the issue of mandatory testing was an increasing threat to the human rights and job security of miners. The repatriation of the Malawian miners had already warned of the huge negative consequences for those diagnosed with the disease.

Another barrier to openness about the disease was the conflictual nature of the labour relations of the era. In 1987 a national mineworkers' strike had resulted in the defeat of the union and a loss of 50 000 jobs. Miners were an embattled community, fighting for their survival on many fronts: a new sexually transmitted disease, with no immediate symptoms, was not one of them.

May Hermanus, who was Health and Safety Officer for NUM at that time, clearly locates the research controversy in this broader context. She sees AIDS as one more flashpoint in the minefield of negotiations between workers and employers. Confidentiality was the hottest issue: workers feared that they would be dismissed if they were known to be HIV positive.

In this climate, the whole subject of HIV was viewed with suspicion, as were those who expressed concern about it.

'Workers felt that it was something the apartheid government had manufactured,' says Hermanus. They were unsure if it was a population control measure, and they were suspicious of where it was coming from. 'Politics made it very hard for them to acknowledge that it was a real threat and that miners must protect themselves. Gender politics was also an issue here.'

Although trade union officials distanced themselves publicly from the research paper, they did continue the discussion among themselves. In acknowledgement of the threat to their membership, they decided that it was time to embark on HIV and AIDS awareness and education programmes in the union. The mining houses followed a similar course of action. Anglo American developed a campaign based on condom promotion, treatment for sexually transmitted infections, education and awareness.

However, there was no concerted effort to strike at the root of miners' vulnerability, and the system of migratory labour and single-sex hostels remained in force.

The implications were as clear in 1989 as they had been

30 years earlier, when Kark was writing about the syphilis epidemic:

'Without an understanding of the economic factors involved, and the historical development of the vast social pathological changes brought about during the last 70 years, no treatment will save the spread of syphilis in South Africa,' he wrote. 'Treatment of individuals... cannot succeed in any but a few cases. The first line of treatment must be to remedy the unhealthy social relationships which have emerged as the inevitable result of masses of men leaving their homes every year.'

It was several years before academics found the courage to return to this troubled subject. In the 1990s epidemiologists began to re-examine the link between migration and HIV. One three-year study compared levels of HIV between migrants and non-migrants and found that migrants were more than twice as likely to be HIV infected than their stay-at-home peers.

Others sought to understand how the life world of mining and migration has moulded notions of masculinity, sex and gender roles. One authoritative study conducted by Professor Catherine Campbell in a Gauteng mining community showed that the qualities needed to survive the work underground — the physical strength and courage — contributed to a particularly macho construction of masculinity. In the words of an interviewee: 'There are two things to being a man: going underground and going after a woman.'

In her book *Letting them die*[44], Campbell describes how this notion of masculinity drives men to risky behaviour even though they may be well informed about HIV. 'Linked to this masculine identity,' she writes, 'were the repertoires of insatiable sexuality, the need for multiple sexual partners and a manly desire for the pleasure of what is locally called flesh-to-flesh contact.'

This study confirmed the dire predictions made by the Witwatersrand University researchers a decade earlier. Despite the existence of comprehensive AIDS education and prevention programmes, levels of HIV in the area continued to soar. By 2001, 36 per cent of miners in the area of Campbell's study had HIV.[45] But more shocking still was the evidence of an epidemic of crisis proportions among young women in the neighbouring township. Here, HIV prevalence among women in their mid-20s peaked at nearly 70 per cent.[46]

The virus emerges

By the end of the 1980s there was already mounting evidence that South Africa's heterosexual population was bound to experience the epidemic that was devastating the countries to the north.[47] Not only was HIV prevalence on the mines increasing, but men and women began arriving in township hospitals with symptoms of the disease.

The Chris Hani-Baragwanath Hospital in Soweto was just one site that bore witness to the beginnings of the heterosexual epidemic. Their records show that their first patient with AIDS was admitted in the spring of 1987. By November there were so many people requiring treatment that a specialised outpatient clinic was established. By 1991 the clinic was seeing 45 to 60 adults and 10 to 14 children per year.

These were the people already ill with AIDS-related diseases. This meant that there were many more people infected with the virus who remained undiagnosed.

From mid 1987 the hospital began offering HIV testing and counselling in the maternity unit. It was the first hospital in the country to do so. Within a year, 15 out of every 100 women passing through its doors were testing positive

Ongoing monitoring also revealed an increasing prevalence of HIV in inner-city Johannesburg. One analysis of over 6 000 people attending clinics for family planning and the treatment of sexually transmitted infections (STI) found that around 1 per cent of black men and women were HIV positive. (In the same survey more than a fifth of gay men were HIV positive.)[48]

Researchers were stunned. From a zero statistic in 1986, HIV was now present in the general population. And it seemed to be doubling every year.[49]

Writing in a medical journal in 1989, virologist Dr Reuben Sher summarised the incontrovertible evidence from across the country that pointed to the coming crisis.[50] It concluded:

'We need to seriously ask ourselves: "How many more people must die before we do something about this disease?" A pre-emptive strike is needed now; in five years time it will be too late… Future generations will judge whether we were civilised or not by the manner in which we manage the AIDS threat.'

But there was no matching concern from the government, or from the general public. Even the medical community viewed the statistics with equanimity.

Dr James McIntyre, who has worked at the Chris Hani-Baragwanath Perinatal HIV Research Unit since those early days, says that HIV was regarded as a sideline in academic medical circles. 'I think for many people this was seen as an epidemic that wasn't going to happen,' he says. 'It was still perceived as a gay, white, male disease, and we were seen as slightly crazy for moving ahead on it.'

In the popular media there was confused talk. 'People began to say that AIDS was moving over from the gay community to the heterosexual community,' says Dr Denis Sifris. 'I couldn't quite understand how. Because the last person a gay white man is going to sleep with is a rural woman.' There was not a scrap of evidence that gays were infecting heterosexuals.

Scientific evidence later clarified that the two epidemics were entirely separate. The first epidemic was linked by sexual networks to the gay community[51] in the US and Europe; the second heterosexual epidemic was linked to that in Central and East Africa. The evidence was in the fact that the two epidemics were characterised by infection with a different subtype of the virus. Subtype B of the virus is most common in gay men in South Africa as well as North America and Europe, and extremely rare in the rest of Africa; while subtype C is most common in Southern and East Africa.

By 1990, the reported number of heterosexuals with HIV in South Africa outstripped that of gay men for the first time. In some groups HIV prevalence was doubling every six months.

The authorities were doing little to make the crisis known. Dr Clive Evian, who was running the Community AIDS Centre in Hillbrow at the time, claims there was a concerted effort on the part of the government to keep the statistics quiet. He found the government's chief epidemiologist evasive.[52] When asked, he played down the seriousness of the matter by saying that there were only one or two cases. 'The bulk of the problem was HIV, not AIDS, so it was very easy to distort,' says Evian. 'People were keeping it secret for all sorts of stigma reasons.'

Sher, who was one of the founders of the SAIMR AIDS Centre, agrees. 'It was a silent disease for many years. We were very worried about disclosing increasing numbers being infected because of the alarm. But now I think that may have been wrong.'

THE SECOND EPIDEMIC

Questions remain over the timing of South Africa's heterosexual epidemic. Although HIV was known to be present in neighbouring countries for many years, why did it only arrive in the country in the late 1980s?

South African epidemiologists have long argued that it was the migratory labour system on the mines that introduced the virus into South Africa and scattered it across the land. But this system, although undoubtedly an important driving force, cannot entirely account for the epidemic's late advent and explosive growth. After all, migrant mineworkers had been recruited from high prevalence countries for many years before the second heterosexual epidemic emerged.

The explanation must be sought in the far-reaching social and economic changes that predicated the demise of the apartheid state. The late 1980s was a period of political reform in South Africa: no less than a shifting of apartheid's tectonic plates. It was also a period of violent conflict and dramatic social change. In this turmoil, the virus flourished.

As the apartheid government lost its stranglehold on the region, South Africa began to realign with the greater community of African nations. Despite economic sanctions, trade with African countries as far north as Kenya was on the rise. People from countries to the north, lured by visions of impossible wealth, found new and creative ways of breaching South Africa's hitherto impenetrable borders. Although there were concerted efforts to keep foreign 'illegals' out, increasing numbers of refugees and economic migrants from high HIV-prevalence countries poured into the cities and industrial areas. With them came HIV.

Hitchhiking its way across the continent, the virus also had ready help from truckers and traders who frequented the busy roadside bars. The connection between long-haul truckers, sex work and HIV has been demonstrated in many countries, and South Africa was no exception. One survey[53] at a truck stop catering for trans continental truckers in KwaZulu-Natal found that more than half the people there were HIV positive.

There were other, less obvious ports of entry for the virus too. Ironically, the very soldiers engaged to defend South Africa from democracy and change were holed up in one of the highest HIV-prevalence areas of the region: northern Namibia. For a decade or more, the South African Defence Force (SADF) had been waging a secret war to the west, and by the mid 1980s parts of neighbouring Namibia had become one large SADF camp. Army headquarters were in the town of Katimo Mulilo[54] in East Caprivi. By the time regular HIV monitoring began, Katimo Mulilo was at the epicentre of the region's epidemic.[55] When apartheid's illegal wars came to an end in the late 1980s, thousands of SADF soldiers came home. With them, surely, came HIV.

Caprivi was the military frontier of the region, a narrow strip of land wedged between the countries of Namibia, Angola, Botswana, Zambia and Zimbabwe. Its local population was host not only to the official soldiers of the SADF, but also to the guerrilla forces of the African National Congress (ANC) and the Namibian liberation movement, Swapo.

In this period, the armed struggle against apartheid was escalating, and increasing numbers of ANC cadres were crossing into the country to take refuge in safe houses across the land. This invigorated underground railway of military cadres provided another route for the virus. Many of the guerrilla soldiers came from military camps in the high HIV-prevalence countries of Uganda, Tanzania and Zambia. Although the extent of HIV among these cadres was not documented, by 1988 ANC leaders openly acknowledged that there had been deaths from AIDS in their military camps.

Although there is still much to know and understand, there is scientific evidence for the hypothesis that HIV entered South Africa from different points at different times. Investigations of the genetic structure of the virus in South Africa's blood provide many of the answers that we seek. The extreme diversity[56] in the genetic structure of the subtype C virus among heterosexuals in South Africa suggests that HIV arrived independently from the neighbouring countries of Zambia, Malawi, Botswana and Zimbabwe.

Once inside the country, the virus found fertile ground in the dramatic changes brought about by the reform of the apartheid state. Until 1986, a large proportion of South Africa's own workers were migrants who had no legal right to live permanently in the towns, or at the place of their employment. Like the migrant mineworkers, many of them stayed alone in single-sex hostels or backyard rooms and saw their rural families infrequently. More than three million South Africans were thus caught up in a cycle of permanent oscillation between rural homes and urban hostels. Their movement was curtailed by a rigorous system of influx control, vigorously policed by a dedicated squad that prowled the urban areas by night. Ironically these extreme controls over freedom of movement (then known as the pass laws) may have actually retarded the initial spread of HIV.

But in mid 1986, as a prelude to political reform, President PW Botha's government surprised the world by abolishing influx control. For the first time in a century, black South Africans had the freedom to move across the land that was their own, choosing where they might live and work. And move they did! Large numbers of men and women flocked to the cities — to find work, to reunite with family members, to escape rural poverty.

Unlike many other African countries, South Africa was equipped with a sophisticated transport network linking mine and country, town and township, squatter camp and inner city. Good roads and trains, and well-heeled passengers with the money to use them, provided the virus with unfettered movement across the land.

Thus it was that the abolition of apartheid's notorious influx control laws unleashed decades of pent-up urbanisation. And in the margins of this rediscovered freedom lurked a new virus, uniquely adapted to thrive on human frailty and exploit the turmoil of the times.

Toni

Twenty-two-year-old Toni Zimmerman was on lunchtime switchboard duty when she received a telephone call that changed her life. It was her family doctor, informing her that her partner was HIV positive. 'Do you know?' he asked. 'And what are you going to do about it?'

Toni went for an HIV test and found that she too had the virus. 'Just that feeling,' she says. 'It was incredible. You know the saying "A train went over me"? Well, this one went, and stopped. It just stayed still.'

Because her partner was reluctant to reveal his HIV status, Toni was obliged to keep hers quiet too. Soon their relationship began to fall apart and Toni was alone with her secret. And then she discovered she was pregnant.

Toni went for help at the new AIDS Testing and Counselling Centre in Durban. She also confided in her father, who was a minister in the Christian Reformed Church. He immediately got in the car and made the long journey from Ladysmith to see her. 'My parents were very sad,' says Toni. 'Afterwards I heard that my mom cried for three days.'

The doctor tried to persuade her to have an abortion, but Toni decided to take the risk. The statistics of the day gave the baby a one-in-three chance of being HIV positive. 'I cancelled and went for counselling,' she said. 'I realised that this was probably the only chance for me to have a baby and it was also against my religion to have an abortion.'

But when the baby, Calvin, was tested for HIV, he too had the virus. 'I thought: This is my fault. I made the choice and now my son is going to die of AIDS. I was devastated. But you know he has been so well and he is living such a happy life and he is making everyone else so happy...

'A lot of people ask me if I don't feel guilty about it and I don't think so. I believe he is going to grow quite old because he's just doing so well.'

Despite her fears and her sadness, Toni decided to go public about her HIV status. 'I just knew I wanted to make a difference,' she says. 'I wanted to shake up my peers because I knew that whatever I did wrong, they are doing the same thing. It was a huge shock to my system to suddenly realise that you can die of AIDS. I don't want other people to feel this way.'

Telling her friends was one of the most difficult things she had ever done. 'Every time I decided to tell a friend I was in a terrible state of depression, because you never know who is going to be the weak one and say, "OK I'm backing off". But it didn't happen.'

Toni was interviewed in 1996.
Calvin died in 1999. [57]

Chapter Three
Sex in the city

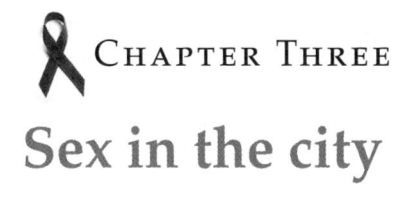

HIV IN THE CITY

Outside the mining industry, the first systematic surveys of HIV pre-valence were conducted in the inner-city Johannesburg area of Hillbrow.[58] By the late 1980s researchers were sure they were seeing the beginning of a serious heterosexual epidemic there. This densely populated triangle of high-rise buildings seemed to provide the perfect meeting place for the virus and its unwitting hosts.

Since its foundation, Hillbrow, with its busy shopping streets and cheap lodgings, had been home to new arrivals to the city — first the waves of young Afrikaner families fleeing the poverty of the countryside in the 1930s, and later, immigrants from post-war Europe. Then, as the apartheid government's segregationist strategy crumbled, black people began moving into the area.

The abolition of the influx control legislation in 1986 was a turning point in Hillbrow's history. Now that black South Africans were free to migrate, they fled from the overcrowded rural bantustans to the cities, which held the promise of prosperity. Hillbrow also provided a refuge for people escaping the violence and poor conditions in the Reef townships. As apartheid's *cordon sanitaire* disintegrated, these new urban dwellers were joined by refugees, immigrants and economic migrants from all over Africa. Soon Hillbrow became the beating pulse of a new nation in the making.[59]

In 1989, in response to the rising prevalence of HIV, the Johannesburg City Health Department established a dedicated AIDS Centre in Hillbrow. This would provide walk-in HIV services, such as testing and counselling for Johannesburg residents. Dr Clive Evian, already a volunteer at the Johannesburg General Hospital's AIDS clinic, got the job of running it. Almost at once he found himself up against some serious opposition from the other tenants in the building, even though it was mainly a medical block.

'The doctors wouldn't allow us to put up a sign saying there was an AIDS Centre,' says Evian, 'because they thought the building would become tainted or contaminated, or they thought their patients would think that.'

Soon the centre was forced to move to the more hospitable terrain of Esselin Street, which already housed the reproductive health services for the area. The Community AIDS Centre, as it became known, was a walk-in service that also saw referrals from the clinic for sexually transmitted infections (STI) next door.

Even so, there were problems. 'There was a lot of resentment from Family Planning because we were seen as privileged,' says Mary Crewe, one of the centre's first staff members. The nurses from the STI clinic felt that the AIDS Centre had all the funding and went out and did interesting things, and they were just stuck in their offices grappling with social disease.

Many of the Family Planning and STI clinic staff members were long-standing employees from the apartheid era, with attitudes to match. They resented this new breed of service provider who was committed to care and counselling, and the empowerment of their clients.

By contrast the STI clinic had a special stamp reserved for the cards of clients who came back a third time. It read 'repeat offender'. 'We struggled to get them to see that this was just not acceptable, but they never got it,' says Crewe.

Despite the challenges, the Centre went from strength to strength. When Peter Busse, now a trained and experienced counsellor, joined them to coordinate the counselling services, he found the atmosphere welcoming. The staff and clients were a mixed bunch — black, white, gay, straight, men, women. The fact that clients didn't need an appointment meant that confidentiality was preserved. For the first few years, though, the majority of clients were white men, and from this it was hard to avoid the perception that HIV was primarily a gay disease.

From the start the Centre was busy, helping the many anxious people who wanted HIV tests to set their minds at rest. But infections were mounting. 'Very gradually it changed, from it being a rare experience to give people a positive result to it being more and more common,' says Busse. One day he sat down and did a rough calculation: prevalence was one-in-ten among those coming in off the street, and one-in-four among the referrals from the STI clinic. The majority of the new clients were black.

Within a short space of time the Community AIDS Centre was stretched to capacity. Demand for testing, for condoms and for educational materials was soaring. Counsellors were seeing clients back to back, from early in the morning until eight at night: these sessions were 55 minutes with just a five-minute break in between.

'It was tough work,' says Busse, 'and most of it was done by volunteers. So even then, there were a lot of people who wanted to do something to help.'

In the evenings they would get together and discuss the increasing caseload. When counsellors found themselves giving out two or three positive diagnoses a day, staff morale began to suffer.

The rapid demographic transition in Hillbrow made it difficult for the Centre to understand the nature of the community it was serving. 'All the rich whites had moved, except for some intrepid Germans, but there was not a sense of a new community coming in with the relaxation of the laws,' says Crewe. 'It was too transient. It was also fascinating to see how rapidly it got run down.'

From an initially gay, male clientele, the Centre began to see increasing numbers of women.

'If I really start getting in touch with that time,' says counsellor Pierre Brouard, 'the main thing was the lack of treatment and the real helplessness when you diagnosed people. What could you offer them — a pamphlet, a bit of nutritional advice… and exercise?'

Working lives

Throughout the years, Hillbrow's transient people had taken comfort — and found employment — in the hotels, brothels and bars that dotted the area. This period was no exception. The late 1980s witnessed a massive growth in the Hillbrow sex industry. The scrapping of the legislation that had criminalised sex between black and white gave new life to an already established sex industry. The demographic transition meant that landlords were searching for a new clientele, and they found that sex workers were lucrative and reliable tenants. Hotels that had formerly catered for immigrants, transients and tourists turned readily to the trade in sex.[60]

By the early 1990s, about 1 000 women were selling sex in Hillbrow. The Dorchester, the Summit Club, the Golden Key, the Quirinale were among the many venues that explicitly catered for sex workers and their clients. Some had bars, clubs and dance floors. Live music, food and sex were on offer seven nights a week.

It was a layered industry, ranging from women who worked the streets to high-class escort agencies. The women who worked in the hotels were free agents, relying on hotel security guards instead of pimps to protect them from unruly clients.

In 1990 the local authorities added a sex-worker programme to the existing services at the Community AIDS Centre. The programme, led by the young Afrikaans sociologist Herman van der Watt, struggled to establish a presence in the city. But within a year there was a dedicated clinic for sex workers on a Thursday night, and an outreach team that worked in the hotels. They were seeing 250 people a day.

It was a mixed group. New to the city, many young women had been drawn into the game by the push and pull of material life. Others were selling sex to support their drug habits. The clients were from everywhere.

'I've seen clients from politicians to the farmers of the Free State,' says Van der Watt. 'You had the massage parlour guys who were different from the crawlers. They came from all walks of life. I've seen people that today are in the highest positions, black and white, everyone. In Hillbrow you could almost be faceless — across the colour line.'

The women were extremely vulnerable. Their desperate need for accommodation meant that they were exploited and abused by hotel managers and security guards. They lived from hour to hour. Their working lives were short and brutal.

'It seems you start on top, with a fur coat,' says Van der Watt, 'and at the end of the day you have nothing underneath. They were just used. They became commodities.'

The sex-worker programme offered HIV and general health education, as well as counselling and testing. It also tried to equip the women with the skills they needed to keep safe, and to maintain their self-esteem. Busse remembers attending the annual party at the Summit Club, which was held during downtime, in the late afternoon. 'It was basically, how to change your hairstyle in four minutes between clients,' says Busse, 'so they had hairdressing demonstrations and shows of exotic lingerie interspersed with safer sex and condom use. It was brilliant.'

Consistent and correct condom use was one aim of the programme, and the women were more than amenable to this idea. But their success was hampered by clients who used persuasion, bribery and violence to get their sex 'flesh to flesh'.

An even more intractable problem was the one they faced at home: although the majority of women were committed to using condoms with their clients, few used condoms with their regular partners. This is a common problem for sex workers around the world, and has been widely documented in the AIDS literature.

Studies done in a later period have sought to understand the relationship between HIV and sex work in Hillbrow. One survey in 1997 showed that 45 per cent of sex workers were HIV positive; two years later it was 53 per cent. While almost all of women said they used condoms with their clients, none did so with their boyfriends.

'He really hates a condom,' said one woman about her boyfriend. 'He always beats me and has taken out four of my teeth. Even if I can run away, when I come back he will say I am his. That's the problem that I have.'

Understanding the risk, some older women preferred to live alone. 'Our spinners (boyfriends),' said one, 'have girlfriends in most of these hotels. They don't use condoms. He comes back to infect you.'

By 2000, there were between 5 000 and 10 000 commercial sex workers in Hillbrow. Many of them were children.

Back in the late 1980s, the brisk trade in sex was a catalyst for the new epidemic of HIV, but the context in which it was taking place greatly magnified the risk. Not only was Hillbrow home to increasing numbers of immigrants from high HIV-prevalence countries in the north, but it was also the chosen spot for the covert military forces of both left and right.

ANC guerrillas, who were entering the country in increasing numbers, found refuge in the anonymity of the place. The Community AIDS Centre bore witness to this. As the years drew on, increasing numbers of their clients were returnees from the liberation struggle. Brouard particularly remembers counselling a soldier and his partner. 'It was a devastating thing for him to realise that he had come home as a liberator, but he was dying.'

The covert forces of the extreme right wing were also well established in the area. Their members owned many of the hotels, restaurants and bars there, and the faded European-style cafés that lined the main streets had long been the haunt of the apartheid police death squads.

The sex industry catered for members of both left and right wing military groups, whose members had journeyed oft and far through high-prevalence countries to the north. This was confirmed by the many references to Hillbrow hotels, brothels and bars during the amnesty hearings of the Truth and Reconciliation Commission.

One case that came before the Truth and Reconciliation Commission suggests a more active role for the political underground in the seeding of the epidemic during those early years: the right wing may have deliberately used HIV in their dirty war.

Two security policemen made a statement to the Truth Commission alleging that there was a conspiracy to infiltrate HIV-positive askaris[61] into Hillbrow brothels in 1988. The policemen claimed that the notorious third-force killer Eugene de Kock had tasked them with finding jobs for four HIV-positive men as security guards at the Little Roseneath and Chelsea hotels. They alleged that the men were instructed to spread HIV among Hillbrow sex workers. De Kock later dismissed[62] these allegations under oath, saying that everyone knew that it was mainly white men who visited the brothels, and therefore such a plot would backfire. The testimony was withdrawn and the case was never investigated.

For someone who knew the terrain as intimately as Van der Watt, this was not a far-fetched allegation. It was clear to him that the mobsters of the right were running Hillbrow, and had complete control over the hiring of the security guards.

'They were specifically placed there,' he says. 'Their superiors knew they were HIV positive and planted them there in order to have the desired effect. If a woman wanted protection from them, she would have to have sex with them.

'Actually we discovered many of these security guards were HIV positive. I have experienced many years of this... They came to us because they had STIs — they slept with everyone. And when we treat an STI we have to counsel for HIV. We knew what was happening behind the scenes.'

Whether it was a deliberate conspiracy we may never know, but it is probable that hotel owners did use askaris as security guards. And the exchange of sexual favours for protection, between sex workers and security guards, was well known.

Later, during the dying days of apartheid, the death squads of the right wing openly used the sex industry for business and for pleasure. Journalist Jacques Pauw's research into this dark world places third-force[63] agents at many venues with hookers and strippers. Pauw described how De Kock gave a friend R35 000 to set up a brothel in the suburbs and recruit sex workers who 'did not mind sleeping with black men'. According to Pauw, this brothel — in Waverley, Johannesburg — became a major rendezvous for Military Intelligence in the early 1990s. Later, policeman (and convicted assassin) Ferdi Barnard[64] was hired to establish a string of brothels in the inner city to entrap the ANC leaders who were now legally living in the country. Barnard soon earned the title 'the King of Smut'.

Third-force killer Paul van Vuuren described the zeitgeist of the covert forces in the crudest possible terms when he told Pauw: 'It was exciting days, those years. They say to kill is like sleeping with a woman. It is true.'

Alpha male De Kock, however, was more of a prude, and was said to have assaulted one of his closest confidants when found in the lavatory of a Hillbrow hotel with a black sex worker.

In love and war

If Hillbrow was the urban hotspot for HIV, the green hilly province of KwaZulu-Natal was its rural stronghold. The first heterosexual person with HIV in the province was identified at Edendale Hospital, Pietermaritzburg, in June 1987.

Between the appearance of this case and the start of the annual antenatal HIV survey in 1990, KwaZulu-Natal had become the epicentre of South Africa's epidemic.

There are many factors to explain this: the presence of two major truck routes, the high numbers of migrant workers in the province and the high levels of poverty and unemployment are the most commonly cited.

But there is another piece of the puzzle that needs to be considered. During the 1980s, KwaZulu-Natal was also the epicentre of a violent civil war. Cadres from the Zulu nationalist group, the Inkatha Freedom Party (IFP), were waging war on the ANC-supporting United Democratic Front (UDF). By December 1988, over 60 000 had been displaced by the violence and 1 000 people had lost their lives.

Many wars in other times and places have been the catalyst for burgeoning epidemics of sexually transmitted infections. Armed forces, for example, were central to the epidemics of syphilis during the two world wars. During wartime priorities change and safe sex is not one of them. When communities are destroyed and large numbers flee as refugees, sexual mores shift and turn. This war was no exception.

While there is no in-depth research on this subject, NGOs have long understood that the high level of HIV in KwaZulu-Natal is a legacy of those violent times.

In a 1996 interview, Sam Nxumalo, then director of an AIDS prevention programme in the north of the province, explained some of the ways that young people were affected. On the one hand, he said, women displaced by the violence were vulnerable to HIV because they were 'forced to be in love with men, just to get accommodation'. On the other hand, notions of masculinity[65] forged in the struggle years favoured the transmission of HIV. Years after the conflict had ended, struggle machismo continued to put ex-fighters at risk. When Nxumalo tried to speak to young comrades about HIV, they regarded him with scorn. 'They are not scared of death. So if you warn them and say, "Some time you are going to die of AIDS," they say "Nobody lives forever."

'If you die you are considered a brave man, and if you are scared of death, you are a coward.'

Along with a contempt for death, this form of masculinity promotes — and significantly reshapes — traditional sexual mores. 'People say it is in our culture, that as a Zulu male you must have more than one girlfriend or wife,' says Nxumalo. 'If you have one, people will say that you are living like a dove.'

While struggle machismo created favourable conditions for the rapid transmission of HIV, the virus may have had an even more precise agent: martial rape. We now know that many Inkatha fighters received military training from the apartheid forces in Caprivi. Not only was this a high HIV-prevalence district of Namibia, but their training included 'defensive and offensive strategies of war'. In plain speaking, this meant rape and murder.

The records of the amnesty hearings of the Truth Commission[66] give a chilling insight into the horror of those times. Daluxulo Luthuli, Inkatha commander and Caprivi trainee, told the Commission: 'I can say that the situation was bad... People were fleeing the area, fleeing the violence. They were choosing to become UDF members instead of joining the Inkatha, which was involved in killing, kidnapping, rape, stealing, burning and the shooting of people in broad daylight.'

In early 1988 some of these Inkatha paramilitaries were inserted into the KwaZulu-Natal police force to bolster Inkatha's dirty war. Israel Hlongwane was one such policeman. He told the Commission that the rape of young women was a common ploy on both sides of the conflict. 'If they were looking for (an enemy) and they did not find him,' he said, 'they would rape whoever was in the house.'

When asked by a Commissioner what political objective these rapes were intended to achieve, Hlongwane replied:

'It was not a political objective, but objectives of war. I was fighting with a political enemy. The UDF would tell their female members to spy on IFP areas and they would not want to do so after this incident because they would know what had happened to the other girls. Therefore this was a message being sent to the UDF.'

At the time, KwaZulu-Natal communities gave a Zulu name to the hit squads of the apartheid state. The name was *mashayabhuqe*, meaning 'it hits everything'. Ten years after the war ended, they christened the virus with the same name. Like the hit squads, AIDS destroyed everything in its path. It was more than just a metaphor.

'Rape as a weapon of war' featured prominently in the proceedings of the international tribunals for genocide in both Yugoslavia and Rwanda, but rape is yet to be fully acknowledged as a war crime. Certainly the South African Truth Commissioners were wary of engaging with it. The widespread use of rape during apartheid's dirty wars has never been systematically documented, and thus an opportunity to understand its role in the spread of HIV has been lost.

In the case of Israel Hlongwane the Commission dismissed altogether the idea of rape as a political weapon. The musings of the Amnesty Committee provide a fascinating insight into South

African perceptions of sexual violence in wartime.

While trying to get to the bottom of the story, a commissioner asked Hlongwane's attorney: 'If a commander orders his soldiers to get an erection they won't get an erection because there is no self-stimulation, but with rape there has to be that element of self-satisfaction… You know how can you physically rape a person and your motive is purely political? How can you do it?'

Later, a second commissioner underscored his team's failure to understand the concept of martial rape when he said to Hlongwane's attorney: 'What governed the day was love and fear, and the most powerful of the two was fear. And I say, taking that fear and looking at it in the context of rape — you must first have that love, and if that love is preceded by fear would you in the circumstances say rape was political?'

After several minutes of meandering discussion the commission's Judge Khamphepe concluded that the rape was not politically motivated. She said:

'There has not been a single instant wherein the applicants, who we know have been operatives and were performing their tasks sterlingly for their political organisation — there hasn't been a single incident where rape has been an issue.'

But the good judge was not quite correct. There were over 400 statements to the Truth Commission that mentioned sexual abuse of women during the broader political conflict. And this was deemed a gross underestimate by the Special Women's Hearings of the TRC.

Writer Antjie Krog has commented on the 'mutterings of rape behind closed doors'.[67] From her vigil at the Truth Commission hearings, she concluded that many high-profile women were raped and 'no one will utter an audible word about it'.

During the political struggle in South Africa, as in other conflicts internationally, rape was used by both sides as a means of destroying enemy women and humiliating their men. And, as in other conflicts, this war-within-war was largely ignored and soon forgotten. But the legacy of rape has a longer memory.

Much has been written about the links between rape and HIV. But the most compelling evidence comes from an understanding of human biology. In ordinary circumstances, HIV transmission is impeded by the intact tissues of the reproductive tract. But when these are torn or damaged, the likelihood of HIV infection is greatly increased. It follows, then, that a woman who is brutally raped by an HIV-positive man is more likely to become infected than during consensual sex.

The Truth Commissioners' ambivalence aside, political sensitivities have prevented us from getting to the bottom of the complex links between rape, HIV and the liberation struggle.

When an academic at the University of the Western Cape, Professor Robert Shell[68], attempted to dissect the role of the military (left and right) in seeding HIV, he was excoriated by critics from the left who raged against the notion that ANC guerrillas may have been among those who brought HIV to the land. In a piece that expressed the feeling of the time[69], a group of senior AIDS analysts dismissed the idea as 'a favourite piece of apartheid misinformation'. They also rejected the theory about HIV-positive askaris in the Hillbrow sex industry. 'If one wants to find the roots of our epidemic,' they wrote, 'one need look no further than the system of migrant labour in Southern Africa'.

EVERYDAY LOVE

It is easy to see how the fractured social landscape of late-1980s South Africa would have provided a welcoming environment for the new virus.

The movement of miners, travellers, traders and soldiers across the borders, the to and fro of migrant workers, the sexual violence and the destabilisation of apartheid's wars all combined to import the virus and disperse it across the land. And exacerbating all of this were the socio-economic upheavals of the reform period leading to rapid urbanisation, poor living conditions and a booming sex industry, all of which provided fertile ground for HIV.

But there were other forces that contributed to the near-exponential growth of the epidemic in these early years. Then, as now, the new virus found the catalyst it required in everyday notions of masculinity, sexuality and gender roles.

Unequal power relations between men and women are thought to be at the heart of the HIV crisis across the globe. South Africa is no exception. But here, power inequalities between the sexes have been hugely amplified by the harsh world of apartheid — and the struggle against it.

Today a growing number of academics are engaging with

this subject in new and different ways. 'The fact of the AIDS epidemic has started to push in the direction of sexuality studies,' says Suzanne Leclerc-Madlala, professor of anthropology at the University of KwaZulu-Natal. 'It is an important body of study that moves us away from simply gender studies to look at sexuality issues and sexual socialisation and try to understand what role that plays.'

The challenge of this inquiry is to understand the historical construction of sexual culture, how the particular historical conditions shape ideas of masculinity and gender roles and how this has heightened risk for HIV. Understanding the machismo that enabled men to survive the trials of life under apartheid is but one aspect of this complex puzzle. Another that demands attention is the epidemic of sexual violence that has gripped the land. This is a crisis that has coincided historically — almost exactly — with the epidemic of HIV. Recent years have seen a proliferation of academic research that aims to understand the particular construction of a masculinity that allow for rape and non-consensual sex.

Its most extreme form is gang rape. One early study by sociologist Steve Mokwena[70] describes the origins and modus operandi of the violent gangs that emerged in the townships in the late 1980s. The Jackrollers were a gang that specialised in violence towards young women, and gave their name to the growing phenomenon of gang rape. Writing about his in-depth, qualitative research on this subject[71], Mokwena describes how jackrolling, or gang rape, popularised sexual violence among township youth. Jackrolling, he says, was different from ordinary rape in that it was primarily a youth phenomenon. It was always committed openly, often in public places. In time, jackrolling came to be seen almost as a fashion, or a game.

Mokwena is at pains to emphasise that jackrolling must be understood as a historical phenomenon, emerging from the crisis in the education system, from youth unemployment and the social ruptures of the late 1980s. All this against the backdrop of a racist society that emasculated black men.

As Mokwena explains, it is the conjunction of these factors that 'leads to a situation where violence is used as a means of increasing self-esteem. Women, as less powerful persons, become the victim of displaced aggression, the victims of a symbolic reassertion of masculinity and control. Thus, the use of physical force against young women has found widespread acceptance.'

Apart from this rise in gang violence, there has been a huge increase in rape[72] in South Africa since the early 1990s. The country is now said to have the highest level of rape in any country not at war. The streets are no longer safe places for young women to walk alone, and in some areas schools have become places of danger. A recent report of the South African Medical Research Council revealed that almost one-fifth of South African men had raped a woman at least once in their lives.

Less newsworthy than rape, but far more common, is the phenomenon of intimate partner violence. Much has been written about gender violence and non-consensual sex in the context of HIV. One survey of 600 teenaged women in Cape Town found that 60 per cent had been beaten by a male partner. Physical assault was so commonplace that some women saw it simply as an expression of 'everyday love'. In a later piece of research, the same researchers tried to quantify the relationship between gender-based violence and HIV. Interviews with over 1 300 women at antenatal clinics in Soweto confirmed that women who had experienced physical or sexual violence from their male partners were almost twice as likely to be HIV positive as those who had not.

The boundaries between rape, non-consensual sex and everyday love are sometimes difficult to see, as the 2006 rape trial of former deputy president Jacob Zuma[73] revealed. His testimony illuminated the links between struggle machismo, cultural concepts of masculinity, non-consensual sex and HIV. Zuma, a former ANC guerrilla and important role model for the nation's youth, was accused of raping a young HIV-positive family friend. Crowds of supporters, young and old, gathered outside the court. Some chanted struggle slogans like *'awu leth'umshini wam'* (bring me my machine gun). Others wore T-shirts proclaiming: '100 per cent Zuluboy'. Inside the court room, Zuma maintained that the sex was consensual, and justified the incident with recourse to Zulu culture. Much of the time he spoke in Zulu, referring to his accuser's genitals as *isibhaya sika bab'wakhe*, meaning her father's kraal. He admitted entering 'the kraal' without her father's permission, explaining that the young woman was in a state of arousal. He told the court that he had been taught that 'leaving a woman in that state was the worst thing a man could do'.

Historians and cultural activists were quick to point out

that such behaviour is not intrinsic to traditional Zulu sexual culture. For example Professor Sihawu Ngubane, Director of the isiZulu programme at the University of KwaZulu-Natal, told the *Mail & Guardian*: 'Our culture is not written and there are no books that we can go back to for reference on such issues. JZ's statement on Zulu culture is new to me. I'm not aware of such a thing in Zulu culture…'.

The histrionics surrounding the trial were as much to do with the politics of succession as they were to do with sexual culture. However, the extent of Zuma's support demonstrates the acceptance of non-consensual sex as a man's natural right.

At the time AIDS activists expressed the concern that the Zuma trial would set back the AIDS response by many measures. Although he was the former head of South Africa's National AIDS Commission, Zuma told the court that he did not think he was at serious risk of contracting the virus from unprotected sex with an HIV-positive woman. And in any case, he said, he took the precaution of having a shower.

AIDS IN THE CITY

Back in the late 1980s, levels of HIV in South Africa continued to soar. And as the epidemic matured, Chris Hani-Baragwanath[74] hospital in Soweto began to see the signs of what was to come. By the end of 1990, the hospital had treated some 278 people with AIDS-related symptoms — 208 of these in 1990 alone. Hospital staff found this crisis so traumatic that they needed counselling to deal with it. In some cases ward attendants were too afraid to clean the rooms or bring food to those who were ill, and mortuary attendants refused to open body bags to allow relatives to identify bodies. Some members of the medical staff were reluctant to touch or treat the sick, or even to tend to HIV-positive mothers in the delivery wards.

'There had been at least three cases of real medical neglect based on fear,' says Dr James McIntyre who was then a specialist obstetrician at the hospital. 'One woman had a bleed after delivery and because she was positive, nobody wanted to touch her. Another thing was the nurses would put them (HIV-positive women) right down at the far end of the labour ward where nobody would ever see them, so monitoring wasn't happening… that kind of thing.'

It was HIV-positive mothers who were at the cutting edge of Soweto's epidemic. For many, they were the first family member to have been diagnosed, and their babies were the first family members to show symptoms of HIV infection. To deal with this growing crisis, McIntyre and his colleagues established a dedicated antenatal clinic for HIV-positive pregnant women. Without medicines or resources there was little else they could do but offer support and counselling

The unit soon came to represent much more than a medical intervention. Its supportive environment helped women take control of their lives. Mercy Makhalemele was one of the first to pass through this unit. She relied heavily on the doctors, and the positive women that she met at the Perinatal HIV Research Unit of the hospital.

'We decided we needed a group,' says Makhalemele, 'basically to support each other emotionally, but also to talk about HIV, and what we were going to do, and to understand all the issues around breastfeeding, etc.'

The women met regularly, and from an ordinary support network the group grew and developed. The women became active participants in managing their own disease. 'We became women who were very optimistic about life in general and how things were done for women in the clinic,' says Makhalemele. 'By discussing with our doctors and understanding what was happening, the feeling of taking action came.'

In time the group found ways to raise money so that the women could afford to buy the breastmilk substitutes they would need once their babies were born. They called it the 'Forty Rand' scheme — the hospital provided the first R40 as well as free tea, water, milk, sugar and cups. Each group member had a turn to make healthy snacks, which were sold to the women waiting in the long queues for antenatal care. The profit was then hers to keep, and the capital was passed on to the next woman.

Participating in the group also helped the women deal with the inevitability that some of their babies would be born HIV positive. 'We just prayed... I wish mine... I wish mine...' says Makhalemele. 'But from the support group you were already prepared; at least you knew your child would die being cared for.'

Shaun

During the years following his diagnosis in 1986, Shaun Mellors became increasingly frustrated with the media coverage of HIV and AIDS. 'It was always portrayed as if you could immediately tell if someone had HIV, because they were frail and they had that particular look.'

Shaun knew that this imagery was creating a credibility gap among members of the gay community, who by and large were still free of symptoms. Something had to be done.

Shaun had already begun revealing his HIV status at small gatherings, and it was after one of these occasions in 1988 that a member of the National Party government's AIDS unit asked him if he would be willing to feature in their forthcoming AIDS awareness campaign. Assuming that this would entail a simple testimony in the standard educational leaflet, Shaun readily agreed to be interviewed and photographed.

A few weeks later he opened a national Sunday newspaper to see a full-page public service advertisement. 'There was a big picture of me that was not very flattering... it seemed as if they had tried to find one that would make me look victimised,' says Shaun. Even more worrying was the use of his full name, and his life story (complete with inaccuracies).

It was the first time an HIV-positive person had been identified in South Africa's mass media, and it had a huge impact, not least of all on Shaun's friends and relatives who were unaware of his HIV status. His stunned parents answered the constantly ringing telephone with the words, 'This is the first we have heard about it.'

The campaign seemed to take on a life of its own, and the advertisement continued to appear in other newspapers and magazines. As Shaun's notoriety grew, it began to ruin his life. People recognised him in the street and former friends avoided him. He struggled to find a job and the dentist was suddenly too busy to give him an appointment.

Having been involuntarily 'outed' by the government, Shaun continued to disclose his status. Surprisingly, there was hostility from the gay community. Many shunned him, for complex reasons imbued with fear and denial. 'I asked one guy years later why he did that, and he said that he had just discovered that he was HIV positive... He just couldn't cope with his own diagnosis and couldn't understand how I could be so vocal about such a shameful thing, because it was obvious that, as a gay man, you got it from unprotected intercourse.'

Chapter Four
Bad behaviour

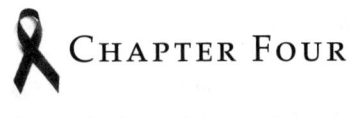

Dangerous disinformation

During the early years of the gay epidemic, the apartheid government had tried to avoid any responsibility for curbing the spread of the disease. But as the heterosexual epidemic began to threaten all South Africans, the government engaged in its own inimitable way. Now that homosexuals and foreigners could no longer be blamed, politicians soon found a new culprit: bad behaviour.

In January 1988, the health minister Willie van Niekerk announced: 'Promiscuity is the greatest danger, whether one likes it or not. We have to say that. It is a fact. There is no way one can say "I still want to sleep around but I don't want to get AIDS."'[75]

In April that year, AIDS was the subject of a lively parliamentary debate.[76] A senior National Party[77] member read from an article that slammed the 'dangerous disinformation' that condoms can prevent the transmission of HIV. He claimed that this advice was only given by doctors who had lost the moral courage 'to tell a hedonistic world that sodomy and other forms of extramarital sex is morally and medically harmful, even fatal, and that the best method of avoiding AIDS, or for that matter any sexually transmitted disease, is to practise virginity before (marriage) and remain totally and exclusively faithful to your spouse.' Another member of parliament wanted to know when legislation would be introduced to 'authorise the Honourable Minister to remove such persons from the community'.

It was against this moralising backdrop that the health department's first mass AIDS awareness campaigns were launched. Government-sponsored posters began appearing in 1988, with a variety of messages. One told its audience: 'Don't sleep around. One-partner relationships are safe. If in doubt, use a condom.'

This message shared the flaws of many of the early international public education campaigns: they stigmatised people who were HIV positive by implying that they were promiscuous. Not only were they counterproductive, but they were also factually incorrect. As many studies have subsequently shown, it is married women, involved in what they believe to be monogamous relationships, who are often the most at risk. Abstinence and monogamy messages are not much use in this scenario.

True to the logic of apartheid, separate educational materials were devised for black and white audiences. And, like apartheid, they were not equal.

In one campaign the white audience was shown a wall covered with graffiti that showed how one youth's multiple sexual contacts created a large sexual network in which the virus would spread.

The advertisement aimed at the black population showed mourners lowering a coffin into a grave. As there had been no known deaths from AIDS in the black community, this was a confusing message. A survey later revealed that most viewers thought that the subject of the poster had died in political violence.

By June 1989, the health minister was expressing his fears about AIDS in the clearest possible terms. He warned that the epidemic had 'the potential to lead to chaos in Africa and South Africa, not only destroying the social and political structures but to lead to economic chaos'.[78] The government ratcheted up its response, and funding was found to reinvigorate the AIDS campaign. Condom use was promoted and a free telephone advice line established. Nearly a million rand was spent on printing and distributing a new round of leaflets. By 1990 the government was distributing 25 million free condoms a year.

AIDS Training, Information and Counselling Centres (ATICCs), which provided free HIV testing and counselling, were also established in several cities and in all provinces with varying degrees of success.

These had a fair degree of independence from the national Department of Health, and some, like the Community AIDS Centre in Johannesburg, managed to establish good relationships with the communities they served. The Hillbrow centre developed innovative programmes, which included an educational play taken to mines and other workplaces around Johannesburg. The feedback from the play provided valuable experience about effective messaging for HIV prevention. Centre staff soon realised the limits of conventional drama as an educative tool. Although the audience was engaging with the plot, the essential health messages were not always getting through. Dr Clive Evian, the Centre's first director says that the play was more of a discussion-starter, not a take-home message. 'In a way you couldn't win, you would always offend someone.'

'What it did do was highlight what a complex and difficult issue this was to address,' says Mary Crewe, the Centre's second director. 'There were some wonderful moments in the play. But there were also some moments which people completely misunderstood.' One such event occurred during a demonstration of condom use. It was usual for men in the audience to gasp and cross their legs when they first saw the gigantic wooden penis on which the condom was to be placed. But on one occasion, Crewe remembers, the actress ran into unanticipated difficulties. 'She said, "It's very simple, when you have finished you take the condom off. And she got it three-quarters of the way off, and there was some sort of vacuum that was created and it just stuck. By the time she got the condom off, it made such a resounding thwack that you could see 500 miners thinking "Oh no, not me, not me."'

Despite the fact that the AIDS testing centres were part of the apartheid local government structure, there was useful work going on. Rose Smart, who worked in one of the earliest AIDS testing centres in KwaZulu-Natal, remembers the good atmosphere that their open-door policy created. Smart doubled her budget with contributions from local businesses and they developed outreach programmes in the townships and informal settlements. Although the civil strife between Inkatha and the ANC was beginning to abate, the AIDS effort still had to find its place in the general post-conflict chaos. 'There were many displaced persons and many places where we couldn't work,' says Smart. 'Even where we could work we had to help to build clinics, organise rubbish collection. It was a hard lesson on how to do development.'

However, many black people shunned the centres because they associated them with the National Party's aggressive family planning policy. For decades the apartheid government had sunk a large share of the public health budget into a black family planning programme that was widely seen as a population control measure. Youth movements from 1976 onward encouraged their members to procreate to counter the effects of what they feared was a mass sterilisation campaign. 'A lot of black people felt that (AIDS campaigns) were a conspiracy to get people to use condoms, which would reduce their fertility and power,' says Evian. 'There was a generalised suspicion. Whatever the National Party did would not have been accepted. People would have looked for some ulterior motive in it.'

The late 1980s and early 1990s saw the growth of a large number of non-governmental organisations (NGOs) specialising in HIV and AIDS. Anxiety about the inadequacy of government prevention programmes, coupled with new international funding opportunities, allowed these organisations to flourish and establish good bases in the townships, informal settlements and rural areas. The NGOs represented a combined workforce of anti-apartheid professionals from the health, education and legal sectors, as well as activists and concerned community members. These organisations developed skills and experience in HIV prevention and care — from printed and audio-visual materials to community theatre; from workshops to income-generating schemes; from home-based care to support groups for people living with HIV.

In 1992, 45 NGOs working in the field came together to form the AIDS Consortium, which had the remit of promoting and protecting human rights in the context of HIV and AIDS. By 1996, there were more than 600 AIDS service organisations working across the country. White gay men who had had first-hand experience of the epidemic comprised a large part of the leadership.

Despite — or because of — the gravity of the issues that were their currency, this was a querulous community with complex politics. 'There were all kinds of territories, and huge toes to stand on,' says Evian. 'There was the gay world and the non-gay world, there was the white world and the black world... everyone thought it was their territory.'

'COME BACK AFRICA'

Back in 1990, in the heady climate of secret negotiations with the exiled African National Congress, a major health conference took place in the Mozambican capital of Maputo.[79] Organised by a grouping of exiled, anti-apartheid health academics in the US, the meeting brought together South African health activists, exiled health professionals and members of the ANC. The purpose was to discuss a strategy for democratising health care in a future liberated South Africa. AIDS was high on the agenda.

It was clear that AIDS was already an issue for the ANC participants, and that they had been seeing illness and death among the exiles in their camps in other African countries for quite some time. South African Communist Party leader Chris Hani[80] addressed the conference with the prophetic words:

'Some of us might regard AIDS as a diversion from the important task of transfer of power to the people... Those of us in exile are in the unfortunate situation of being in the areas where the prevalence is high. We cannot afford to allow the AIDS epidemic to ruin the realisation of our dreams. Existing statistics indicate that we are still at the beginning of the AIDS epidemic in our country. Unattended, however, this will result in untold damage and suffering by the end of the century.'[81]

Alfred Nzo[82], who was later to become the minister for foreign affairs in the ANC-led government, issued a document on behalf of the ANC Health Desk acknowledging that there might be up to 60 000 HIV-positive people in the country. The document recommended abstinence and condom use and condemned stigma and discrimination against those who were HIV positive. It also called for an end to taboos about discussions on sexuality.

The conference delegated an existing health NGO, the National Progressive Primary Health Care network (NPPHC), to take the AIDS agenda forward.

'It was an exciting time,' says Dr Ivan Toms, who attended the conference. 'If you think back, it was really a progressive, proactive response. It was people-centred. We were asking, what can we do for our people?'

Not all participants were as enthusiastic. Dr Liz Floyd, a health activist in the South African delegation, recollects a feeling of unease about how the conference had been run and organised. According to Floyd, in the months prior to the conference, the US organisers had sent a team on a lightning tour through South Africa, interviewing assorted experts and activists about the health problems of the country and the AIDS epidemic. From this, they developed a paper on strategies for HIV and AIDS control which was presented at the conference. This 'outsider' approach did not go down too well with members of the South African contingent; they had their own views, based on many years of active experience in the health system.

'Already there was the politics of ownership,' says Floyd. 'We reacted by saying "Look, if you want South Africans to get involved, don't treat us as people who don't know what is going on."'

Floyd's concerns were shared by many in the large, vibrant NGO sector within the country. This tension prefigured the serious conflicts that would later develop between the exile and 'inzile' community, in which issues of territory and ownership would become the fulcrum around which the AIDS response hovered.

By now there had been a significant shift in the apartheid political machinery, and FW de Klerk's reform-minded cabinet was in charge. The AIDS programme received a boost from a new, more progressive health minister, Dr Rina Venter.

Stricter blood control measures were implemented and plans were announced to expand the ATICCs across the country. By 1992 the AIDS budget had increased from R5,4 million to R20,9 million. Venter established an AIDS Advisory group[83] that included NGOs, and a specialised AIDS unit was established within the health department. The new Unit was headed by psychologist Dr Manda Holmshaw, assisted by Dr Wilson Carswell, a veteran of the successful Ugandan AIDS prevention programme.[84]

Holmshaw and Carswell's team designed an AIDS awareness package[85] for schools that was jointly launched by the ministers of health and education in March 1992. It comprised a 'First AIDS Kit' of literature and audio-visual media, and was available in eight languages. This programme, as well as the one developed later by the ANC-led government, was to face many obstacles in the form of conservative attitudes towards sexuality education. For example, in early 1993, two safe-sex educational videos were banned[86] by the apartheid censorship machine, the Publications Control Board. Even where materials were available the programmes were seldom implemented in the schools. It would be a further six years before such a programme, despite being so desperately needed, would be on offer in the nations' schools.

The AIDS Unit engaged the professional services of an advertising agency to re-brand the government campaign against AIDS. Since 1988, the red ribbon had been an international symbol for the AIDS response, but perhaps because the colour red is associated with communism, this symbol was rejected by the Unit. Instead they chose a hand with fingers outspread in a 'stop' gesture. The hand was yellow, to avoid any unfortunate racial or political associations.[87]

It didn't work. Four years, and R6 million later, there was little evidence that the campaign had made an impact. One survey found that, in rural areas, the symbol was recognised on only 15 per cent of occasions. And in urban areas it was jokingly dismissed as the wagging finger of 'the madam' in her yellow kitchen gloves.[88]

Making a plan

After the release of Nelson Mandela from prison and the unbanning of the ANC in February 1990, the country headed into a new phase that, for the first time, favoured a coherent AIDS policy. Active in this new environment was a group of newly returned exiles with both political credibility and HIV and AIDS expertise.

Among them was Dr Nkosasana Zuma, one of the most outspoken AIDS advocates in exile circles who had worked with exiles living with the virus in the ANC camps. While she mobilised the ANC Women's Movement in KwaZulu-Natal, she took up a contract with the Medical Research Council. Her research, which remains unpublished, focused on the way in which opinion-makers and political leaders regarded HIV and AIDS.

Dr Manto Tshabalala-Msimang, who had also been a central figure at the Maputo conference, became active in the NPPHC, which was coordinating the national NGO AIDS response.

During the early 1990s, the nation and its leaders were absorbed in political negotiations that began in triumph, halted, stumbled and resumed again. The pace of HIV, on the other hand, was steady and relentless, an emergency that would not await the outcome of peace talks and the establishment of a new government.

Dr Zuma and her comrades-in-struggle were influential in placing the AIDS issue on the political agenda. Soon the health desk of the ANC and the ruling government's Department of Health and Population Development began to talk about a united campaign against HIV. This led to the formation of a cross-party think-tank on HIV and AIDS, which was to draft a national plan for a future South Africa.

The first meeting to discuss a coordinated response was held in October 1992. The National AIDS Convention of South

Africa (Nacosa)[89] was a huge affair, attended by more than 400 representatives from a wide cross-section of political and civil groupings, including political parties, NGOs, religious groups, businesses, trade unions and youth groups.

The conference was opened by Nelson Mandela[90], who warned that AIDS threatened the socio-economic fabric of South African society and called for a collective effort to engage in the battle against it. Mandela noted that the current government lacked the credibility to lead the campaign. 'Efforts by the government to introduce preventative measures are viewed with suspicion and as a ploy to control the population,' he said.

Mandela urged parents to find ways of talking to their children about sex and HIV and called for an AIDS Charter that would educate and protect the rights of people living with HIV. He also emphasised the need to address the socio-economic context that was enhancing risk and vulnerability to HIV.

'Compatriots,' he said, 'we have an obligation to move decisively to remove all those obstacles which limit our capacity to deal effectively with this scourge. Do we really have any justification for perpetuating such practices as the migrant labour system, single-sex hostels, which not only destroy family life, but certainly limit our capacity to establish stable self-reliant communities that can be the core of a dynamic society able to cope with this and other problems?

'Is it not time we address the problem of illiteracy and poverty, and empower our womenfolk — all crucial factors for an effective intervention strategy?'

Participants at the two-day meeting agreed to form an umbrella body to coordinate the AIDS response, and to come up with a National AIDS Plan. Dr Zuma was voted chair of the AIDS strategy group. Other convenors included health professionals such as Tshabalala-Msimang and Floyd, as well as prominent members of the AIDS fraternity, such as Peter Busse and Mary Crewe and human rights lawyer Edwin Cameron.

The one grouping notable by its absence was the Democratic Party (DP). This party, which for so many years had represented the only parliamentary opposition to apartheid, was finding itself increasingly marginalised in the new climate of negotiations. Mike Ellis, health spokesman for the DP at the time, says that they were not invited to the launch of Nacosa and were not invited to comment. 'We were pretty miffed. We have said on numerous occasions that AIDS transcends party lines and if you really want to fight AIDS it's got to be a non-political issue.'

One of the conference speakers, Dr Quorraisha Abdool Karim remembers otherwise. 'It was an open meeting. Nobody specified that you can't come in. If anybody didn't pitch up it was by choice, by accident or lack of knowledge. I don't know. The National Party was the dominant party — they were there.'

In the circumstances, the failure to include a small political party was understandable. However, this oversight may have laid the basis for a serious party political conflict that would haunt the AIDS response in years to come.

After widespread consultation and research, the final writing of the National AIDS Plan fell to Crewe. She drew on her experience of running the Community AIDS Centre to decide what was realistic and achievable. 'It was a good benchmark,' says Crewe, 'because we were well resourced and had a lot of capacity. It wasn't a bad thing to use.'

The National AIDS Plan was comprehensive, covering all the areas and sectors of an integrated AIDS response: education and prevention, counselling, health care, human rights and law reform, welfare and research. Each of these had two or three priorities for immediate attention.

The plan went beyond practical and strategic thinking to emphasise the importance of protecting the rights of people living with HIV and AIDS. Confidentiality and informed consent, and the vulnerabilities and the rights of women, were identified as fundamental principles on which the AIDS programme would be based. In its emphasis on human rights, the South African plan went further than the World Health Organisation guidelines of the time.

The National AIDS Plan was well received, and later endorsed by the ANC-led government as the basis of its AIDS strategy. Busse, who co-wrote the section on counselling, says proudly: 'The people who have reviewed it have said it was probably one of the best in the world, because there was very wide consultation.'

Bad timing

With a unified plan to beat the epidemic, and a proactive activist government in the wings, the future of the AIDS response may have seemed assured. But the negotiation years of the early 1990s were fraught with complexity and tension, not least of which was a deep ambivalence towards the political settlement among the ruling elite, an ambivalence that nurtured secret right-wing strategies and agendas.

Covert forces were creating havoc and violence across the land, and at times a civil war seemed imminent. The attention of progressive leaders was attuned to the overwhelming importance of the political settlement for the country's future. This was the issue of the day, and in this context the AIDS response suffered.

For their part, right-wing leaders found new and creative ways of using the epidemic to support their segregationist policies. Banners bearing the slogan 'Apartheid, solution for AIDS' were a common sight at right-wing rallies. Pamphlets [91] claiming that the virus could be spread by informal contact were published to justify this argument. One leaflet claimed that the virus could be spread by coughing or sneezing, and by mosquitoes, and advised readers to regularly test their domestic workers 'to save the white race from extinction'.

Much of the focus, now as later, was on the HIV status of exiled ANC members, many of whom were stationed in military camps in high-prevalence African countries. In 1988, anonymous leaflets began surfacing in the townships, threatening that people who socialised with ANC guerilla fighters would 'cry, and die of AIDS'. Right-wing leaders publicly claimed that all the ANC leaders at the Lusaka headquarters of the ANC were HIV positive, and that the ANC was sending infected guerrilla fighters into the country on suicide missions. Veteran AIDS journalist Laurie Garrett was one of those who investigated this story in 1988.[92] She described how Zambian President Kenneth Kaunda laughed at the allegations, saying, 'Those people (the Afrikaners) are sick mentally. Basically, they are the patients, themselves. They can only think in terms of race, that's all. Colour. The truth is that AIDS is everywhere on earth today, in some places more pronounced than others. But to say that South Africa is free of AIDS, and the ANC are taking the disease to South Africa…'.

Thabo Mbeki, then a senior ANC leader in Lusaka, also dismissed the claims. 'Yes,' he said, 'some of our people have developed AIDS. I don't know how many. But it is our specific policy that they should not be sent into South Africa, because it would be wrong. Absolutely wrong.'

During the political negotiations, the return of the armed wing of the ANC became a fevered issue, and the Conservative Party's[93] AIDS propaganda strategy intensified. In 1991 a Conservative Party MP demanded that all returning exiles be tested[94], and refused entry if found HIV positive. This was countered by Health Minister Venter, who said that this would be an abuse of human rights.

It is not unlikely that a significant number of the some 40 000 exiles returning from Tanzania, Zambia and Uganda were HIV positive.[95] But the politicised and irrational nature of the discussion made it difficult to see this for what it was: a public health challenge. ANC negotiators became increasingly polarised and defensive, and the issue of AIDS was in danger of being swept under the carpet.

The right-wing political strategy to demonise ANC guerrillas had long-term consequences. For years to come, neither the AIDS fraternity nor the ANC were able to countenance any discussion of exiles and HIV. This not only distorted the understanding of the epidemic but condemned many to painful, solitary deaths.

Despite their high-level commitment to the Nacosa process, there seemed to be a growing uncertainty within the health department about the AIDS programme. In June 1992 it was reported that as much as a third of the department's budget for HIV and AIDS was being spent on other things. When the AIDS Unit's Holmshaw and Carswell tried to meet with the minister about this, they were rebuffed. Within a week they were told by the deputy director of health that their unit was to be taken over by the Office of Health Promotion, and that they themselves were to be demoted.[96]

Writing later in *The Lancet*, Carswell described how, in a short space of time, Holmshaw was fired and all prevention initiatives closed except for the continued availability of educational pamphlets in English and Afrikaans.[97] He speculated that there might have been sinister motives. Their actions, he wrote, suggested that '... the government is committing genocide by allowing excess mortality from AIDS to decimate black heterosexuals during the impending period of interim rule and political transition.'

Carswell's suspicions were confirmed by AT Viljoen, member of the government's AIDS advisory group who had written earlier to *The Lancet* to say, 'Insidious voices are already being heard saying the government should stop all reform processes and anti-AIDS campaigns and just "sit it out".'[98]

In many ways, the timing of South Africa's heterosexual epidemic could not have been worse. The violence that was wracking the land and the imperative to rapidly negotiate a political settlement to end apartheid were the issues foremost on the great political minds of the time. It could not have been any other way. But under cover of these monumental events, the virus took root. The annual antenatal survey[99] showed that during the negotiation years, levels of HIV among pregnant women increased exponentially. From a national average of 0,7 per cent in 1990, HIV levels increased tenfold to 7,6 per cent by 1994, possibly the sharpest rise in HIV prevalence ever witnessed.

The timing of South Africa's epidemic was also unfortunate in the context of international AIDS politics. By the time the Nacosa process had begun, a turf war within the World Health Organisation had pushed the charismatic leaders of the Global Programme on AIDS (GPA) out of the agency, and the global AIDS response was faltering. The absence of the feared heterosexual epidemic in the rich north also meant that interest in AIDS was waning, and donor funding for programmes in poor countries had dropped to an all-time low. Even a 1990 report by the CIA[100], warning of a global AIDS crisis by the end of the century, was ignored by the US administration. Interestingly this report, which was remarkably accurate in all other respects, saw South Africa's epidemic as following an industrialised-nations pattern, with a large gay epidemic and only a small number of heterosexual infections.

The troubles in the WHO's Global Programme on AIDS had a direct impact on South Africa. Just when the government programme was most in need of good technical advice, there was not much to be found. The National AIDS Plan was now at the stage when it had to be translated from a theoretical strategy into an implementation plan. When the international experts were called in to assess the plan, they complained that it did not meet their specifications. Crewe remembers this as a galling experience.

'I remember (them) picking up the thing and saying, "This is not a plan. At GPA we have the short-, the medium- and the long-term plan. I have it here on the discs — you can take the discs and you work it like this…".'

In Crewe's view, the experts were out of touch with South

African realities and, in their eagerness to make the plan conform to the textbook WHO approach, they destroyed it. 'What happened is over the next six months we took our organic plan and got it into their bloody logjams (sic) and then it became completely and totally unworkable.'

For a start, once the comprehensive plan was costed, it came to R236 million — which was almost 10 times the current AIDS budget — and called for a daunting complement of staff to implement it. 'I think it was an absolutely fascinating example of how international people homogenised developing countries and did not understand the process that needs to be followed,' says Crewe.

The virus continued...

In 1991 the Department of Health and population development released the findings of the first national HIV survey, conducted the previous year. Women visiting antenatal clinics nationally had been tested for HIV, and less than 1 per cent[101] were found to be HIV positive. Although this was a low statistic in comparison with neighbouring countries, it was still cause for alarm: up to 120 000 South Africans were living with HIV.

But few beyond the small group of experts and activists were paying attention to this unfolding tragedy. Evian remembers looking at the graphs and going cold. 'I had images of being in Nazi Germany as a Jewish person, knowing what was going on and everyone else around you not really understanding. Nobody was getting excited about it. It was a country that couldn't respond.'

While the AIDS response was becoming increasingly entangled in the politics of transition, the socio-economic factors facilitating the spread of HIV were also running out of control.

The new, hard-won freedoms of movement and abode meant that residential areas were changing fast. Inner cities and townships became increasingly overcrowded, and vast settlements of corrugated iron housing sprang up wherever there was space. Increasingly, the occupants of these shacks were single women who were new arrivals in the towns. In these times of rising unemployment, the women would have to depend on informal methods to make ends meet — the sale of food and liquor, sexual liaisons with men who were in work.[102]

In many areas the municipal authorities released their

control of the single-sex hostels that had been constructed to accommodate migrant men. Women from the rural areas, who had friends or relatives in these hostels, were able to move in and set up homes and businesses among the men.[103] One study by geographer Professor Glen Elder, in an East Rand hostel in the early 1990s, showed how it became a site of public and domestic violence and 'an important node in the spread of HIV'.[104]

When Elder returned to the site 10 years later to follow up the 30 women in his study, he found that all but one had contracted HIV. Twenty of the women had already died.

Later research demonstrates the link between HIV prevalence and informal housing. A comprehensive national survey conducted by the Human Sciences Research Council in 2005 showed that those who lived in informal housing were almost twice as likely to have HIV as those in proper urban housing.[105]

Back in the early 1990s, the increasing prevalence of HIV among young women was of great concern to researchers in the field. It seemed as if women from all walks of life were at risk — urban women, rural women, women in marriages and monogamous relationships, young mothers-to-be, older matriarchs, unemployed women, students, secretaries and shopkeepers.

One epidemiologist who was becoming interested in this problem was Quorraisha Abdool Karim. She had recently trained in public health at Columbia University in the US, and on her return began to pursue her interest in HIV.

'I contacted the blood bank and found that they were seeing HIV infection among black people and school children,' she says. 'But there was no other surveillance going on.'

Working with the Medical Research Council in 1990, Abdool Karim was able to integrate an HIV component into an ongoing community-based malaria survey in northern KwaZulu-Natal.[106] She found that HIV prevalence was still at a low level, but three times greater among women than men. The youngest HIV-positive woman in her survey was 12 years old, and the oldest, 66. Few young men — and none between the ages of 10 and 19 years of age — were infected.

Six months later, the survey showed that HIV levels had doubled. KwaZulu-Natal was at the beginning of an explosive epidemic, with women at its centre.

To understand more about women's vulnerability to HIV,

Abdool Karim went out to talk to them in person. The results were illuminating: most women had a good understanding of the virus and how it was transmitted, but very few had the knowledge, skills or power to insist on consistent condom use. Women also felt that men had a right to multiple partners. While few of the women admitted to having multiple partners themselves, they believed that it was common practice for women to take lovers for financial and housing security.

'There was a whole notion that the body must be used for survival when you don't have other mechanisms,' says Abdool Karim. 'It's not sex work. It's due to poverty and abandonment, the need to put food on the table. They were worried about hungry kids, they were not worried about AIDS. Only people with a strong sense of future can afford to worry about survival in five or seven year's time.'

Thus it was that HIV took hold of an unsuspecting populace. The reforms of the late apartheid period created the conditions for a burgeoning HIV epidemic, but at the same time, the imploding political landscape delayed the implementation of a coherent strategy to contain the crisis. South Africa's first democratic government was to inherit one of the most serious epidemics known to humankind.

PART TWO

FAULT LINES 1994 TO 1998

When South Africa's first democratic government came to power in 1994, people living and working with HIV and AIDS were filled with hope. The political will and the resources for an effective AIDS response were assured, and large stores of local and international expertise were available for the asking.

But AIDS issues soon became snarled up in the complexities of political transition: the plain challenge of restructuring a divided health sector was compounded and confounded by party politics, vested economic interests and the racialised thought patterns of the past.

By 1996 the fault lines created by apartheid's evil legacy were clear: the widening gulf between the new government and their long-time supporters in the AIDS community was set to shape the decade to come. And against this backdrop, the virus flourished....

Mercy

There was dancing in the street: Nelson Mandela was coming to address the people of Johannesburg. 24-year-old Mercy Makhalemele was watching the celebrations through the window of the shop where she worked. Earlier in the day her employer had offered to close up, so that they could both go over to the stadium and join in the excitement. He was surprised when Mercy said that she would rather work.

Freedom was something precious, longed for, and fought for even, throughout her student days, but now Mercy had other things on her mind.

'Everybody was rejoicing that Nelson Mandela was becoming president. But my life was already gone. I knew I had this deadly disease and I might not live to see the beauty that this man was going to create in our country.'

Throughout her pregnancy Mercy had been too afraid to disclose her HIV status to the family. But when her baby girl tested positive, Mercy knew she had to tell her husband the truth. It took several months before she could pluck up the courage. But instead of giving her the support she needed, her husband blamed her for everything. They had a huge fight and he threw boiling water at her.

'I lost my home that night,' says Mercy, 'because the next morning I went to work and he arrived there and insisted that I come back home and pack my things immediately.'

To compound matters, a colleague overheard the argument and phoned her employer, who arrived with her 'blue book'. Unemployed and homeless, Mercy turned to the hospital support group for help. They found her a job that came with a small room where she could live and care for her two children. 'So from a manageress I became a maid,' says Mercy. 'And that was not my dream, but I had to kick my pride and say well you are not doing this for yourself, but for your children. You can even clean the street, it doesn't matter.'

Some months later, Mercy's husband fell ill. Only then did he believe what she had told him, and he came looking for her. She nursed him throughout his final illness. The funeral was difficult because her parents-in-law demanded an explanation for his death. They couldn't understand why Mercy was saying they both had HIV, when she looked so well. 'It was very terrible,' she says. 'I was just back from the cemetery and I had to stand with that blanket over me and address both families… and they didn't believe me until they saw for themselves that my baby was HIV positive.'

Chapter Five

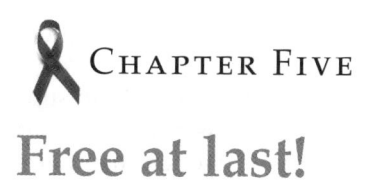

Free at last!

New brooms

By the time Nelson Mandela became president in May 1994, HIV had worked its way across the land, peaking at an alarming high in KwaZulu-Natal where 15 per cent of pregnant women were testing positive.

But in the euphoria that swept the country after the first democratic election, it was difficult to appreciate the enormity of the crisis. For a start, the epidemic was still in its silent, asymptomatic HIV phase, and the small number of people experiencing AIDS-related illnesses failed to dent the nation's good mood. Although the shocking results of the HIV survey were released annually, they were seldom publicised. And with little evidence of illness or death, the press chose not to dwell on an issue that was so out of step with the optimism of the times.

Those who were in the know placed their hopes on the ability of the popular ANC government to avert the catastrophe. The new health minister, Dr Nkosasana Zuma, had a proud record of engagement with AIDS, and President Mandela had spoken with wisdom and insight about the threat of the epidemic. Within the first three months of office, Zuma had endorsed the National AIDS Plan and announced her intention to dramatically hike the AIDS budget. AIDS was named as one of 20 presidential priority programmes.

For the country's AIDS activists this truly was a time of high hopes and brave hearts. With political support, increased funding and a watertight national plan, things had never looked so good.

'We had our new government, and the National AIDS Plan was completed and on Zuma's desk on day one, so that was a very impressive thing,' says Peter Busse. 'During 1994/5 there was collaboration between the government and the NGOs. There was this sense that we were all in this together.'

International observers were also upbeat. 'We felt optimistic,' says Dr Julian Lambert, who was a health adviser in the British government's international aid programme. 'We felt that if any country could do something about AIDS, it's South Africa. It had the infrastructure, it had a pretty effective health system, it had the resources — financial and human.'

But there were early signs that AIDS was an issue whose time had in fact not yet come. Although they had adopted the National AIDS Plan, the new leaders had rejected one of its key recommendations: to place the AIDS programme within the president's office. This recommendation had been based on the experience of successful AIDS control programmes in Uganda and other countries, where top political leadership had provided the critical ingredient for success. But the new government had decided that the Department of Health should continue to take responsibility for the AIDS programme.

From the first day of the new government, Nacosa, the multi-party committee that had drawn up the National AIDS Plan, attempted to meet with President Mandela. But it took six months before a first meeting could be arranged. In his memoir, *Witness to AIDS*, Judge Edwin Cameron (then a co-convenor of Nacosa) remembers how Mandela delegated the meeting to his second deputy president, FW de Klerk.[107]

The sobering truth was that the AIDS crisis was just one of many urgent national priorities. The new government was faced with the immediate imperative of nation-building and the challenge of quelling civil strife to maintain economic and political stability. The new dispensation also required the dismantling of the apartheid architecture of black bantustans and white provinces: from the old order, a quasi-federal system of nine provincial structures and one national government would emerge.

And cutting across these major challenges was the need to redistribute services and resources from the privileged white minority to all of those who needed them. Nowhere was this clearer than in the dual health system inherited from the apartheid regime. This comprised a well-resourced private sector that catered for a fifth of the population (and accounted for nearly half of health expenditure) and an under-funded public sector for the rest.[108]

These then were the issues that occupied the attention of the new government. It was almost a year before Minister Zuma was able to launch the new AIDS unit — the Directorate of HIV/AIDS and Sexually Transmitted Diseases.

The young epidemiologist, Dr Quarraisha Abdool Karim, was the first director. Her expertise in AIDS made her an obvious candidate for the job. She had also established a good working relationship with Minister Zuma when they were both researchers at the Medical Research Council in Durban. Other well-known AIDS activists, like Mary Crewe, Peter Busse and Clive Evian, who had grown their expertise in the forcing ground of the Community AIDS Centre in Hillbrow, would later contribute to the team.

It was with some trepidation that Abdool Karim set off, one morning in January 1995, for her first day in the new job in Pretoria. She remembered all too clearly her first visit to the capital city of apartheid, when as a student in the 1980s she had been turned off a 'whites-only' bus and was obliged to walk up the long hill from the station. Now she was going to her own office on the 18th floor of the Civitas Centre where she would be a director in the new Department of Health.

In some respects, this day turned out to be closer to that nightmarish memory than she could have anticipated. Along with an HIV epidemic that was out of control, Abdool Karim inherited the entire staff and infrastructure of the old apartheid administration. 'They did business as usual,' she says. 'My first executive meeting was in Afrikaans and so I had to intervene and say "I don't mind you doing the meeting in Afrikaans but I would appreciate it if important issues get translated into English every now and again."'

Then there was the matter of the disappearing furniture. As a high-ranking executive, her office was fitted with a comfortable suite and a small boardroom table for meetings. But, like a student initiation prank without the laughs, the furniture kept disappearing and in no time she was left with just a desk and a chair.

Far worse was the lack of even the most basic understanding of HIV and AIDS among her staff. Abdool Karim did a brief survey of the nine staff members and found that not one of them had a comprehensive knowledge of how HIV was transmitted, nor how it could be prevented.

And it was not just the quality of the human resources that was an issue. Abdool Karim had also inherited the contracts and old working methods of the previous regime. For example, when she tried to act on complaints about the poor quality of the free government condoms, she had to argue it out with the tender board. 'They said, "We are not designed for (assessing) quality — we go with the lowest quote." There were already commitments there, and the previous procurements were in place,' she says.

Beyond the struggle to master the bureaucracy was the more substantive challenge of translating the National AIDS Plan into an implementation strategy. 'It ended up quite a monster,' says Abdool Karim. 'It put a lot of responsibility on government structures without taking account at all of what was there. What you had was something that had been developed through a very collective process being usurped, and people felt disengaged. It took responsibility away from people and they lost interest.'

Despite the challenges and the setbacks, Abdool Karim persevered. Staff members who had not left abruptly in her first days pulled together and helped her get the show on the road. She was able to employ consultants who contributed their considerable experience in the field. By the end of the year she had been able to hire more and better trained staff and the HIV prevention budget had quadrupled to R85,5 million. There were plans for awareness campaigns, and to blitz the country with HIV prevention billboards. The condom distribution programme was one of the early successes of the department. By June, the programme had procured 97 million male condoms and 90 000 female condoms for free distribution.[109]

But the very nature of the disease — the stigma and fear that surrounded it — created obstacles for the directorate. For example, the National AIDS Plan had incorporated the agreed international principle of including people living with HIV in all programming. In accordance with this, Abdool Karim tried to recruit people who were open about their HIV status to become 'faces of AIDS' in the provinces, acting as role models for others. But despite high levels of unemployment, there were few who were prepared to be identified. 'We tried to recruit 12 positive people in 1995, and that was an impossible task,' says Abdool Karim. 'Sometimes you forget that.'

Living positively

For their part, people living with HIV were struggling to assert their rights in a hostile environment. After the launch of Nacosa in 1992, a small group formed to represent the rights and needs of people living with HIV. They soon became a formal organisation and named themselves the National Association for People Living with HIV and AIDS (Napwa). From the start it was a huge challenge to organise people who were secretive about the one thing that qualified them for membership. Many of their supporters — like Edwin Cameron and Zackie Achmat — were not yet open about their HIV status.

'Part of the challenge of Napwa... was how we were going to get our membership without necessarily outing them,' says first Napwa chair Shaun Mellors. New members were recruited from the waiting rooms and support groups at the hospitals. Confidentiality was the golden rule.

'Something we always asked was "How do you want me to react if you see me in the street? Do I acknowledge you or do I ignore you?"' says Mellors. 'The majority of the time people said, "Ignore me."'

Peter Busse, a founder member of Napwa, was one of the few who had begun to reveal his HIV status, starting with his closest friends and colleagues. 'You first have to become comfortable with your diagnosis before you can share it,' he says. 'In the 1980s I had this idea that I had very limited time. Then by the '90s, realising that all the Christmases had come and gone and I was still healthy, and there was a future, I wanted to disclose to become complete.'

It took several years before his first public disclosure. While he was attending a meeting to discuss the writing of the National AIDS Plan, he looked around and realised that he was the only person in the room who was HIV positive. When it came to his turn to introduce himself he said: 'My name is Peter Busse. I've been HIV positive since 1985 and I'm living with HIV. I'd like to bring that perspective into the writing of the National AIDS Plan.'[110]

In all parts of the globe where there is HIV, there is also this fearful secrecy that leads to ignorance, which in turn leads to stigma and discrimination against people living with HIV.

From the beginning of her appointment as health minister,

Zuma was among those who were determined to find ways to break this vicious circle. During her budget vote in June 1995, she told the Senate[111] that AIDS must be demystified, and that affected people should be able to speak openly about it. 'They don't do anything that we don't do,' she said. 'They get it from sexual encounters. Who here doesn't have sexual encounters?'[112]

Abdool Karim was also working to try to break the circle. Soon after her appointment she called a meeting with Napwa members. 'She told us that the government thought it was important to support people living with AIDS,' says Busse, 'and that they would give funding if we became a formal organisation.'

The new government's support for people living with HIV enabled Napwa to begin organising with renewed energy. Their focus and membership began to change. 'In the early years it was a majority of white gay men,' says Mellors, 'but then the epidemic itself started changing a lot and it was no longer appropriate to have a white gay man speak or represent issues of a broader constituency.'

At first it was young black women who threw in their lot in with the gay boys. Mercy Makhalemele, one of the first black Napwa members, remembers 'always being the woman amongst gay men', but with a certain fondness.

Alongside their efforts to get the organisation off the ground, the small active membership was also frantically preparing to host a major international conference of people living with HIV. The Seventh International Global Network of People Living with AIDS (GNP+)[113] attracted over 600 HIV-positive people from all over the globe, along with major international donors and several politicians with an interest in the issue, such as Minister Zuma and former Zambian president, Kenneth Kaunda. Mandela had been invited to open the conference, but declined, sending his deputy in his place. Thabo Mbeki told the audience how crucial it was going to be for the new democracy to learn how to support people living with HIV.

'It was an incredible conference,' says Mellors, 'all these people coming together and sitting in one room and trying to develop the global advocacy agenda and 99 per cent of them had the virus.'

After Mellors addressed the meeting, Mbeki came up to him and gave him a big hug, in itself a strong statement in the current climate of fear about HIV. For Mellors, it was an emotional experience. 'In the opening ceremony Mbeki was very emotional as well,' says Mellors. 'He had a tear or two in his eye. The things he said in that speech in comparison with where he is today is mind-boggling.'

This important moment was not covered by the television channels. But even if they had had a mind to report the conference, they would not have been able to film the audience, as the majority were not open about their HIV status.

Napwa continued to face these kinds of challenges. The few openly positive members carried a huge workload, addressing meetings and presenting the views of people living with HIV to the authorities. Several times they made the journey to Cape Town to address politicians. Makhalemele remembers accompanying Busse and others to a meeting with the parliamentary health portfolio committee. 'I saw all these famous people for the first time. De Klerk was there, and Ma Sisulu. I kept on looking at her as I spoke, and I was thinking life is something amazing to be looking at her from so close — I've read and followed and been inspired by the politics of her husband and Mandela. So AIDS did that. I had to be HIV positive to be in close contact with our leaders.'

Makhalemele and Busse spoke to parliamentarians about living with HIV, and many questions were asked and answered. They were daunted by the lack of knowledge of the people in the room. The questions were so basic: How did you contract it? How long will you live? 'I thought, oh my God,' says Makhalemele, 'there is so much work to be done. This is just the beginning.'

ENEMIES IN HIGH PLACES

The AIDS response was just one small part of the health department's mandate. Minister Zuma embraced her entire portfolio with extraordinary energy and zeal, introducing a series of radical reforms that garnered her some powerful enemies. In time, the growing antagonism towards the minister would inflict serious damage on the AIDS programme.

In her first health budget speech[114], in October 1994, Minister Zuma had signalled her intention to radically restructure the racially divided health system. The cornerstone of the new healthcare model was to be a district health system, offering a package of primary health care at minimal cost to users. Although this was textbook public health thinking — and endorsed by the World

Health Organisation — it was not well received by the health professional elite. Among other things, it would involve diverting resources from academic and tertiary institutions to meet the needs of the poorest. Recruiting doctors to under-served rural areas, and giving them incentives to stay there, was another challenge. Zuma therefore signed an agreement on medical cooperation with Cuba, which saw the arrival of more than 100 Cuban doctors in South Africa's rural areas. She also introduced compulsory community service for newly qualified doctors.

Within the first hundred days of the new government the Department of Health had begun providing free health care for children under six years of age and pregnant women. Soon thereafter Zuma took on the powerful tobacco and pharmaceutical industries, and enraged religious conservatives by indicating her intention to allow abortion on demand.

Zuma's concern to strengthen the anti-smoking legislation[115] hit at the heart of Afrikaner capital. For decades there had been a close political relationship between the tobacco industry and the Afrikaner nationalist government. Tobacco giant Anton Rupert had provided massive financial and political support to the National Party, and in exchange there had been almost no control over the tobacco industry until 1993. Under the old dispensation, taxes and cigarette prices had fallen, and cigarette consumption had risen steadily for three decades.

Zuma took this as a challenge, and soon after her appointment she announced big changes. She introduced the first compulsory health warnings on cigarette packs, and raised taxes on smoking. The conflict with the tobacco barons heated up when word went out that Zuma was planning to ban cigarette advertisements altogether. In response, Rupert took out a full-page advertisement in the largest circulation Sunday newspaper criticising the minister.

Another serious conflict — and one that would have a direct impact on the AIDS response — stemmed from the minister's determination to transform the pharmaceutical sector. Like the tobacco industry, the pharmaceutical industry had prospered under the apartheid government. Prices of drugs in South Africa were very high, and they accounted for a huge chunk of health expenditure. Drug company practices, such as sampling and bonuses, gave incentives to doctors to prescribe certain medicines over others, and the lack of a coherent procurement policy meant that large numbers of different drugs were being bought.

This was an expensive and inefficient way of doing business, and Zuma meant to change it. In her early days in office she appointed a committee to come up with a national drug policy. The aim was to promote a more rational use of drugs, to reduce prices and improve licensing and regulation. At its heart was the development of an essential drugs list and standard treatment guidelines for use in the State health system. This strategy had the blessing of the WHO, which had provided Zuma with a technical adviser to advance the policy.

In June 1995, Zuma told parliament[116] that an essential drugs list for common health conditions would be introduced before the end of the year. She also said that the State should have the right to import medicines from other countries if South African manufacturers failed to make their products available at reasonable prices.[117] This, she said, was a fair challenge to the country's manufacturers, who were responsible for producing nearly half of the drugs consumed in the country.

While her reform programme endeared Zuma to public health advocates abroad and anti-apartheid health activists at home, they earned her a line-up of very powerful detractors who would lose no future opportunities to undermine her authority. Her rhetoric and actions, including her much-publicised visits to Cuba, brought her to the attention of conservatives anxiously watching the new government for signs of socialist tendencies. The private health sector and academic health institutions felt under threat and feared for their survival.

The Democratic Party's Mike Ellis confirms that they feared Zuma's reforms would cause the collapse of health care in South Africa.

'We argued long and hard, that while one understood the importance of making health care available to all… (they) were doing it with such speed and such determination that you had the very real prospect of undermining the private health care sector completely, which would have placed a greater burden on the public sector. If the private sector collapsed — you had four or five million people who were on private health care at the time — they would then become extra burdens to the public health sector. But it was being rushed through without any thought at all.'

This then was the political environment in which Abdool

Karim and her small, somewhat dysfunctional team took on the most powerful virus of the modern age.

Although the new staff energised the directorate's work, they were still struggling to come to terms with the unfamiliar bureaucracy.

'I have enormous sympathy for Quarraisha and Zuma, because government was complex,' says Crewe, who worked there at that time. 'I think the decision to just let go all the old bureaucrats who knew the ropes was strategically unwise. It might have been ideologically correct, but it was strategically unwise.

'Some stayed on, but there was a huge haemorrhaging of people who had years of institutional memory. And you would have people coming in saying, "Why does the minister have to have her stuff in a grey file and the director-general in a blue file?" And you didn't know the answers, but the answers were very clear once you saw the system working and realised that it was so that people instantly knew who had to sign, and what they had to sign, and how.'

There were many other challenges: the energy and resources of the new government were finite, and the AIDS programme was struggling to find its place.

This was not a financial problem. Lack of human capacity meant that the Department of Health consistently underspent[118] its AIDS budget until 1998. The new federal system created another set of obstacles. Under this dispensation the provinces were left to implement their own programmes, and here there was little enthusiasm for AIDS.

Lost among competing priorities, the National AIDS Plan faltered. And despite everything that had been learned about the importance of political leadership in the war against AIDS, President Mandela, the one person who held the nation's heart, did not lead.

Florence

Florence Ngobeni was 23 years old when she fell pregnant and discovered that she was HIV positive. She has written a moving account [91] of her experiences:

'I called my baby girl Nomthunzi, the Zulu word for shadow. At the age of three months she became ill. It was only when she was tested for HIV that I found out that I was HIV positive. My partner George, the father of my child, died of AIDS in the same month that I found out that our baby was HIV positive.

'People used to come to my house to see a child who was dying of AIDS. Watching her die slowly every day was heart-breaking. Nomthunzi died in February 1997; she was five months old. I cried day and night, surviving on little sleep and less food. Fortunately, some of the neighbours let me play and read stories to their children, and this was a healing process for me and I continue to be grateful to them.'

Just a few months after her baby died, Florence became a counsellor at the Chris Hani-Baragwanath Hospital's Perinatal HIV Research Unit. Increasing numbers of women were coming to the unit for help, but without drugs there was little that could be done.

'Sharing my personal experiences during counselling sessions has helped both my patients and me. People feel that it is the end of the world when they find out that they are HIV positive. I try to help them continue their lives by sharing some of my past and help them tread this path of survival gently and carefully. I encourage them to find the courage to report cases of rape and violence and to address issues of gender power by inviting their partners for counselling.'

Florence became a prominent spokesperson for women living with HIV, giving educational talks at home and abroad. 'And that's a choice. I dedicate my life to making sure that somebody who's HIV positive can be empowered to know that they can make the difference to their own lives, to make sure that they can negotiate safer sex.' [119]

Chapter Six

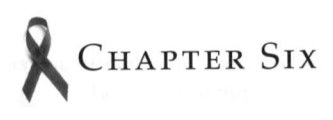

A song and dance

Making a splash

During the first two years of democratic rule, HIV prevalence continued to rise. By the end of 1996 over 14 per cent of pregnant women in the country were testing HIV positive. But the government's AIDS directorate was still struggling to get the National AIDS Programme off the ground. For Minister Zuma and Directorate Chief Quarraisha Abdool Karim it was an ongoing battle. They were up against the conservative bureaucracy inherited from the past, the burden of outdated contractual obligations and even donor ambivalence.

Despite the change in government, it was the NGOs that were still providing the bulk of AIDS services. But in this altered political environment these organisations were losing their strength and independence. Apart from haemorrhaging their top leadership into government posts, NGOs were facing a new funding crisis. Whereas previously they had direct access to huge funding streams from international donors, now the donors were giving their money directly to the democratically elected government. Several leading NGOs were forced to close, among them the National Progressive Primary Health Care network, which had been the driving force of the national AIDS programme.

Although the ANC-led government was more supportive of NGOs than its predecessor, the relationship was damaged by this state of affairs. There was a sense that while the AIDS directorate had displaced the NGOs, it was failing to deliver. Many feared that the AIDS response was grinding to a halt.

Zuma and Abdool Karim were all too aware of this. 'We had this staff that was inherited (from the apartheid era), that had different goals, and they were not always intended for the public good,' says Abdool Karim. 'The Minister was concerned that we had all these strategies in place, but things were slow. She kept asking me: "Can't we take something out there?"'

Against this backdrop of frustrated plans, high expectations and rising HIV, Minister Zuma came up with new plans for a high-profile campaign that included posters, billboards and theatre aimed at raising AIDS awareness among young people. To give it the punch and glamour that would appeal to the youth, Zuma hit upon the idea of engaging South Africa's premier black playwright, Mbongeni Ngema, to produce a musical with an AIDS theme.[120]

Ngema had been turning out box office hits for more than a decade. His popularity with young people, his genius with costume and choreography, and the compelling beat of his scores had the potential to reach into youth culture with new AIDS messages.

With impeccable struggle credentials, Ngema was also the darling of Africa-watchers and exiles abroad, where his plays had toured to critical acclaim. His 1987 play, *Sarafina*, for example, had been a long-running Broadway hit, and had earned several Tony Award nominations. *Sarafina* popularised the plight of young people caught up in the 1976 schools uprising and brought the political struggle against apartheid onto the world stage.

While there were dozens of small NGOs already working in community-based theatre, there had not yet been a project of this magnitude. Judging from Ngema's track record, Zuma felt that he could be relied upon to produce something with more impact than the standard fare of amateur drama groups. Dr Warren Parker, a communication specialist working in the directorate at the time says, 'I think a lot of it was tied to the idea that here we had this great South African playwright who could make a Broadway-standard play, which was now going to do for AIDS what *Sarafina* did for politics. It wasn't a bad idea.'

Thus it was that in June 1995, Zuma and a few members of her team flew to Durban to consult with the man himself.

'I think he was approaching it quite sincerely,' says Parker. 'It was a great honour.'

The group came up with the idea of modelling an AIDS education musical on *Sarafina*, and sending it on tour around the country. It would play in township halls and rural schools, reaching remote areas untouched by television and other media campaigns.

'At that stage it was really conceived as quite a small thing, with a budget of around R800 000. The trucks were going to be donated by Mercedes Benz,' says Parker. 'That was the concept, and then it went through its machinations.'

The meeting was later described by the minister as an opportunity simply to test her idea on an experienced theatre director, rather than to commission Ngema to do the work. Ngema, however, had formed another impression. He later told the *Sunday Argus*, 'When the minister had this idea, it was very clear in her mind that she wanted me to do the play. There is no one else with an international track record and there was no one else who could produce this kind of play and draw in a crowd of black people to the theatre.'

After the meeting, the group flew back to Pretoria and put in place the necessary steps to make the play happen. In a somewhat irregular tender procedure, three theatre companies, including Ngema's, were invited to quote. 'Everyone was new in government and they didn't know what the systems were,' says Parker. 'Things were very much driven politically. Zuma had this idea that *Sarafina II* was the thing to do.'

In August, it was announced that Ngema had won the contract, and the deal was signed. His quote for the play and its national tour was an astronomical R14,27 million. The following week, both Abdool Karim and the new director-general of health, Dr Olive Shisana, wrote to the minister, to alert her to the fact that Ngema's quote exceeded the agreed R5 million budgetary ceiling. But there was no response.

Soon there were other problems. Ngema failed to communicate with anyone in the department about the content of the play. Although he assured them that he was accustomed to doing his own research, there was concern that the complexity of the subject would present too great a challenge. Abdool Karim was responsible for the play's educational messages, but she could never get hold of a script. Ngema kept telling her that he didn't work with a script. It was a work in progress, he said.

'I could see a disaster looming,' says Parker. 'I just worked on other stuff. It was clear that it had political weight behind it, and it kept going.'

A few weeks before the opening night, Abdool Karim, Parker and another staff member flew down to Durban to see a rehearsal. They all felt that the HIV-prevention messages were unclear and inconsistent, and that as an educational project the play was seriously flawed. 'We were really appalled,' says Abdool Karim.

'I phoned Olive and Nkosazana (Minister Zuma), and raised our concerns. There were some discussions with Ngema and he just said: "Let's do the first run and we will work on it."'

'The play was very, very long. Maybe four hours,' says Parker. 'And there were a whole lot of problems and technical inaccuracies. For instance, there was this really effeminate black gay guy with appalling dialogue.'

Parker remembers that Abdool Karim flew back to Pretoria after the rehearsal, leaving him and his colleague to deal with the fallout.

They scheduled a meeting for the following day to discuss changes to the script, but when the time came, his colleague was nowhere to be seen. 'I had to sit down with Ngema and go through all the problems and try to explain how they could possibly be resolved on this short deadline,' says Parker. 'I can't precisely remember if it was two weeks, but the opening night was very close. As I understood it there was a directive that our recommendations would be followed.

'Then we had to fly back and I had to find (my colleague) and he had been hanging out in some pub. He just didn't want to do it. He couldn't face the whole thing.'

By the time the play opened, the most offensive bits had been erased. Despite the fact that the musical was still a long, rambling affair, the kids loved it. It opened to a full theatre in Durban on December 1, World AIDS Day, and all the dignitaries were there, including the European Union Ambassador, Erwan Fouéré.

From the start, AIDS advocates in the NGO sector were critical of the play and of its messages. Pierre Brouard, a trained counsellor at the Community AIDS Centre in Hillbrow, was one of many with educational theatre experience who rejected the work. 'There was a lot of unintended stigmatising stuff going on — unintended consequences from images of sickly people, and death and dying,' he says. 'It also reflected quite an unsophisticated view on what would work to make people change their behaviour. You need much more creative, interesting work that is grounded in an understanding of human behaviour, rather than an expensive play. It was almost like they pinned their hopes on this play… but it wasn't going to do the trick. A play is not going to turn everything around.

'Also Ngema was a bit of a womaniser, and here is he writing about AIDS, and nobody is doing the maths. It's like Mswati (the king of Swaziland) saying you mustn't have sex, and then he has 18 wives.'

Despite their reservations, the NGOs responded constructively, offering to help with a thorough re-write of the script. They met in a large group to watch a video version and come up with solutions. Dr Ivan Toms, who was called in to mediate between them and Ngema, found the playwright open to suggestion. 'He was not an activist or a politician but an entertainer. It was a case of not seeing the bigger picture, and not seeing the consequences of putting in some things.'

Gym slips and pelvic thrusts

For a while it looked as though the situation had been saved. But then, after the play had completed an uneventful two-month run in KwaZulu-Natal, the national press got hold of the story. On January 28, 1996, the *Sunday Times*, South Africa's largest circulation Sunday newspaper, carried an uncompromising attack on the shortcomings of the play — and its huge price tag. The article gave prominence to the views of one enraged health worker who charged that the play represented 'millions of rands worth of gym slips and pelvic thrusts'.

In no time, the musical was on the front page of every newspaper. At first the focus was on the money.[121]

Up until now, state spending on AIDS had been limited, and the *Sarafina II* budget represented a sizeable chunk of the AIDS directorate's budget of R85 million. One KwaZulu-Natal newspaper claimed that the amount was double the entire AIDS allocation for the province — a budget that paid for a local drama group, three counselling and testing centres and several NGOs. Another newspaper exposed to public scrutiny the high salaries earned by the director, his crew and cast. The investment in a luxury bus to transport the cast attracted particular attention. Ngema was criticised for his extravagant lifestyle — one newspaper even forked out for a photographer to take aerial photographs of his house in the Kloof hills. It was a large house, but nothing spectacular.

Accusations of profligate spending came from many aggrieved parties. Theatre directors were quoted as saying that they could produce a similar play for one-seventh of the price;

NGOs complained that they could have made better use of the money; health workers, who were on strike for higher wages, felt that the funding should have gone to them.

And then opposition political parties joined in the fray. 'A frivolous use of public resources'... 'a waste of taxpayers' money'... 'Horrifying, outrageous,' they cried.

The Inkatha Freedom Party took an altogether novel approach for a party with its base in KwaZulu-Natal; its leaders condemned the government for overrating the AIDS crisis. The government, they said, should be spending more money on development issues.

Soon the discontent moved on to the more complex terrain of pedagogy. AIDS activists, who felt their expertise had been impugned, asked why they had not been consulted. Community theatre groups that performed without state funding were particularly aggrieved. Ngema's musical extravaganza flouted all the principles of Freireian participatory theatre [122] on which they based their work. Even the moralists had their say, condemning the play's choice of condoms, rather than abstinence, as a prevention measure.

The anger of the powerful NGO sector was exacerbated by their funding crisis, for which they felt the government was to blame. For the first time, NGOs were being forced to apply for funding through national and provincial channels, and submit their proposals to funding committees. 'You can imagine all the discussion about who was on the committees and who was impartial,' says Peter Busse. 'It was a big source of conflict, and irritation about that, and about *Sarafina*, fed into each other.'

The antagonism of the NGOs to *Sarafina II* was also informed by the old 'ownership' issue. 'There are a few people who are vocal and who set themselves up as gate-keepers of what should be the right messages,' says Abdool Karim. 'For some reason, some AIDS activists and academics have assumed a certain moral high ground. They think they know what is best and I disagree with that approach.'

In the week the story broke, Minister Zuma was in Cuba, making final arrangements for the arrival of the 101 Cuban doctors who would fill the vacant posts in South Africa's rural areas. On her return, on February 7, Zuma confirmed her support for the play and its budget. She told the press that Ngema was well known and she couldn't think of a better person to produce a popular play about AIDS. She also said that she didn't feel she should have consulted

NGOs. 'AIDS doesn't consult,' she said crossly. 'It infects people.'

Shisana was also unrepentant. She dismissed claims that taxpayers' money had been wasted, saying that funds had been donated by the European Union. 'We are not apologetic about what we have done,' she said. 'The previous government paid no attention to the AIDS crisis.' She wanted to know from the theatre directors who claimed they could do the play for less: 'Why haven't they produced anything for that R2 million? Who is to say that a life is not worth R14 million?'

Ngema, too, remained unfazed. He calmly told the *Mail & Guardian* that his services were so valuable that he should have been paid at least three times that amount. But does any director in this country earn those figures, the journalist inquired? 'I don't think you can compare me to anyone in this country,' was his reply.

The persona of Ngema was fuelling at least some part of this controversy. Amid the detritus that this episode had dredged were bitter grievances against the theatre director himself. While his strategy of recruiting unknown child actors from humble backgrounds had earned him a massive following in the townships, his peers on the cultural left were not so keen. There were allegations that he had acquired wealth and fame at the expense of children who were poorly paid and under-schooled. The fact that he recruited at least one of his wives from this pool of compliant youths led to other suspicions.

Zuma, and her colleagues in the ANC who had been in exile during the height of Ngema's fame, may not have known that there had been serious criticisms of the storylines of some of his previous plays.

For example *Township Fever* [123], a musical about the violent 1987 railway strike, was picketed by Cosatu for its factual inaccuracies and its portrayal of popular leaders as drunken fools. There were also allegations that his scripts required a thorough pruning by theatre producers abroad, before the work was fit to go on tour. To some in the world of struggle theatre, Ngema was an opportunist who profited from political crisis.

Though it is hard to rule out the poison that comes from envy, it seems that in the particular case of *Sarafina II*, his detractors may have had a case. 'He never delivered,' says Abdool Karim. 'He put in a couple of million for this bus that was moving around, but he never did those journeys. He fell short of delivering on that.'

Crying foul

In the face of all the criticism and carping, Minister Zuma and her team held fast to their faith in the musical.

But things soon took a more serious turn. Information about irregularities in the tender procedure began to surface, and provoked conflict of a more party political nature: the Democratic Party vs the African National Congress.

Mike Ellis, the Democratic Party health spokesperson explains: 'We were already critical of her (Zuma) then, because we had anticipated that with the arrival of the ANC in power that there would be quite an issue around AIDS. And there wasn't. And it did seem that the minister was going to use *Sarafina II* as an attempt to persuade people that she was actually involved… (but) this was really a kind of showcase that could have no benefit at all.'

The parliamentary health portfolio committee, a multi-party watchdog chaired by ANC member of parliament Dr Manto Tshabalala-Msimang, became increasingly concerned about all the allegations. Zuma and Shisana were called to a meeting. According to Ellis, Zuma was angry and defensive and failed to give a proper account of what had gone wrong. At the time Ellis told the press: 'They were allowed to get away with this because clearly the ANC members of the committee were not going to ask pertinent questions.'

Ellis then called for the immediate suspension of Zuma, but he lost the vote. Instead, the committee passed a motion of confidence in the minister.

After the meeting President Mandela came out in public support of the minister.[124] The ANC issued a statement saying, 'It appears as if those elements within the DP seek to abuse *Sarafina II* to tarnish the image of Zuma whose role in the fight against AIDS and in the transformation of the health sector has been broadly acknowledged. The ANC rejects the call for the suspension of Zuma as little more than sour grapes from a party which failed to win its position within the portfolio committee.'[125]

So two years into the new democracy, AIDS had become a political issue, in the narrowest sense of party politics. From now on, doubts would hang over anyone who commented unfavourably on the government's AIDS programme.

Immediately after the health portfolio committee meeting,

the European Union issued a statement repudiating the claim that it had donated the money for the play.[126] This provoked a further outcry, and the Democratic Party asked the office of the public protector to investigate.[127]

This was the first time the office of the public protector — a new body created to protect the public from government misdeed — had been called upon to act. Ellis expressed his concern that the president's public support for Zuma might result in the matter remaining unresolved.

By the time the public protector, Selby Baqwa, made his findings known[128], the play, and the accounts, had been frozen. Baqwa exonerated the minister and found that the idea of the play was a worthy one. Both Abdool Karim and Shisana were criticised[129] for the way they had discharged their duties. Baqwa said the inexperience of the Department of Health's lawyer, which led to flaws in Ngema's contract, was also to blame. However, only the acting chair of the tender board, and the chief director of departmental support services — both members of the inherited bureaucracy — were found guilty of misconduct. Baqwa found that they had colluded to mislead the minister into thinking that the tender had been approved, when apparently it had not.

On the matter of the funding, Baqwa accepted witnesses' statements that there was genuine confusion around the European Union's funding procedures, which the directorate had subsequently resolved. Nonetheless, he found that the money constituted unauthorised expenditure. This meant that the department had spent money that it did not have, and did not have the authority to spend. Zuma accepted Baqwa's findings without reserve and reported on her actions to strengthen management procedures in her department. She also announced the termination of Ngema's contract. The ANC also welcomed the findings and congratulated the minister for accepting them.[130] The bureaucrats from the apartheid regime had become the convenient fall-guys. 'We note with concern,' their statement read, 'that the minister was misled into taking certain decisions on the basis of misrepresentation by two officials in her department... Only history will tell whether the two had acted with political or sectarian motives...'

But by the time all was said and done, the abortive play had cost the government more than R10 million.[131]

The balance sheet

The public discourse around *Sarafina II* had complex undertones. What seemed, on the face of it, to be serious mismanagement of a well-meaning project became tainted with resonances of corruption and wrongdoing. This was reinforced when the minister and her staff closed ranks, became defensive and gave misleading explanations.

President Mandela was later to say that *Sarafina II* was one of the major errors of his government. In his January 1997 address to the nation, he said: 'Let us not be defensive… I have recently made this point in regard to how we handled *Sarafina II* and the issue of funding for the ANC. The question is not so much whether one makes mistakes or not, but rather whether, as an organisation, we are prepared to admit mistakes, and above all to learn from and quickly rectify weaknesses in our work.'[132]

But it was impossible to estimate the damage done to the government's relationship with the AIDS fraternity in the country. Most serious was the trust that had been broken between the minister and the AIDS research community.

'I suspect that both sides didn't really understand where it was heading,' says Dr James McIntyre, founder of the Perinatal HIV Research Unit at the Chris Hani-Baragwanath Hospital. 'I don't think the activist community thought the government would get so upset, and I don't think the government thought the activists would take it as far as they did in terms of public criticism. That was the first time this government had been criticised. Whether it had been *Sarafina* or housing, the government's response would have been the same. I think for me that was the beginning of the end of the relationship.'

McIntyre's personal relationship with the minister of health was permanently impaired, and this would dent her confidence in his research. 'The minister was very upset, because I was quoted on the front page of some newspaper criticising her, and her response was that I could have picked up the phone and talked to her directly. And so she kind of stopped talking to me,' he says. '*Sarafina* really broke apart the trust that existed between the medical community, the AIDS community and the government. Completely. It then became very hard to push for anything because there was always seen to be an ulterior motive for trying to push something forward.'

This mistrust must have been significant in the later political struggle over access to treatment for pregnant women, in which

McIntyre's research formed the basis of the activists' demands.

So the *Sarafina* episode marked a turning point for the AIDS fraternity and the government. Writing in an academic journal four years later, Mary Crewe summed it up: '*Sarafina* introduced the beginnings of AIDS orthodoxy — the government line was the one orthodoxy, and the NGO line the other... This division came at the time when a united response could have worked to shift public perception about the disease and about people who were living with HIV. Instead, the general public was largely excluded from the AIDS world — instead of creating a climate of inclusiveness, the AIDS orthodoxy drove people away.

'AIDS became a world of exclusion, both by the government — who shunned at all times local expertise and experience looking to outsiders to generate an African response — and by AIDS organisations who fiercely guarded who was "in" and who was "out", who could talk and who could not.'[133]

The biggest loser was the National AIDS Plan. Instead of using the failures of the play to focus on the escalating HIV crisis, and to stimulate debate about how to respond, the discourse was all accusation and acrimony, superficial point scoring and moralistic judgements about money and who had the right to earn and spend it.

'I thought people were fixating wrongly on the R14 million, that wasn't the issue,' says Crewe, who was working in the directorate at the time. 'We had just got a grant for R14 million for the lifeskills work. It was not a lot of money for eight-and-a-half million schoolchildren.'

Instead of receiving praise for the massive hike in AIDS spending, critics lambasted the government's expenditure on *Sarafina* by comparing it to the previous apartheid-era AIDS budget.

The *Sarafina* episode represented a missed opportunity to start a fertile debate about appropriate mass communication strategies that would reach the nation's youth. Levels of basic AIDS literacy in South Africa were already high, but young people remained unconvinced that they were at personal risk. There was an urgent need to break through this first barrier to behaviour change.

The episode was also to set a pattern for the way the mass media would deal with AIDS in years to come. Instead of treating AIDS with the seriousness it deserved, the media's treatment of *Sarafina* turned AIDS into a political farce, a standing joke.

But there was something more disturbing about the news

coverage, which seemed to hark back to former times. Zuma was not merely criticised, she was vilified. She was not merely satirised by cartoonists, but caricatured as a stout, fat-lipped, ugly satyr that danced and threw money across the stage. The dividing line between disrespect and a good cartoon may be hard to find, but the wordsmiths also went at her with a fervour that seemed out of place for serious journalists. 'She reminds me of a middle-aged Staffordshire bull terrier or two I have known,' wrote a journalist from the *Mail & Guardian*. 'She is stolid, doughty, thickset and low-slung, unfashionable but powerful; wilful and driven; self-contained, diffident and sometimes downright crabby.'[134]

It was almost as if the *Sarafina* crisis had opened the floodgates to a torrent of suppressed anger, disappointment, envy and hostility towards the country's new leaders. For two years now the new government had trodden lightly over the wreckage of the apartheid past. President Mandela's statesmanship had earned him admiration and respect from all quarters. But now the grace period was over. It was time for the real thing to begin.

ENTER BIG PHARMA [135]

There is yet another dimension to the vitriol that greeted the minister's AIDS education debacle. The *Sarafina II* episode was not playing on an empty stage, but against the backdrop of Zuma's radical health reforms.[136] The feisty health minister's attempts to democratise access to health services, her pro-abortion bill and her anti-smoking laws, had stoked a chorus of angry of voices.

The Democratic Party was closely involved in monitoring the new health legislation, and their response to these reforms, and to *Sarafina II*, soon became entwined. By the time of the public protector's report on *Sarafina II*, relations between the Democratic Party and the government had dived to an all-time low. Ellis, who was watching both stories, explains: 'There was a huge standoff between Zuma and myself, because at the same time we were starting to deal with all this other contentious legislation,' says Ellis. 'The minister was trying to revolutionise health care in South Africa… It had the potential to really force the collapse of health care in South Africa.'

The Democratic Party's opposition, which went to the heart of its political mandate, was crudely understood. 'I was just seen by the ANC as a white racist,' says Ellis, 'and every time I got up to challenge Zuma it was said, "You are challenging a black woman because you are a white man."'

The most contentious of the minister's proposed reforms concerned access to affordable medicines. Zuma's new drug policy sought to radically reduce the cost of medicines and included measures to promote the use of generic drugs rather than the more expensive branded versions. The policy was revealed around the time that the *Sarafina* scandal broke, and provoked the ire of the powerful pharmaceutical industry.

President Mandela was among those who felt that the outcry over *Sarafina* was related to this wider political and economic environment. In September 1996 he openly suggested that the uproar over the play was part of a broader strategy to discredit Zuma.

'What is being fought in this country by traditionally white parties and white interests,' he said, 'is the fact that for the first time, we have a minister who has decided to take on the multinationals monopolising the market dealing with drugs. What the minister is doing is to try and ensure that medical services are affordable to the poorest of the poor. That of course is going to mean the market that is monopolised by big foreign conglomerates is now going to be exposed to competition. That is the battle that is being fought.'[137]

The pharmaceutical industry reacted angrily to this accusation. Their representative, chief executive officer of the Pharmaceutical Manufacturer's Association (PMA), Mirryena Deeb, told the press, 'It is both unfair and unfounded to blame the multinational pharmaceutical companies for an issue that has only to do with bad governance and nothing to do with issues of health policy.'[138]

This was the first exchange of fire in the long battle between the government and the pharmaceutical industry, which would have its denouement on the world stage in 2001.

Within two years of office, Zuma had a powerful array of enemies to the left and to the right. She had offended legions of former political allies, threatened the Afrikaner establishment and taken a stab at the multinational pharmaceutical industry. No wonder she felt that her back was against the wall.

She told a *Mail & Guardian* journalist that the 'enemies of transformation'[139] of the new era were far worse than the enemies she encountered as an underground operative in the liberation struggle.

Despite her bad press at home, Zuma's commitment to health reform and to fighting HIV had earned her considerable credibility in international circles. She was by now serving as vice chair of the governing body of the Joint United Nations Programme on HIV/AIDS (UNAIDS), the agency established to coordinate the United Nations' response to the virus.[140] In 1996, she was invited to give the keynote address at the XI International AIDS Conference in Vancouver, which was a major event on the global AIDS calendar. This conference was the first to bring any encouraging news for those living with HIV. Trials of a new class of anti-AIDS drugs were showing positive results when used in combination with other medicines. Antiretroviral therapy (ART) comprised three separate drugs whose combination had been found to clear the virus from the blood. This new therapy was not an unqualified success, as the drugs did not cure, and they had to be taken continually to prevent the virus from rebounding. In addition, ART was a complex regimen of up to 20 tablets a day, a regimen that required ongoing monitoring for efficacy and side effects. And even for rich countries, the cost was exorbitant.[141]

Nonetheless, early trials were showing miraculous results. Many people who were near to death at the onset of treatment had returned to good health in what came to be known as the Lazarus effect.

There was still more good news. Another new study showed that treatment with a single drug, AZT, could radically reduce the incidence of HIV transmission from mother to child. This, too, was an expensive regimen, but promising trials in West Africa indicated that a shorter (and thus cheaper) course of AZT might be effective.

This moment in 1996 was a significant milestone. For the first time in the history of the epidemic, the multinational pharmaceutical industry held the key to the survival of the some 21 million people living with HIV.

In her keynote address at the conference, however, Minister Zuma was at pains to remind her audience that the majority of HIV-positive people were in countries too poor to contemplate these remedies. She warned that AIDS was changing the population structure of many African countries. By 2010, life expectancy in Zambia and Zimbabwe was expected to fall by over 30 years. 'These countries will lose an entire generation of elders,' she said.

But the minister was unable to enjoy her moment of authority and fame. In the middle of her speech she was interrupted by the shouts and chants of angry South African AIDS activists, calling her to account. *Sarafina II* had followed her halfway across the globe.[142]

Mercy

Although Nkosi Makhalemele was healthy at birth, by the time she was two years of age her small body was feeling the effect of the virus in her blood. For her mother, Mercy, it was a time of anxiety and pain. There were frequent episodes of acute illness that ended in late night dashes to the nearest hospital. 'It would be a fight', says Mercy. 'Some hospitals did not want to admit a baby that was HIV positive. They didn't have enough beds... they didn't have enough oxygen. Oh, you know...'.

Many times Mercy had to call Glenda Grey, the doctor from the Perinatal Unit at Chris Hani-Baragwanath, to help her fight her case. 'My child went through hell with this thing. The Jo'burg Gen, Edenvale... I will never forget... I would call Glenda in the middle of the night and say "Look Nkosi is not breathing, what will I do?" And Glenda would get up and come to the hospital and help me to get her admitted.'

One day Nkosi was tearing around the house in high spirits, when she began to sweat profusely. Although Mercy was not worried, she decided to take her to the hospital.

'Twelve o' clock midnight, she died. She still had her hair in these little bunches and I had to undo them when I came to the hospital at two o'clock in the morning. Still very healthy and fat. The chest just decided to close. She had no pneumonia, she had no asthma, she had no bronchitis. The only thing was, she had a problem with her heart.'

A few months after the death of her child, Mercy was offered a job as the Napwa regional coordinator in KwaZulu-Natal. She jumped at the chance, arriving in Durban on the day of her 26th birthday. That night she took herself out to dinner, alone.

One of her first engagements was to address the annual Miss Durban competition. As a Napwa representative, she needed to reach young people with her message of living positively with HIV.

'Before the crowning I had to talk,' says Mercy. 'There were about 2 000 people and they wanted to see Miss Durban and they didn't give a shit about me. I said I am not getting off this stage until you keep quiet and hear what it is that I have to say. I just stood and stood. I was not even embarrassed. I just kept standing there until there was silence.

'Then I said to them: I am not terminally ill with AIDS. I am just like you, but I am HIV positive. And this is a message from HIV-positive people. You cannot identify us. You live life with us and even though you say you are scared of us, whatever you are doing, we are always there. Today I have been sitting with you, we have been dancing together. You say you are scared of touching us, but I have touched many of you today. Don't worry, I cannot infect you in this way.

'And there was silence. Silence. Silence.'

Chapter Seven

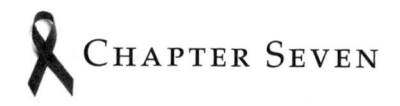

Of hearts and minds

A cure for Africans by Africans

One Wednesday morning in January 1997, South African cabinet ministers met to discuss a matter that would shape the future of the country's AIDS response. With permission brokered by Deputy President Mbeki, the health minister had invited some unusual guests. Among them was a slight, dark-haired woman who was introduced as Olga Visser.

To the rapt group, Visser described the chance occurrence that led her to stumble upon a cure for AIDS. In the course of her research at the University of Pretoria, she had discovered a chemical that could kill the virus without damaging the cells of the host. This ingredient, she told them, was now patented as Virodene PO58.

After her discovery, as the story went, Visser engaged the help of her colleagues Professor Dirk du Plessis and Dr Kallie Landauer, to advance the research. When *in vitro* tests looked hopeful, they began testing this substance on a dozen people seriously ill with AIDS-related illnesses. She had brought two of them with her to talk about their experiences.

Later Mbeki would write about how moved he was by the testimonies of Visser's patients on that day.

Under conditions of anonymity, these patients told their stories to the press. 'John', a self-employed Soweto resident, spoke about how he had been diagnosed as HIV positive a few years previously. Before starting Visser's treatment, his body was covered in boils and he was in a bad way. 'Really I was so weak I couldn't even lift a mug,' he said. After just three doses of Virodene, administered as a skin patch, he had gained ten kilograms and his boils had gone. 'John's' wife 'Emma' had a similar tale. She had herpes sores and was dangerously thin, but the way she told it, after just one dose of Virodene the infection cleared up and she gained weight. Her diarrhoea had also stopped.

Visser summarised the test results, giving statistics that showed that after just a few doses, the amount of the virus in the blood dropped dramatically, and the immune system cells rebounded.[143]

The most encouraging thing about the drug, said Visser, was that it was able to fight the virus in the brain and lymph system. This was an advance on the recently discovered three-drug cocktail, she said, which could only eliminate the virus from the blood.

Even more encouraging was the cost. One dose of Virodene was estimated at around R80, and the researchers thought that a cure could be achieved within just six weeks. By comparison, the triple-drug cocktail was a lifelong investment of over R7 000 a month. Visser told cabinet that they needed a further R3,7 million to complete their work.

After the presentation, the entire cabinet stood up and applauded. Years later, cabinet secretary Jakes Gerwel could still remember the excitement in the room. He told a journalist, 'It was like a church confessional. The patients said they were dying, they got this treatment, and then they were saved! The thing I will always remember is the pride in South African scientists.'[144]

Later that day Mbeki told the press that the government would look favourably on the scientists' request for funding. 'We would be interested that the research continues,' he said.[145]

The story dominated the news headlines and billboards across the land. Virodene was hailed as a major breakthrough, a wonder cure for AIDS. Many column inches were devoted to interviews with Visser, her team and patients.[146] Complex explanations were given for the way the wonder drug worked, and elaborate diagrams tracked how the tiny molecules of Virodene were able to penetrate the body's cells and attack the virus lodged within.

The newspapers also provided an explanation for the mysterious way in which this breakthrough had been made public. Visser's husband and business partner, Zigi[147], told the *Sunday Independent* that their research had been blocked by the big drug companies and powerful people in the AIDS world.

'We then decided to take the study underground,' he said. 'Once we started clinical trials it was top secret and only the minister (Zuma) and some members of her department knew anything about it.'[148] According to Zigi Visser, they had approached Zuma eight months previously, and she had helped them circumvent the red tape and gain access to the laboratories and hospital facilities they needed to do their research.

Olga Visser's characterisation of the Virodene story chimed with the patriotism of the era — the rainbow nation, the new South Africa. It was, she said, 'a cure developed in Africa, for Africans'.

Waking up on Thursday morning to this barrage of media triumphalism was a shock for people working and living with HIV. For them the story had a surreal quality. 'I seem to remember we were stunned,' says Mary Crewe, who was then director of the Community AIDS Centre in Hillbrow. 'It was this very strange mixed feeling… Is it true? How exciting if it is true… on the other hand, how could this possibly happen? And then there were the incredible levels of hope that were raised.'

Crewe and her colleagues at the centre were inundated with queries from the public, people calling to find out more about the cure and asking how they could lay their hands on it. Their replies were cautious: apart from what they read in the press, they had no details about the drug. Nor was there any information forthcoming from the government's Directorate for HIV and AIDS in Pretoria. Neither the new director, Rose Smart, nor her team of AIDS advisers, had been briefed about the cure that had been embraced so wholeheartedly by their minister.

The instinct was to mistrust the news. For Peter Busse, who had attended medical conferences on AIDS for several years, the fact that it came out of a complete vacuum was cause for suspicion. 'This is not the way the world works,' he says. 'You don't have a breakthrough like this when nobody has even heard of any promising trials.'

From the start, members of the large expert research community voiced their concerns. Without knowing the active ingredient of the drug, they were sceptical about such dramatic claims from a group of unknown researchers whose work had not been submitted for peer review. There was no published information on their research at all. Nor had the drug regulatory body, the Medicines Control Council, approved the research protocol.

As more details emerged, it became clear that the research had been in serious breach of medical ethics. Visser and her team had by-passed the standard research protocols and experimented with a dozen desperately ill 'human guinea pigs', five of whom had been 'lost' to ongoing research. Not only was their approach unethical, but it was also unscientific. While this kind of preliminary small-scale trial, known as a Phase 1 trial, is standard in pharmaceutical research, it gives neither definitive results nor an indication of long-term side effects.

As the furore unfolded, the scientists were challenged — and failed — to produce evidence of controlled clinical tests. The medical community was up in arms.

The Medicines Control Council kicked into action. Within three days of the cabinet meeting, the council chair, Professor Peter Folb, met with Visser and her team. They agreed to suspend the human trials for ten days while the research results were being scrutinised.

The Olga and Zigi show

The aspect of the story that most puzzled members of the scientific and medical community was the absence of AIDS expertise in Visser's team.

So who were these path-breakers, and how had they come to headline-grabbing fame in such a short space of time?

Du Plessis, whose academic qualifications lent gravitas to the enterprise, was a cardio-thoracic surgeon, and Landauer was his clinical assistant. Both were based at the University of Pretoria. In an interview printed later in the *South African Medical Journal*[149], Du Plessis confessed that they knew 'sweet nothing' about medical research. Although they had experience in cryopreservation (the preservation of living tissue), this was their first encounter with drug research. He expressed regret that the story had reached the media in the way that it had.

Olga Visser, the focus of most of the media attention, was a medical technician who worked for Du Plessis. Her job involved operating the heart-lung machine during open-heart surgery, but she had also been experimenting with preserving heart tissue at low temperatures.

Visser also had prior media exposure. In 1995, the *Sunday Times* reported that Visser had made a major breakthrough in cryobiology by finding a new compound that would allow her to freeze heart tissue with virtually no damage. She claimed that, when warmed, the treated heart (of a rat, not a human) resumed beating normally. These advances would of course open up exciting possibilities in the field of transplant technology, and have great significance for cryonics — the speculative preservation of human life. Cryonics, though not considered a science, is supported by a large, well-funded international research fraternity.

Olga Visser's rat heart story was picked up by international experts in cryobiology, who attempted to engage her in a discussion about her methods. She was invited to write up her research for the journal *Cryobiology*. This would subject her methods to peer review, as is customary in scientific research. Nothing was heard from her until August 1996, when she joined an online discussion in which, among other things, she railed against the scientific orthodoxy, accusing them of conspiring against her and her work.

'Cryonicists beware where you take your business!!!!!' she wrote. 'You might end up in a dead end… My technology will be made available at a low cost to all other cryonic companies… I have succeeded where all others have failed!'

In a later correspondence she advised cryonicists to 'entertain and make friends with the press and media above all else — they are more powerful than all governments and academics put together, they get you heard where it counts… they also give you the leverage you need when it comes to bureaucrats. Before you know it, cryonics will be (as) recognised as cornflakes and you will have achieved your goal.'

Later it emerged that she had been contracted by one of the leading US cryonics companies which was using her work to campaign for unrestricted donations. The world of cryonics, already riven by competition and hostility, was divided into two camps over Visser's research. One of the doubters raised Visser's ire by asking that her US backers provide more than verbal assurances that the experiment worked.

'Perhaps (his) say-so does not make it true, but your contention therefore most certainly does,' she replied. 'Rather crawl back in your miserable hole life has provided for worms like you, than insult those who contribute to life what you can never understand, and suffer humanity no more of your ignorance.'

On February 1, 1997, just one week after her meeting with the South African cabinet, Olga Visser was given the chance to prove to the world what she was worth. She was the leading attraction at Alcor's cryonics festival in Arizona, US.[150] On the first day she submitted to a detailed Q&A session. One of the things she made clear was that her combative emails had not been written by her, but by her husband Zigi and 'an employee of the South African government who protects me from my critics and keeps me away from journalists'.

So it seems that just one week after her meeting with the cabinet, Visser had a public relations officer in the South African civil service, although, apparently, not a very good one.

According to a detailed account written by cryonicist Charles Platt, by 10 am the next day Olga Visser was hard at work, freezing a fresh rat heart in her secret potion. An audience of 30, all world leaders in the field of cryonics, were in the adjacent room watching the experiment on a video monitor.

After 20 minutes, before the eyes of the watching crowd, Visser removed the frozen heart, which was a healthy red-brown colour, and began to warm it to room temperature. She prodded, tapped and massaged it and then pierced the heart with three EEG probes, which translated their signals into audible beeps. Visser told her audience that the beeps indicated muscular contractions, but Platt and other observers suspected that the beeps were caused by the heart being moved. Visser continued to claim success, even after the heart tissue began turning grey — a typical sign of post-freezing injury.

Undaunted, Visser got to work on a second heart, and this one proved an even worse failure than the first. By the end of the day, the audience had dwindled to seven; the fourth heart, when removed from the solution, was cracked and damaged beyond repair.

Platt, who had been present until the bitter end, agrees that the four failed attempts did not disprove the claim, but the demonstration had given him worrying insights into Visser's experimental technique.

'She worked impulsively, changing parameters like a chef deciding to add a little more salt, or a little less sugar, each time she cooked a particular dish,' he wrote. 'There seemed to be no standardised protocol for mixing, filtering and storing chemicals, cleaning equipment and handling the solution… There was no permanent record of EKG signals (other than shaky video) from the re-warmed heart, and there was no one affiliated with the experiment who had the necessary training to evaluate the EKG.'[151]

Mike Darwin, another cryonicist in the audience, later wrote the words that must have been on many people's lips that day: 'Mrs Visser and her husband Zigi were complete frauds… I can

Side effects

Unfortunately the news of Olga Visser's unconvincing performance in Arizona did not filter back to South Africa. Nonetheless, the mass media had swung from their early, uncritical praise to angry denunciations of the bogus cure.[153] The researchers and those who had been taken in by them, particularly Minister Zuma, were condemned and vilified. Some newspaper had even nicknamed the new scandal 'Parrafina' to rhyme with the previous year's AIDS debacle. Much was made of the news that Virodene's active ingredient was a simple industrial solvent. The substance dimethylformamide (DMF) was the same mixture that Visser had been using in her cryonics experiments. And it was known to be harmful to human life.

Soon after Olga Visser's US sojourn, there was a second meeting with the Medicines Control Council to take up the issue of clinical trials. The council was concerned enough about toxicity to impose a moratorium on further research until safety issues had been resolved. They and the researchers reached an agreement that the current research regimen was incapable of 'producing meaningful results'. The main stumbling block, and it was a pretty intractable one, was the toxicity of the drug, DMF.[154]

Folb's dealings with the team had not instilled confidence in their skills. 'I was so appalled,' he says. 'Was this their team? Is this what they know?' At one point during a meeting he turned to Du Plessis and asked, 'What would you think if I started doing cardiac surgery? You know as much about this as I know about cardiac surgery, and it's showing.'

Zigi knew nothing about the science, he didn't pretend to, Folb remembers, but neither did his wife. 'Olga didn't even know what chemical she was dealing with. She was just swept up in it all.'

Despite their reservations, Folb and the council agreed to support the minister and continue working with the team. In a private fax on to Zuma on February 6, Folb wrote that he had been impressed by the sincerity and dedication of the researchers, and stressed his commitment to assist them. 'I'll do everything to provide the necessary support,' he wrote.[155]

Later that day, Zuma issued a public statement in support of the Virodene team. She prefaced it with a vivid picture of what awaited South Africa if an affordable cure was not found — a death toll of 500 a day within ten years. 'I am very concerned about this situation,' she said, 'and any glimmer of hope to get treatment should be encouraged by us all.'[156]

Zuma expressed confidence in the collaborative process between the Medicines Control Council and the scientists. 'We have to race against time for the sake of saving lives.'

On the toxicity question, she commented that every drug has its side effects. 'If the benefits far outweigh them, you use the drug,' she said. When asked whether she was concerned that the team had not cleared the research with the university ethics committee, she said it was not her role to establish their procedures.

'I take that as "a given" from scientists who come from an institution of higher learning,' she said.

This interview gave rise to speculation that Zuma had not known that the researchers had breached protocols.

Towards the end of February, a joint committee comprising the Gauteng Health Department and the University of Pretoria confirmed what Folb and other researchers had been saying: the active ingredient of Virodene was a toxic substance and there was no scientific evidence for its effectiveness against HIV. In fact, the chair of the committee, Professor Henk Huismans, was reported in the *British Medical Journal* as saying that the preclinical trial research and experiments were so 'sloppy' that the results of the clinical trials could not be determined with any degree of certainty.[157] The committee criticised the Virodene team for pursuing the research without the permission of the Medicines Control Council and the ethics committee of the university. They also found that Visser's company — Cryopreservation Technologies — had little scientific standing, and its association with the university was unauthorised.[158]

The researchers, it seems, were undeterred by this setback. In May they launched a fund for their research in the belief that it would soon be approved.[159]

Zuma continued to support the team in the face of mounting opposition. The Democratic Party criticised Zuma's attitude to ethics, and the National Party called for her to be sacked. The 'call and response' lines between Zuma and her critics followed the pattern established during the *Sarafina II* scandal. However, while the conflict over the play stemmed from a political disagreement about how government money should be spent, in this new saga the principles of the scientific method were at stake.

COMPASSIONATE RELEASE

Despite the February ban on human trials for Virodene, there was mounting evidence that the Pretoria researchers were continuing to experiment with their home-grown AIDS cure.

Pierre Brouard, a counsellor at the Community AIDS Centre in Hillbrow, was one of many who came across people with the characteristic red welts caused by the patch used to administer the drug. One of these people had been a charismatic and energetic man, the kind of person who was always the centre of attention at any social event. But he was growing weaker and sicker as the months went by. He gradually lost his eyesight until he was almost blind. 'I didn't challenge it,' says Brouard, 'because it seemed to me to be the last gasp of someone who was desperate. He was convinced that this was going to work.' But, inevitably, the patch did not save him and the man passed away.

By early July 1997, the Virodene researchers were facing disciplinary hearings for continuing their research without the permission of the ethics committee. But reports of their ongoing work continued. There were even stories that Visser had established a private clinic in Portugal where she was working with the drug.

Right from the start of the Virodene episode there had been pressure to allow the researchers to continue with human trials. Newspaper articles published the pleas of dying men and women, begging to be allowed to participate. Desperate people were reported to be putting their names on a waiting list that was circulating in the hospices. Some had even signed statements to say they would not hold the researchers responsible for any negative side effects. 'We're dying anyway,' they said, 'so why not give us the bloody Virodene.'[160]

In the absence of any other affordable treatment, people were willing to try anything. And the fact that Virodene was supported by the minister of health counted strongly in its favour.

'Compassionate access' to an unregistered drug on a named-patient basis is an international practice, employed mainly for seriously ill patients for whom conventional therapy has failed. But this practice is strictly controlled by the established medicines regulatory procedure of the country in question: it is not a free-for-all.

In South Africa, in the case of Virodene, the Medicines Control Council would not budge. 'There is no one in the world who knows if it can offer a glimmer of hope,' said council chief Peter Folb. Nonetheless, Minister Zuma continued to exert pressure for compassionate release. In mid July Folb wrote to Zuma, briefing her against 'compassionate use' of the drug. 'In the worst cases,' he wrote, 'patients could be seriously, even fatally poisoned for no good reason.'[161]

Folb's opinion was shared by the World Health Organisation. As an industrial solvent, the active ingredient of Virodene had been the subject of rigorous testing by the WHO, and its toxic effects were by now well known. The Department of Health had even been provided with a copy of the WHO report on this subject.

But nothing could shake Zuma's confidence in Virodene. Soon after the briefing on compassionate use, Zuma telephoned Folb to try to get him to change his mind. When he refused, she asked him to argue his case with Mbeki. The three met for over two hours, a meeting that ended after nine in the evening.

Folb was received with the greatest interest and cordiality. 'I explained to him all the issues. Basically, it was a dialogue with Mbeki. Dr Zuma, literally and figuratively, was on the side,' says Folb. 'I explained to him how antiretrovirals work and I told him about the experimental/scientific basis for their action. I told him what work had and had not been done with this chemical. He was totally captivated by the science of it and at the end of the meeting I said to myself, "I've done it, he's got it, and I can trust him with this."'

Folb was moved by the sincerity of Mbeki's appreciation. Despite the fact that Folb had been through all these issues with the Virodene team, he readily agreed to the deputy president's invitation to meet them again.

The second meeting at Mbeki's house took place a few weeks later. This time the Virodene researchers were invited. Their team numbered around 20, and according to Folb they seemed most at home in these surroundings. 'I couldn't believe their self-confidence in the home of the deputy president, and dealing with the deputy president who had called them together to meet with me. They were very arrogant. I found it remarkable.'

The tone of this meeting was decidedly different from the first, and harsh words were spoken. The Virodene lawyer threatened to sue Folb for his public statements about the drug. Folb welcomed this as an excellent opportunity to expose the issues.

One of the proposals made at the meeting was that the research be managed by a neutral third party, a professor of medicine at the University of Pretoria. But the researchers would not agree to this. Attitudes were clearly hardening on both sides.

Soon after this meeting the Medicines Control Council made a final decision to refuse compassionate release of the drug. In a fax to the minister, Folb added new doubts to his original fears about the safety of the drug. 'The probability of liver toxicity is all the greater,' he wrote, 'for the reasons that the investigators have miscalculated the dose by a substantial margin and the chemical is formulated in a manner that is unstable and not dependable.'

Themba

Themba[162] was 20 years old when he went for the medical check-up required by his employer's insurance scheme. Like many young people in the late 1980s, Themba was tested for HIV without his knowledge or consent. And like many, he was confronted by his positive HIV status without any preparation.

'To me, HIV positive, it was AIDS, it was death the next day or very soon… I was sent for counselling but when I reached there I couldn't talk with the counsellor. I said, "No I'm fine, I'm just angry." And I went back to work.'

At work he received another shock. They were going to let him go.

Themba lay awake at night trying to work out what to do. He was too confused and afraid to tell his parents or his friends. He contemplated suicide but felt that it might make people suspicious. Instead he turned to a life of violent crime. 'I decided to put myself at risk to be killed by other people. So I was living a risky life in the hope that I would die, like my friends who were dying in those incidents we were involved in.'

Themba was wounded several times, and on one occasion was so severely injured that he remained in a coma for several months. After regaining consciousness he reassessed his life. He decided to confide in his mother, and ask for her help.

'I worried that she would reject me after I had lived that kind of life, but I broke the news to her and told her why I was dismissed, and why I lived alone on the streets.' To his surprise his mother seemed to know a lot about HIV and AIDS. 'She hugged me and supported me. She took me for proper counselling where I found out that a person can live for even twelve years with HIV.'

By 1996, seven years after his diagnosis, Themba was working as a counsellor, helping young people come to terms with HIV. 'I am trying to help people to live positively with HIV. I tell them about the issue of re-infection — because you know some people get angry and they decide to sleep around and spread the virus… They need to get proper counselling and to join support groups. If not, I think the economy of the country will fall down because these are the young people who should be building the country.'

Chapter Eight
Drug wars

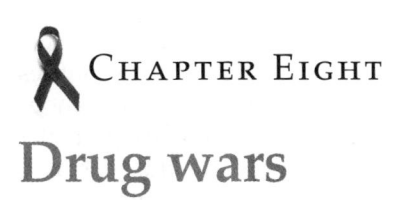

Zuma vs Big Pharma

At the heart of the Virodene controversy was the desire on the part of the government to find an affordable and accessible cure for HIV and AIDS.

The intensity of the support for Virodene, and the commitment to an indigenous cure, can only be understood in the context of the health minister's ongoing struggle to reform the pharmaceutical industry. The new indigenous drug, if it could be made to work, would be the government's answer to Big Pharma's high prices and patents.

In these times there was a general feeling of mistrust about the giant multinational pharmaceutical industry in South Africa and abroad. Several exposés in the 1970s and 1980s had contributed to a growing suspicion that the interests of Big Pharma were in opposition to the health needs of the poor. Influential popular books[163] argued that the commercial practices of the multinational drug companies were leading to widespread waste, suffering and even death in the less-developed countries. They documented cases of price-fixing, experimental testing of medicines in poor countries, and the prescription of inappropriate, inefficient and unsafe drugs. In some of the writing (then as now), there was a sense that standard industry practice was shaped by elaborate conspiracies to profit from the ill health of others.

By the mid 1990s the debate had moved on to include more complex issues to do with drug pricing and patents, or intellectual property rights.

By now the World Trade Organisation's patent agreement, called TRIPS, had strengthened the position of Big Pharma, giving the research-based pharmaceutical industry far greater intellectual property rights over prescription drugs.[164] Under the new dispensation, although it was still legal for poor countries to make and use cheaper generic drugs, the conditions under which they could do so were more limited. For its part, Big Pharma argued that patents, and the high profits they ensured, were necessary to fund the enormous research costs incurred in developing new drugs.

Nowhere was this debate more complex and more acute than in South Africa, where the bulk of prescription drugs were provided by the local subsidiaries of multinational pharmaceutical companies.

From day one in office Minister Zuma had set her mind to rationalising drug use so that she could make best use of public health funds. The endorsement of a smaller range of cheaper generic drugs was at the core of her new National Drug Policy, but from the moment that policy was revealed, the local pharmaceutical companies had opposed it.

Things came to a head when the minister began to try to implement her new drug policy.[165] The first regulations to deal with mandatory generic prescribing evoked such strong reactions that public hearings were held and the minister was forced to withdraw them.[166] But she did not back down.

In March 1997 local newspapers reported that the minister was still determined to do battle on high drug prices.[167] She complained that South Africa was one of the top five most expensive countries in the world for medicines, and that some medicines were priced 4 000 per cent above the world average.

The Pharmaceutical Manufacturers' Association of South Africa (PMA), which represented the local branches of pharmaceutical multinationals, was angered by the statement. Their chief executive officer, Mirryena Deeb, vehemently denied it, choosing the occasion of a public function to acquaint the minister with her views. The PMA even went so far as to ask the public protector to investigate what they deemed false allegations about drug prices.

In May 1997 a bill that aimed to give legislative force to the goals of the National Drug Policy was tabled in parliament. The Medicines and Related Substances Amendment Bill[168] outlined far-reaching changes to the whole drug chain — the procurement, distribution, selection, pricing and rational use of medicines.

The new bill's most contentious and best-publicised clauses

concerned new rules about the manufacturing and importing of medicines. Not only did the bill promote generic medicines for drugs that were out-of-patent, but it also contained a clause that would allow the importation of branded medicines from other countries where they were cheaper. This practice, called parallel importation, would enable the government to take advantage of the best prices on the international market.

The South African pharmaceutical manufacturers were naturally inclined to oppose any legislation that exposed them to greater competition. They objected strongly to the practice of parallel importation and turned to their parent companies abroad for help. By the end of May, US and European pharmaceutical companies were involved in the dispute.[169] In early June, for example, representatives of several US pharmaceutical companies met with South Africa's ambassador, Franklin Sonn, to discuss the proposed law.[170] The day after this meeting, they complained hyperbolically to the US Secretary of Commerce that the new law would have 'grave consequences for not only the US pharmaceutical industry, but all US investment in South Africa'.

The government's political opponents at home were also vigorously opposing the bill. Health spokesperson for the Democratic Party, Mike Ellis, had a somewhat apocalyptic vision of its consequences. 'If it had gone through in the form it was in,' he says 'it would have chased the pharmaceutical industry right out of South Africa. They just said we can't operate.'

Concerned about the adverse responses to the bill, the government held open hearings in parliament, inviting submissions from divergent groups. The bill was largely welcomed by speakers drawn from the progressive, anti-apartheid health community. But as expected, the Pharmaceutical Manufacturers' Association rejected it in plain terms, as did the representative of the US government's trade department.

The reaction of these powerful stakeholders was so unequivocal that the bill was withdrawn. Zuma sent her drafting team back to rewrite the legislation. It was important to get it right: until this law was passed, access to affordable medicines would be a distant dream.

While the minister's team was busy drafting another version of the bill, the pharmaceutical industry continued its campaign against parallel importation. The most vigorous opposition was mounted by the PMA and their US parent companies, which appealed to Congress to intervene. PhRMA, the organisation representing Big Pharma in the US, planned to make the bill a hot issue during the forthcoming high-level US-SA Bi-national Commission. Indeed, when Minister Zuma flew to Washington to attend the meeting in July 1997, she personally met with representatives of PhRMA to discuss the implications of the law.[171] The minister tried to assure them that the South African government was not intending to throw out all the rights of patent holders. Parallel importing, she said, would only be allowed for selected drugs, and when it was most needed. 'It is unacceptable for South Africa to pay higher prices than Australia,' she said.

Around this time a group of US consumer advocates became interested in the dispute. Led by Ralph Nader and his colleague James Love, they embarked on a campaign to support the South African government. In July they wrote to US Vice President Al Gore[172], pointing out that parallel importation was a legal practice in the European Union, accounting for up to 10 per cent of the Netherlands and UK drug market. They requested that 'the US should be supportive of the South African government's thoughtful initiatives,' and use this opportunity to show that US foreign policy would subordinate commercial concerns to broader health interests.

BAD MEDICINE

Round One of Zuma vs Big Pharma received modest but favourable publicity in the press. Even the conservative *Business Times*[173] railed against the 'vested interests' resisting the reforms proposed by the Medicines Bill.[174] But behind the contest between the minister and the pharmaceutical industry was a second narrative that was not getting the attention it deserved.

In their enthusiasm for knock-down drug prices, the usual whistleblowers had failed to notice other sections of the proposed new legislation. These concerned the structure, functioning and governance of the Medicines Control Council, and had a disturbing significance for the minister's Virodene campaign.

The new legislation would give the minister of health much greater powers over the Medicines Control Council, enabling him or her to reduce its size and intellectual weight. For example, the law proposed to do away with the previous stipulation that council members be professionally qualified. The appointment of the executive committee would now be subject to the minister's approval. The legislation was also clear that people associated with the pharmaceutical industry would be precluded from council membership.

The council's embattled chair, Professor Peter Folb, therefore found himself at the centre of yet another controversy. Despite his leadership of a government body, his academic qualifications and his 18-year experience on the council, he had not been consulted about the legislation until the month before it was tabled. Understandably he was concerned about the clauses that related to the council.

'It was very crudely drafted legislation,' says Folb. 'I didn't think it was in the interests of the public for the minister to be interfering. In fact there was an even greater risk than that. The way it was written, the minister could run her own little side show.

'The original drafting would have allowed the minister to make regulatory decisions. So if the minister decided that it was in the public interest to register a medicine or deregister it, she could do it. Presumably her advisers could do it for her. So I could see the potential for ignorant decision-making and corruption.'

In May 1997 Folb wrote to Zuma expressing his concerns. He was also critical of the wording, though not the substance, of the parallel importation clause, which he felt could lead to an unregulated drug market. The letter explained that that the bill contained a number of serious and fundamental flaws. 'It will seriously undermine the National Drug Policy,' he wrote, 'and we advise that it should be reconsidered and withdrawn. May we meet?'[175]

Folb was now in something of a predicament. As chair of the council, which was a government body, he would be expected to speak in the parliamentary hearings, and it would be tricky for him to reject a bill initiated by the Department of Health. In the run-up to the hearings he discussed his concerns with the director-general, Dr Olive Shisana.

'I told Olive I can't agree with this, and Olive said "All your objections will be dealt with. If you object to something it won't go through",' he says. 'So on the basis of that, I spoke and I pointed out my concerns and I said, "I have been given an assurance that they will be changed in the legislation." And on the basis of that assurance I endorsed the rest.'

Folb was very clear then, as he is now, that he was not opposed to the entire substance of the law. 'There were things about it I liked very much, like parallel importing and the special attention paid to generic medicines and affordable medicines,' he says. 'I was very clear what I supported and what I didn't support. Anyway, Olive gave the undertaking that all would be put right, but she wasn't of course writing the legislation, the advisors were, and they weren't having any of that.'

In August, less than two months after the controversial Medicines Bill was withdrawn, a new version was tabled in parliament. This bill differed very little from the previous one, and the changes promised to Folb and others were not reflected in the new wording.

It seems that despite their meetings with all the stakeholders — the Medicines Control Council, industry groups, legal academics and international consultants — the drafting group had been unable to come up with an iteration that would accommodate their critics. There was, however, a new section replacing the original offending paragraphs on parallel importation. But instead of placating the pharmaceutical industry, this clause took the government into deeper water.

Section 15C appeared to go even further than the previous bill.

Its opening sentence read: 'The minister may prescribe the conditions for the supply of more affordable medicines in certain circumstances so as to protect the health of the public.'

This confirmed all the pharmaceutical industry's worst fears. They interpreted the new bill as written proof that the South African government was contemplating an uncontrolled trade in generic medicines. In fact they suspected that this new clause could be interpreted as enabling generic drug manufacturers to make copies of drugs that were still under patent. In the view of the pharmaceutical industry, this practice, called compulsory licensing, would be illegal under the international TRIPS agreement of the World Trade Organisation.

Others argued that the bill would also flout South African patent law. Low- and middle-income countries that had signed up to the WTO had been given until 2000 to comply with the new TRIPS rules. However, the newly democratic South Africa had prematurely amended its patent laws in its eagerness to comply with the WTO. And section 15C of the Medicines Bill sat uneasily with this new commitment.

In mid September the second version of the Medicines Bill was brought before the parliamentary health portfolio committee. This time the hearings were organised differently. Presenters were limited to ten minutes, and only five minutes were allotted for questions and discussions. Observers felt that this was a deliberate strategy to push the bill through. Thirty-two submissions were presented from a wide range of interested parties, the majority of whom were critical of different aspects of the bill. The Pharmaceutical Manufacturers Association predictably rejected the intellectual property rights clauses in section 15C. The Hospital Pharmacists Association argued that other sections would hamper drug access in the public sector.

Folb, who was shocked by the blanket rejection of his previous comments, made an impassioned plea[176] to redraft the bill. His particular concern was with the clauses that restructured the Medicines Control Council. 'I have seen the end of the tunnel described in this draft bill, and it is dark. It is a Third World trap against which the World Health Organisation has repeatedly warned...', he said. 'Failure to act on this draft bill will result in the introduction of ministerial veto and the arbitrary imposition of ministerial will in medicines control.'

By now it would be reasonable to assume that Folb and the government's relationship was in jeopardy. His rejection of both Virodene and the Medicines Bill would appear to have cast him completely in the Big Pharma camp.

This fevered debate, about what was to become a significant international issue, was given little attention by the local or international media. The substance of it was way too complex for non-experts, and when there was coverage, it tended to stick to platitudes and sensational headlines. As with the reactions to the first version of the bill, the clauses affecting the restructuring of the council went almost unnoticed.

The Pharmaceutical Manufacturers' Association continued to lobby the minister, and in a private meeting with her in October requested that she withdraw the controversial section 15C. Big Pharma was also assiduously courting people and groupings that they thought might be on their side. For example Dr Andy Gray, pharmacist and senior lecturer at the University of KwaZulu-Natal, described how he was approached immediately after he spoke critically about the bill at the parliamentary hearings.

'There was a tap on my shoulder and there was this young American who said "That was intriguing, can I speak to you afterwards?"' Gray remembers. The man, who turned out to be a representative of Merck and PhRMA, invited Gray for dinner, an event that went on very late. 'There was this long table so carefully arranged. I was surrounded by people from industry... Mike Ellis and the MCC deputy chairman, etc. You could see those who were opposed.' As the evening wore on it became clear that Gray would not be going home that night. 'They said, "It's too late to get you back. We have booked a seafront suite in this five-star hotel." That man was a real operator,' says Gray.

It's the wording!

After the parliamentary hearings, critics and supporters continued to write to the minister with complaints and advice. The US Ambassador to South Africa, James Joseph, even wrote a letter[177] to the chair of the portfolio committee describing his government's objections to section 15C of the bill.

'My government opposes the notion of parallel imports of patented products anywhere in the world. We argued for a prohibition of such parallel imports in the TRIPS agreement. They are illegal in the United States, both as an infringement of patent rights, and because in the case of medicines, our Food and Drug Administration believes it cannot adequately monitor quality.'

By now James Love, an economist with expertise in intellectual property rights and pharmaceutical polices, had been invited by the minister of health to comment on the bill. He faxed the minister detailed information about parallel importation practices in the European Union and in Japan[178], and outlined how these were permissible under the TRIPS agreement. Love included information on the different prices of drugs being sold by the same manufacturer in the UK and Europe.

'Should South Africa permit or encourage parallel imports of pharmaceutical drugs?' he asked. 'Of course! South African consumers are poor, and high prices for drugs will present terrible barriers for access to medicines. Certainly South Africa should avail itself to the benefits of market competition and purchase drugs as cheaply as possible in world markets.'

The minister's own team, including the WHO adviser Dr Wilbert Bannenberg, were also in agreement that both parallel importation and compulsory licensing were practices permitted by the TRIPS agreement.

The big question was, if all these experts were correct, and both parallel importation and compulsory licensing were allowed under TRIPS, why and how was Big Pharma able to mount such a strong attack?

An indication of the 'why' was given later in PhRMA's annual submission to the US trade department. Writing about the dispute over the Medicines Bill, they said 'It is one of the first "test cases" for interpreting the scope of protection offered by TRIPS to all fields of technology. And thus has importance far beyond its own borders.'[179]

It was clear that the South African medicines case was being used to explore the scope and limitation of the new international agreement on intellectual property rights.

The answer to the 'how' question lay in the sorry truth that the legislation itself was technically flawed. Many felt that section 15C was so loosely worded as to allow for a range of interpretations. In the early stages of the bill Zuma had received advice from the WHO that it needed to be rewritten, and the example of the French legislation was given to her as a model. But this advice was ignored.

'Section 15C was so difficult to understand because it was so badly worded,' says Gray. 'It appeared to give the minister the ability to override the whole Patent Act. It's like, wow, she can do anything she likes.'

Whether the wording of the bill was deliberately vague, or a product of the inexperience of its authors, is not clear. However, some of the conflict over the bill may have stemmed from the conduct of the minister's special adviser, Dr Ian Roberts, who seemed to be personally motivated by a strong antagonism towards the pharmaceutical industry. Folb says, 'He put himself forward as knowledgeable... He didn't know what he was doing, and he was determined to do it. He wanted to dismantle the legislation.'

Even members of the drafting team had problems with the way Roberts worked. On one occasion Dr Bada Pharasi, a chief director in the Department of Health, wrote to the director-general: 'I would be failing in my own conscience if I did not point out that the conduct of the minister's special adviser throughout the entire process of finalising the amendments was at best intimidatory towards the rest of the task team, and at worst insulting. This is borne out not only by his usage of insulting language, but the throwing of tantrums when his viewpoint was not shared by the rest of the team.'[180]

At times even the minister was in a quandary. She was known to remark: 'I am surrounded by knowledgeable people, but I don't know who to trust.'

More side effects

It is worth noting that in these early days of the Medicines Bill dispute, the only drug mentioned by name was the new cancer treatment, Taxol.

Zuma had indicated her intention to licence a cheaper generic version of the drug that cost over $2 000 per injection. The issue here was that the manufacturer, Bristol Myers Squibb, did not hold a patent on the drug, but was using a provision in US law to get five years' excusive rights on it. At the time this was also was being contested by several other countries, including Canada and the Netherlands.

Despite the severity of South Africa's HIV epidemic, the issue of AIDS drugs was not on the table. At this time, the triple drug antiretroviral therapy was in its infancy, and regarded as something of a luxury, for use largely in high-income countries with sophisticated health systems. Minister Zuma did not believe that antiretroviral therapy would ever be affordable or practicable for use in poor countries[181], and this belief was shared by many others in the international health and development community.

There were many reasons for this, quite apart from the high price of the drugs themselves. The regimen was complex, required sophisticated monitoring, and represented a lifelong commitment by health services and users alike. In the rich countries, antiretroviral therapy had rendered AIDS a long-term chronic disease, but in the end it was a treatment, not a cure.

The fact that antiretroviral therapy held so little promise for South Africa's poor gave weight to the government ministers' ongoing commitment to their own cheap miracle cure — Virodene. Throughout 1997 they remained steadfast in their support for Visser and her team. Although the Medicines Control Council had vetoed the Virodene trials, there was evidence that the researchers were continuing to test the drug.

Towards the end of 1997, a young man arrived for treatment at a Pretoria hospital with worrying symptoms. He was short of breath, he said, his throat was swelling, and his body felt as if it was on fire. After discovering that these were the side effects of the AIDS medication he was taking, he sought legal help.

It turned out that the poison department at the hospital had seen many such cases. They all had the tell-tale red marks on their arms, characteristic of the Virodene patch. The doctors concluded that their problems were a result of having applied 'poisonous substances to the body'.[182]

The AIDS Law Project[183], a programme run out of the law department at the University of the Witwatersrand, began to collect the evidence, taking statements from several HIV-positive people who had been treated by Olga Visser and her colleagues. They claimed that Visser had informed them that Virodene was a cure for AIDS and that it was being tested by a doctor in France who approved of the drug.

One person made a statement to the AIDS Law Project that Visser had claimed 'Virodene is a cheap cure, and therefore the research of Virodene as an HIV/AIDS cure/drug is being hampered by the medical authorities in South Africa in an effort to ensure that consumers purchase other more expensive drugs, which are registered and available in South Africa.'[184] Several of the complainants had been referred by Visser to a private doctor who had administered the patches.

On November 20, 1997, the AIDS Law Project went public with the story. One of their clients told the *Sunday Independent* that he had had bought a patch for R200, from Olga Visser, which he had administered himself. His symptoms began shortly after this.

'I felt completely betrayed,' he said. 'The side effects are not what she said they would be, and there has been no change in my condition.'[185]

The AIDS Law Project laid a complaint with the Medicines Control Council, and by the powers vested in them, the council investigated. A raid on the home of the Vissers failed to produce any of the chemical, and both the Vissers and the named doctor denied any knowledge of further trials.[186]

Zigi Visser dismissed the whole story as 'a desperate attempt by the MCC, pharmaceutical companies and AIDS activists who are trying to bury Virodene before the new Health Bills come into effect.'

By now the Medicines Control Council had turned down a third protocol for testing the drug. The grounds were always the same. In a private letter to the minister on December 5, Folb reminded Zuma that their research and expert reports on the drug ran into hundreds of pages. He gave a lengthy description of the dangers of the drug and the way it was being used. According to Folb, the researchers were using industrial grade material that contained known contaminants. On top of this, the raw material was unstable in the form in which it was being used, and though the drug was toxic, the researchers were miscalculating the dose.

'Until now,' he wrote, 'there has been no meaningful evidence provided that dimethylformamide is effective in HIV infection (expert advice suggests the contrary); the risk-benefit relationship for human use must be regarded in the meantime as unfavourable.'[187]

Folb was also concerned about a private meeting that Zuma had had with members of the council who were more sympathetic to her cause. Usually polite, he complained to the minister: 'I am not able to dispel from my mind the possibility that your intent at that meeting (or even the unintended but inevitable result) was to disrupt the normal decision-making process of the council.'

Around this time an internal dispute developed within the Virodene team. Papers were placed before the courts that revealed irregularities in the company's conduct. Some members of the team alleged that trials were continuing and that the drug was being exported and used in illegal trials in Portugal.[188] This was to be the first of several court actions during which certain members of the team requested the liquidation of the company in which they were shareholders.

The in-fighting became so bitter that the government got involved in the dispute. Deputy President Thabo Mbeki intervened personally, bringing together the opposing factions in a series of pre-breakfast meetings.[189] Finally a proposal was made: that the government would appoint and pay for an independent manager who would see to it that the business dealings were regularised and that the research agenda was on track.

The Medicines Control Council was prevailed upon to support the new arrangement. On December 9, a joint statement was released by the council and the Virodene team saying that they had reached consensus on how the drug might be tested.

At last it seemed that Minister Zuma had got her way. She had held out against all the allegations as well as the ongoing refusal of the council to license Virodene. (Or was it because of it?) The more the medical community railed against the Virodene team, the more determined Zuma appeared that they should continue with their work.

Her disregard for Virodene's critics may well have been strengthened by her antipathy to Big Pharma and the intensity with which they were currently opposing her reforming Medicines Bill.

It is not difficult to imagine how the controversies over Virodene and the Medicines Bill would blur, and contaminate responses on all sides. The players began to mistrust one another, perhaps even to regard one another with that snide suspicion that comes from an appreciation of one's own mixed motives. Conspiracies were imagined and battle lines prematurely drawn, as opponents plunged deeper into untenable positions from which there would be no escape.

On December 1, 1997, Zuma addressed a World AIDS Day rally saying, 'It breaks my heart to see the number of letters I receive from patients who are dying, wanting Virodene to be administered to them,' she said. 'I often cry in my office as I feel powerless.'[190] She told the crowd of ANC Youth League supporters that there should be nobody on earth with the power to refuse a patient access to their drug of choice, if it would make a difference to their lives. 'One day I will have the power to overrule the Medicines Control Council,' she said. 'One day — I can't say when — I will take a firm decision on the matter. The new health law soon to be tabled before parliament will enable me to take that decision.'

This day would be coming sooner than her audience might have thought. On December 12, President Mandela signed the much-contested Medicines Act into law. The Act gave the minister new powers that would enable her to control the council as she wished.

Nonhlanhla

It was a Sunday evening and 18-year-old Nonhlanhla Mbokazi was coming home from church when she was approached by three men. They asked her name, and when she refused to speak to them, they pushed her into a drain and gang-raped her.

Later at the hospital, she was given an HIV test. It was negative. She was advised to return for a second test in three month's time — the second test was positive.

'I sat there silently, I couldn't talk. I couldn't do anything. It took some days before I could say, "This really has happened and I can't go back."'

Later she joined a support group for HIV-positive people. It gave her so much courage that she decided to become a counsellor herself.

'I am quite interested in helping our community,' she says 'because I have seen quite a lot of people dying in front of me, dying beside me. Even my lovely ones....

'I tell them they must use condoms. They must remember that life comes only once. If you lose your life you never get it again.'

Nonhlanhla died in 1999. [191]

Chapter Nine

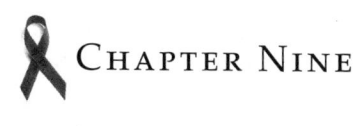

Poisoned barbs

Behind closed doors

On New Year's Eve of 1997, Peter Folb was pleased to receive a telephone call from an international colleague, Professor Graham Dukes. But apart from season's greetings, Dukes had called to say that he had been appointed to lead a team that would review the role of the Medicines Control Council.

Folb knew about the review, which had been discussed earlier in the year. In fact he had welcomed it as a way of giving the health minister greater confidence in the council. But what Dukes had to say came as something of a shock — the review team had been instructed by the minister to complete the report without speaking to either Folb or members of the pharmaceutical industry.

The official reason given by the minister for the review was that the council was too involved in policy issues; it needed restructuring so that it could simply fulfil its technical mandate. But there were clearly other problems, not least of which was the fact that the council was an apartheid-era creation and had retained staff from its early days. It was irksome to many in the new South Africa to see Afrikaner men remaining in positions of power and authority. For example, when asked about the conflict between Folb and Zuma over the Medicines Bill, one of the minister's international advisers, Dr Wilbert Bannenberg, commented to the *Mail & Guardian* that it was a power struggle, an issue of transformation.[192]

The bitter struggles of 1997 over Virodene and the Medicines Bill had put the minister and the council on something of a collision course. Although the Medicines Control Council was a government body, in its current form it had a considerable degree of independence. In Folb's[193] eyes this was its strength, but there were those in the ministry who believed the council was open to undue influence from the pharmaceutical industry.

The Medicines Control Council's function was to register and control medicines and regulate medical research, and a robust council was needed to ensure the quality, efficacy and safety of drugs. But serious differences were now emerging over the way the council should be constituted, and how it should do its work.[194]

Whatever the motives, the review was to begin immediately. In Folb's opinion[195], most members of the review team were too closely connected to the health department to have independent views, and were lacking in knowledge and experience of drug regulation.

Although the review team did later conduct a short interview with Folb (and representatives of the pharmaceutical industry), he had little to do with the proceedings.

Zuma under attack

Throughout that long hot summer, the Virodene controversy simmered. Despite their new commitment to work together, the Virodene researchers and the council were unable to find a way forward.[196] In early February the Medicines Control Council rejected the Virodene team's research protocol for the fourth time. Two weeks later, the minister of health received another blow. The controversy over the Medicines Bill returned with a vengeance. Although President Mandela had signed the law, it had not yet been promulgated. Thus it was that on February 18, 1998, the Pharmaceutical Manufacturers' Association and 41 co-applicants were able to seek an interim interdict in the Pretoria High Court preventing President Mandela from bringing the Medicines Bill into effect.[197] Among other things, they claimed that section 15C of the Act was unconstitutional. This law, they said, would give the minister unrestricted powers to revoke patent rights.

The applicants represented all but one of the major multinational pharmaceutical companies operating in the country. Clearly they, and their parent companies, were not going to give up easily on their mission to change the new law. Papers were then served on ten respondents. Nelson Mandela, who was the only person with authority to promulgate the law, was top of the list. Yet far from being headline news, this dramatic turn of events passed almost unnoticed by all but the business papers.

After this setback it could be assumed that the health minister would be in no mood to trifle with her opponents. Yet this was the very moment that the Democratic Party chose to fire the next round in the Virodene war. In early March, Mike Ellis told the press that he possessed papers alleging that the government stood to benefit financially from the sale of the drug. According to these documents, the Virodene team had agreed to pay the government 6 per cent of their profits.[198]

'I called a press conference and had various facts and figures and copies of the document,' says Ellis. 'We accused the government of being in collusion; they had no right to the 6 per cent… everything pointed to the fact that there was collusion between the ANC and the researchers. It was a very fiery time.'

The ANC and the government furiously denied any knowledge of the matter. Zuma told the press: 'The DP hates ANC supporters. If they had it their way, we would all die of AIDS.'[199]

The allegation arose from the Supreme Court papers presented in the in-house Virodene dispute late in 1997. They included a document by Zigi Visser claiming that the ANC would receive a share of the profits from the drug. There were also references to an office-bearer of government being paid a fee for introducing the researchers to the government.

Folb had known about the documents for some months and had written to the minister for clarification. 'I am advised on the highest authority that these papers raise at least the suspicion of impropriety and vested interests on the part of the office-bearers concerned who hold high office in government,' he wrote. 'These matters are of such seriousness that I would appreciate, by return, your reaction to them. If you are able to give me an explanation and reassurance I would value it highly.'

In this fax, Folb had assured the minister that he had not discussed the substance of the matter with other members of the council, and made it clear that he was simply waiting for her assurances that the allegation was untrue.[200]

When Zuma's response finally came it was an angry one. She said she found Folb's 'insinuations unacceptable and offensive'.

But by then, what had been an unsupported statement made by Zigi Visser had become the international news story of the day. And the ANC's political opponents were playing it for all it was worth.

The court papers did indeed contain the statement that 6 per cent of the profits from the sale of Virodene would accrue to the ANC, as a party, but Zigi Visser explained this away as an error on his part. He claimed he had already written a correction to the ANC's legal desk explaining: 'The description "ANC" was the wrong choice of phrase, and "RDP" (Reconstruction and Development Programme) might have been more accurate in this instance.'[201]

Like the *Sarafina* issue before it, the Virodene issue, particularly the scandal of the 6 per cent, was to inflict lasting damage, undermining the seriousness of the AIDS crisis and perceptions about the integrity of the government's response.

For their part, the ANC and the government were increasingly suspicious of the motives of those who opposed Virodene. This story came so soon after the Big Pharma interdict that it played into a growing sense of siege. The ANC issued a statement[202] that accused Ellis and his party of opposing all efforts at transformation. Most telling, the statement made a personal attack on Ellis, claiming that he was in the pay of the pharmaceutical companies.

'It is public knowledge that Mike Ellis has in many ways benefited materially from his association with pharmaceutical companies, including trips abroad and holidays,' the statement read. 'More significantly, and we have it on reliable authority, that some of the questions he poses in parliament in fact originate from some of these companies.'

Ellis resented being cast as an errand boy of the pharmaceutical industry, and demanded an investigation to prove that he was not in their pay. 'A year to the day,' says Ellis, 'Mr Pahad had to stand up in parliament and apologise unconditionally to me, which was quite a nice little victory.'

'It was Zuma's hatred of the private sector', he says. 'I was seen to be a protagonist of private health care, and that would have added dramatically to the clash that I had. The other political parties seemed unable to grasp the issue… it was very much DP and ANC. It was great days, I loved them. I believed in what I was doing and it gave me a lot of courage to take them on.'

'UNBOUNDED CONTUMELY'

The government, however, did not seem to share in Ellis's enjoyment of the rough and tumble of parliamentary politics. The story of the 6 per cent profit was the first time that the liberation government had been directly accused of corruption, and the accusation was met with unprecedented rage.

Deputy President Mbeki saw fit to write a personal denunciation, which in its tone presaged his future contributions to the AIDS debate. In an article sent to the Sunday newspapers he summed up the opposition to Virodene in such a way as to strongly suggest that it was a conspiracy. The researchers have had 'unbounded contumely' heaped upon them, he wrote. 'As expected, the minister of health has not been spared the poisoned barbs.'[203]

Mbeki commented with anger on the publicity around the ongoing illegal use of Virodene. He said he deplored the 'provocation by a person who falsely claimed to have fallen seriously ill as a result of being treated by Virodene', and the night raids on the Vissers' home that he said were illustrative of this campaign. 'How alien,' he wrote, 'all these goings-on seem to be in the pursuits of medical research! In our strange world, those who seek the good of all humanity have become the villains of our time.'

Mbeki wrote also about his frustration with the Medicines Control Council, saying that it became increasingly difficult to understand their attitude. He claimed that the 'world scientific community' had subjected the Virodene protocol to a detailed assessment, and quoted from several researchers who apparently had given their approval. The fact that the council continued to reject the protocol was evidence of its obduracy.

'To confirm its determined stance against Virodene, and contrary to previous practice, the MCC has, with powers to decide who shall live or die, also denied dying AIDS sufferers the possibility of "mercy treatment" to which they are morally entitled,' he wrote.

Within a matter of weeks, the Medicines Control Council's future was in question and two of its most senior full-time officials had been sacked. Although Zuma and her staff were at pains to emphasise that this had nothing to do with the Virodene episode, the timing and the manner of it were so sharp it is difficult to avoid this interpretation.

This is how it happened: on March 23, 1998, the review team delivered a final report to the minister. They concluded that there had been a serious breakdown in communication between the council and the government, which had allowed for misunderstandings to arise. Among other things, the report commented on conflicts of interest that had weakened the council.

'A medicines regulatory authority exists to serve the public health interest, and no other. Inevitably, however, its most intensive day-to-day contacts are with the pharmaceutical industry, the interests of which do not always run parallel with public health needs.'

The report went on to warn that 'individual experts are also likely to be confronted daily with industrial activity and some inevitably have a degree of financial involvement, eg in the sense that some of their own scientific research receives industrial support.'

The review team recommended that the council be dismantled and replaced with another body and officials. Though the review team found no individuals guilty of misconduct, it also recommended that top officials be placed in other jobs in the health system.

However, after the finalisation of the report, and against its recommendations, a decision was taken to fire the council's registrar Johan Schlebusch and his deputy, Christel Bruckner.[204] The day the report was released, the pair was called to the office of the director-general of health, Dr Olive Shisana, and given letters stating that there would be no room for them in the new body. Various allegations of incompetence and maladministration were made[205], and they were advised to leave voluntarily, and with the government's sincere thanks for their contributions and long service. After this, they were escorted to their offices to fetch their belongings. Their offices were then placed under guard and the locks were changed.

On the same day, Folb received telephone calls, first from Dukes, and then from Zuma, to say that he had been relieved of his chairmanship of the council. Although Minister Zuma rejected the review team's recommendations to dismantle the council entirely, she did appoint a second team to work on its transformation.

As for Folb, he stuck it out as an ordinary member of the council for just two months before deciding to step down.[206]

Sanctions loom...

In March 1998 Bill Clinton made history by becoming the first US president to visit South Africa. Invited to speak in parliament, he pledged to support the country in its efforts to deal with the legacy of apartheid. 'The courage and imagination that created this new South Africa,' he said, 'inspires all of us to be animated by the belief that one day, humanity all the world over can at last be freed from the bonds of hatred and bigotry.'[207]

To generous applause he stressed that the US government was committed to developing closer ties with South Africa through trade and cooperation.

But while Clinton was wowing parliament, his commerce secretary William Daley was having behind-the-scenes talks with Minister Zuma about the Medicines Act.

It was just one month after the court interdict, and Clinton had been under domestic pressure to raise the thorny issue of the Medicines Act during his visit. Although Clinton declined to personally pursue the topic, Daley had been included in the large party travelling with the president across the country. And Daley used the stop in Cape Town to meet with Zuma for a discussion about the implications of section 15C of the Medicines Act. After their 45-minute meeting, Zuma's spokesperson, Vincent Hlongwane, told the press that 'the minister was able to explain the rationale behind what we are doing and assure them that South Africa was not violating any international agreements.'[208]

The report from the US State Department was not so upbeat. According to them, Daley used the meeting as an opportunity to emphasise the US government's resolve that section 15C would undermine pharmaceutical patent rights.

The next day, a representative of the US Pharmaceutical Manufacturers' Association (PhRMA), who was also in the country at the time, was interviewed on SABC radio. Tom Bombelles told South African listeners that the Medicines Act was 'the single most important economic or trade issue'.[209] Bombelles alleged that the Act was being used by India and Argentina as a test run to see how worldwide intellectual property rights agreements could be broken.

From the moment the Medicines Act was passed, PhRMA had been briefing the Clinton administration about the dangers it posed to US trade relations. In a 1998 document for the US Trade

Department, PhRMA wrote that 15C constituted a violation of TRIPS and was a serious threat to the viability of American pharmaceutical investment in South Africa. 'Numerous PhRMA member companies,' they wrote, 'have already indicated that new investment in South Africa, in some cases valued at more than $50 million, have been suspended as a result of the new legislation.'[210]

In May 1998, South Africa was placed on a US government list of countries that represented a threat to intellectual property rights.[211] This list, the Special 301 Watch List[212], was drawn up every year by the US Trade Representative (USTR) to identify countries that denied adequate protection for intellectual property rights. Countries on the 301 Watch List ran the risk of bilateral trade sanctions. In addition to this listing, the USTR began withholding trade benefits from South African companies.[213]

In days past, the ANC had played a starring role in the sanctions campaign that had brought the apartheid government to its knees. For the tables to be turned, so suddenly, and over such an unexpected problem, must have been a blow to the liberation government. What had begun as a conflict with local drug manufacturers had blown up into an international trade dispute. In its determined campaign to rejoin the global economy, this was the last thing South Africa's new government needed.

One week in Geneva

In early May 1998, Minster Zuma boarded a plane bound for Geneva to attend the annual meeting of the World Health Assembly.[214]

Although her Medicines Act was on ice and the threat of sanctions loomed, Zuma had grounds to feel optimistic about the future. This year the Assembly was to debate a resolution in support of rational drug policies for low-income countries.

Called the Revised Drug Strategy[215], this resolution had already been approved by the WHO's Executive Board. Now it was to be debated before a full committee of the world's health ministers.

The second clause of this resolution urged member states to 'ensure that public health rather than commercial interests have primacy in pharmaceutical and health policies, and to review their options under the Agreement on Trade Related Aspects of Intellectual Property Rights to safeguard access to essential drugs'.

Although the adoption of the Revised Drug Strategy would not give South Africa any legal grounds to dismiss Big Pharma's court challenge, it would give a much-needed boost to the health minister's cause.

Zuma, and her director-general Shisana, would have been fairly confident of support in this forum, in which the world's poorest countries were well represented.

According to US consumer activist James Love, members of the US pharmaceutical industry had asked the US government to oppose the resolution.[216] And when the time came, the US position was supported by Japan, Australia, Switzerland and a number of EU states, including the UK and Germany.

Because of the controversy over this particular resolution, a small drafting group was convened to reach a compromise on new wording. Sessions lasted well into the night without agreement. The US delegation was particularly offended by the phrase concerning the primacy of public health over commercial concerns, referring to it as 'objectionable language'. After four days of disagreement, the drafting group finally came up with a compromise (though rather a flawed one), which contained bracketed clauses on which there was no agreement. The strategy of the US and its allies was to refer the resolution back to the executive board to deal with the detail. This would avoid a debate in the full committee of 191 member states, where the US and its northern allies would be unlikely to have majority support.

The South African delegation was becoming increasingly impatient and was pushing for the original resolution to be debated in the full committee. Harsh words were spoken, but eventually the assembly voted for the deferment, and the issue was put off for yet another year.

A confidential US memo[217] on this meeting, apparently written by Ambassador George Moose (representative of the US to the European office of the UN), was later posted on the Internet by the Consumer Project on Technology. In it, Moose claimed that the hard line taken by the South Africans made it impossible to reach consensus over the wording. The memo made it clear that, although neither the US nor the South African delegation referred explicitly to the dispute over the Medicines Act, it had haunted the discussions.

In the memo, South Africa's director-general of health was

singled out for special attention. 'Dr Olive Shisana… one of the authors of the Medicines Act, led the charge for Africans in the drafting group debate,' Moose wrote. 'She clearly has a vested interest, and can present convincing arguments, especially when talking to health rather than trade officials. And her previous tenure as a health officer in the Washington DC health department has given her good insight into the US negotiating style.'

Moose commented, rather plaintively, that it was clear that South Africa, Namibia, Zambia, Botswana and Zimbabwe were committed to the exact wording that the US found the most problematic. His memo urged the US to engage actively in the next stage of the process. He concluded that the US government had a 'responsibility and opportunity to develop a position on the revised drug strategy resolution that will enable health and trade to move together in a compatible manner not be used to foster a north-south trade dispute using health as a proxy.'

In a later document, PhRMA suggested that the South African delegation was intent on shaking up global intellectual property rights. 'From the recent remarks and actions,' they wrote, 'the apparent intent of the Government of South Africa is to not only defend its diminishment of the effectiveness of patent protection in South Africa, but to urge other countries to similarly weaken patent protection for pharmaceutical products.'

Shisana's performance at the World Health Assembly meeting earned her many enemies. At one stage the US delegation even threatened diplomatic pressure to remove her from the negotiations altogether.

From the other side, the picture looked quite different: Shisana's debating skills had prevented the rich nations from undermining the resolution. Not only was she forceful and convincing, but unlike most other delegates, she had a good command of the issues.

But this success was not to be rewarded by Shisana's own government. While Zuma and Shisana were attending the meeting in Geneva, the newspapers at home had leaked a report that the minister was planning to let Shisana go.[218]

This came as no surprise: the week before Shisana had left for Geneva, she had testified before the Parliament's Public Accounts Committee on the *Sarafina II* debacle. Observers alleged that Shisana had been expected to take the blame and apologise for the debacle. Instead she delivered a comprehensive report that showed that other senior officials had been responsible for many irregularities.[219]

An article in *The Star* newspaper made an additional curious allegation. It claimed that Shisana had also been incorrectly blamed for mislaying critical documents concerning the controversial Medicines Act. The missing file, the story went, had delayed the promulgation of the Act, thus creating the opportunity for Big Pharma's legal challenge of the new law.

Something new out of Africa...

Back home, there were new developments in the Virodene story. Despite the fact that there was no permission to continue trials of the drug, the saga was not over.

In June 1998, the newspapers revealed that the company had been bought by a new group of investors and that the government-appointed interim manager had resigned.[220] Renamed Virodene Pharmaceutical Holdings, the company was now being managed by Joshua Nxumalo, a former member of the ANC's military wing, who was said to have headed the organisation's intelligence operations in neighbouring Swaziland before turning his talents to commerce. The articles played up his shadowy background, alleging, among other things, that he had been involved in car theft and drug dealing rings.

The new investors, who apart from Nxumalo declined to be named, now owned 60 per cent of the shares alongside the original shareholders' 30 per cent. The Vissers had allegedly been paid R5 million in cash. The new investors undertook to cover further costs of bringing the drug to market, including the cost of securing Virodene's international patents, which now fell due.

It was also clear that the government was still committed to seeing that the drug was tested in clinical trials.

The new chair of the Medicines Control Council, Dr Helen Rees[221], told the *Mail & Guardian* that the council had established a team of top medical experts to help prepare the protocol that would clear Virodene for human trials. This was being paid for by the government. Rees said that it was unusual for a special committee to be created to assist a private company, but as the government had identified the treatment of AIDS as a priority, the council was duty-bound to help. 'The committee has spent an enormous amount of effort giving them scientific feedback,' she said.

Yet even this more sympathetic grouping could not come up with a protocol that would justify testing Virodene on human beings. By the end of the year they too had rejected applications for clinical trials on the basis of science and public safety.

'The unanimous decision that has now been reached has involved some of the best scientific and clinical minds in the country,' they said.[222]

After this, the Virodene researchers gave up on official approval for their experiments with human life. They simply continued their work underground.

The controversies over Virodene, the Medicines Act and Medicines Control Council were intricately linked in a complex web, in which timing was often as important as ideology, and personalities as important as facts. But unlike Escher's impossible geometry, this puzzle was not floating free in space, but grounded in the matrix of the country's transformation to democracy. It both drew on and fed into the challenges of governance and nation-building, which were at the heart of the new state.

As the first decade of freedom advanced, it seemed that Mandela had become more content to play the role of statesman, while Deputy President Mbeki governed. Nowhere was this clearer than in the AIDS story. Since *Sarafina II*, Mandela had taken a back seat, leaving Mbeki to deal with the Medicines Control Council and the Virodene researchers.

And while Mbeki was preparing to take over the presidency, he was also working on an Africanist treatise designed to give hope and inspiration to all Africans: the idea of the African Renaissance.

In April 1998 Mbeki addressed the United Nations University with his first major speech on the African Renaissance. He began it by quoting the Roman philosopher Pliny — in Latin: 'Ex Africa semper aliquid novi' (Something new always comes out of Africa).

Mbeki argued that the moment for Africa to shake off the legacy of centuries of slavery, colonialism and imperialism was long overdue: now was the time for the continent to experience cultural, political and economic rebirth. And in this rebirth the new South Africa would play a leading role.

The realities of warfare, dictatorships and underdevelopment must change, along with global perceptions of Africa as a hungry, conflict-ridden continent, he said.

'Out of Africa reborn must come modern products of human economic activity, significant contributions to the world of knowledge in the arts, science and technology, new images of an Africa of peace and prosperity.'[223]

In the Q&A session after his speech, Mbeki referred specifically to the role that the World Trade Organisation could play in unlocking African markets, thereby promoting African trade and development.

It is not difficult to see the relevance of African Renaissance thinking to ideas about the AIDS epidemic and its solutions. For a start, the Western media's visualisation of 'African AIDS' was inimical to the idea of an African renaissance. Imagery of emaciated, disease-ridden Africans had long been a source of annoyance not only to Africanists, but to all HIV and AIDS activists all around the world.

But it was the disease itself that was the deal breaker. Instead of re-birth, the burgeoning AIDS epidemic was threatening the continent with social chaos, declining longevity and economic disaster — a development process in reverse.

Renaissance thinking also explains the government's intense commitment to Virodene — a drug invented by Africans, for Africans, which had the power to save the world from the new disease.

The tragic irony was that 'something new' had already come out of Africa: this was the conquering virus of the twentieth century, and not its cure.

Mercy

As Mercy Makhalemele's profile as an HIV-positive activist grew, it began to affect her family life. One day she came home to find her six-and-a-half-year-old son, Thabang crying. 'As a mother you always want to know what is going on with your child,' says Mercy. 'He said "No, no, no, Mum, don't touch me. At school they told me you have got AIDS and you've got germs."'

He was afraid of getting AIDS from his mother, and the children at school refused to play with him. 'He didn't want to go to school, he just dropped out and I had to take him to therapy, and for that six months we had to deal with his feelings.'

After help from a counsellor, Thabang came to understand more about HIV, but he developed other concerns. 'He couldn't cry in front of me. He would cry alone in the room, and when the social worker asked him he said, "I don't want to hurt my mum. That is why I'm crying that side."'

When Mercy took a job in Durban she decided it would be better for Thabang to stay with his auntie in Johannesburg. They missed each other badly.

'But he understood why I had to go. When I left, he gave me these two stones and he said: "Mum, if you are going to KwaZulu-Natal to educate people about the disease that killed my sister and my father, take these stones and hold them very tight, and just talk."'

Chapter Ten

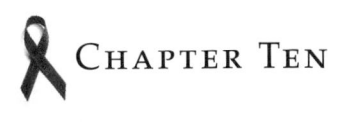

'Pills cost pennies'

Suffer the children

Flattened cardboard boxes cover the red cement corridor outside the paediatric ward of Grey's Hospital in Pietermaritzburg. On one, a plump mother lies sleeping. Paediatrician Dr Neil McKerrow is working in his office next door. All is quiet until a faint wailing begins. When the sound rises to a crescendo McKerrow knows, without inquiring, that a baby has died and a counsellor must be called. The death of a baby with HIV is sudden, an unpredictable yet common event on the wards these days.

By the late 1990s, hospital wards are filling up with babies and small children with AIDS-related illnesses. These little ones stay longer and come back to the hospital more often than other child patients. They are also more likely to die on the wards. One academic paper describing the situation at Chris Hani-Baragwanath Hospital in Soweto charts a 42 per cent rise in in-hospital child mortality in the five years between 1992 and 1997.[224]

Most women discover they are HIV positive during pregnancy — diagnosed with a terminal disease while preparing to bring a new life into the world. And how much more devastated the mother when she realises she may have passed HIV on to her baby.[225] Approximately one-third of babies born to HIV-positive women are HIV positive themselves[226], but without expensive testing their HIV status cannot immediately be known. For the mother, it means months of anxious waiting.

For counsellors like Florence Ngobeni at the Chris Hani-Baragwanath Perinatal HIV Research Unit, this represents a daily challenge. 'Every pregnant woman is worried about whether they'll have a premature baby, or a child born with a disability,' she says, 'and now they find they are HIV positive and there's no medication. It just brings lots of fears and stress.'

Dying babies, bereaved mothers, these are stories that the world does not care to know. But those on the frontline wonder at the long-term effects of such a tragedy.

New research suggests that children are damaged by AIDS in the family even when they are neither infected nor orphaned. Their problems seem to be caused by their mothers' depression.

'These children have been found in some studies to have significantly more attentional and behavioural problems,' says an international team of child psychologists. 'Uninfected children whose mothers have HIV are important because they form the largest sub-group of young children.'

For South Africa, struggling to emerge from the damage of apartheid, this new scourge is hard to bear; the despair of HIV, one new stone in the pond, with side effects that will ripple through the generations to come.

During the late 1990s, new research conducted in Thailand brought hope to HIV-positive mothers. A short course of the drug AZT (zidovudine) given to the mother after 36 weeks of pregnancy was shown to halve the likelihood of transmission of HIV from mother to child. Unlike the triple-drug cocktail used to treat HIV-positive adults in Europe and the US, this regimen was relatively inexpensive. Because of the short duration of the treatment and the simplicity of the regimen, this was the first HIV treatment to be even remotely affordable in low-income countries. In March 1998, UNAIDS and the WHO welcomed the study, describing the Thai regimen as akin to 'vaccinating the children of infected mothers'.

A large group of South African public health advocates had been watching these trials closely. Drs Glenda Gray and James McIntyre, two global leaders in perinatal HIV research (who themselves were conducting drug trials), called a meeting to prepare for immediate action.[227] Fareed Abdullah of the Western Cape provincial health department was an enthusiastic participant. 'I was the only senior government official there and I was asked to say a few words,' Abdullah recalls. 'I said, "We are convinced that this is the right thing to do and we will not let the grass grow under our feet."'

But there were problems. The first was the price of the drug. Even though it was a short course, the cost would still come in at over US $200 per woman. Then there were additional costs to make the programme work — testing, counselling, breast-milk substitutes. Given the high HIV prevalence in South Africa, this programme would come with a huge price tag.

While the minister of health was considering her options, two provincial health departments went ahead with their own plans to deliver the treatment. 'Within two weeks we had a task team and we began implementing it in Khayelitsha,' says Abdullah. The regional health department for Gauteng also planned pilot projects at five sites, and was ready to move with the therapy within weeks.

AZT — A BACK STORY

Like Virodene, AZT had been a troublesome drug from the start, and as we shall see later, its controversial nature was the catalyst for President Mbeki's revisionist construct of AIDS.

Used initially as a cancer drug, AZT was registered in the US as a treatment for adults with HIV in 1987. And it was very expensive. Pharmaceutical manufacturers justified their prices by referring to their enormous research and development costs[228], but the AZT regimen had been trialled by government researchers and was only acquired later by the manufacturer in what many saw as a reprehensible patent-grab. These goings-on brought AZT into the sights of HIV-positive activists in the United States. The activist group ACT UP[229] lobbied fiercely to have costs reduced, and more than once they stopped trade on the New York Stock Exchange. Protesters dubbed the manufacturer the 'evil empire'.

Next, there was a controversy over the side effects and toxicity of the drug. HIV clinicians and activists in the US argued that the recommended dose caused serious side effects, even death. In 1990, after much debate, the Food and Drug Administration halved the recommended dose.[230] Although early results from the use of AZT monotherapy were encouraging[231], a study in 1994, called the Concorde study, showed that when used alone, AZT did not have lasting effects.[232]

By contrast, from the early 1990s ongoing trials using AZT to prevent mother-to-child transmission of HIV were more promising. The first results of these were published in 1994 and showed that the drug administered to pregnant women at

14 weeks of pregnancy and to the baby for six weeks after birth, dramatically reduced perinatal transmission of HIV. Because the dose was small and the regimen was limited in duration, the harmful effects of the drug were minimised. As in chemotherapy for cancer, the benefits of the treatment outweighed the side effects. Within three years of this research being applied in the United States and Europe, transmission rates between mothers and infants dropped dramatically.[233]

Research then began with ever-shorter AZT regimens that would be more affordable in low-income countries. By 1998 one of these, the Thai regimen, was producing encouraging results, showing that it was now possible to halve the number of HIV-positive births at a much lower cost. But even for a middle-income country like South Africa, this cost was not insignificant.

These promising results presented a serious challenge to the manufacturer Glaxo Wellcome.[234] Peter Young, then a senior manager at Glaxo's UK office recalls the predicament. 'It was very clear to me that up to that point, what was only an academic policy issue around the disparity between purchasing power, prevalence and access, was going to flip directly into a major public health issue and therefore a political issue.'

Young, who felt both professionally and personally challenged by this, had been working on a strategy that would allow drugs to be sold at lower prices to countries that could not afford them.

'I had the fairly simple view that if you are in the business to develop medicines, and most of the people who need the medicines can't use them,' he says, 'it is a business problem as well as a public health problem and you should have an active interest in trying to figure it out.'

Young pitched a concept of tiered pricing to the company, where it found favour, with the proviso that it would be possible to prevent the discounts given in poor countries from seeping into the wealthy markets. The idea was to reverse the business model of low-volume, high price that had worked for rich countries.

Thus it was that Young began to travel the world to discuss the situation with Glaxo's regional managers. They were given the discretion to cut prices of AZT and a second drug, 3TC, but despite endorsement and encouragement from the top, nothing much happened. Company managers were not actively resistant to the idea, but felt there were too many obstacles for such a venture in low-income countries.

'Some of them viewed me as a bit naïve,' says Young. 'They thought it was going to take more than a discount to get government acceptance. There may have been a bit of passive resistance on that basis. Not because they were venal about it, but they were sceptical.'

Glaxo's South African medical director, Peter Moore, was one of those who took the idea seriously. Some time in mid 1997, Moore offered a deal to the South African government.[235] What was proposed was not a discount but a complex arrangement where a fund of money, equivalent to a discount, could be used to train counsellors and develop other infrastructure necessary to deliver the treatment. The actual figures could only be determined later when the official results of the Thai trial would allow a precise calculation of the cost of drug per person.

The health minister's spokesperson, Vincent Hlongwane, confirmed that she was taking the proposition seriously — they were just waiting for Glaxo to state its price.

In March 1988, two weeks after the results of the Thai study were announced, Young went public with Glaxo's global discount offer on AZT.[236] He told the US media that the company felt an obligation to make the drug more widely available. It was not an act of charity, he said, but an 'ethically sound' undertaking. He later said he was hoping to galvanise regional managers and governments into action.

But Health Minister Zuma still did not bite.

There were good reasons for her lukewarm response. The pharmaceutical industry's opposition to her reforms had provoked her displeasure and mistrust — by now Big Pharma had already gone to court to freeze the Medicines Act. The pending trial would inevitably muddy the waters for any cooperation between the government and the industry. Under these conditions, accepting a discount from Glaxo could possibly undermine the government's case, and the minister's advisers were likely to be telling her so.

Ironically the announcement of the success of the Thai research had been made on February 18 — the same day as Big Pharma's interdict against the Medicines Act.

Yet again, the AIDS response in South Africa had fallen victim to the vagaries of time — chance calendar events that determined the course of history.

Bridging the gap

This wrangling over drugs, legislation and discounts in South Africa was taking place against the backdrop of a rapidly changing international landscape for AIDS treatment.

Since the new combination therapies had hit the headlines in 1996, a growing mass of evidence testified to their effectiveness. In the US, for example, combination therapy had seen the death toll from HIV decline by 70 per cent between 1995 and 1998.[237] People who had been in the final stages of AIDS-related illness had shown such remarkable recoveries on the therapy that it had been dubbed the 'Lazarus effect'.

Antiretroviral therapy had its drawbacks. It was a complex regimen — up to 20 pills to be taken each day, some with food, some without — and the price of the drugs, up to $15 000 per patient per year, was exorbitant. But with the correct monitoring and care, HIV was now a manageable chronic disease. Most rich countries with small epidemics weighed the cost against the economic and ethical burden of AIDS deaths and found that the use of the therapy in the public health system was justified.

Not so in low-income countries.

In Africa, where the epidemic was most entrenched, no government had the resources to make the drugs available, and few individuals could afford the purchase price in the private health market.

This created a particularly cruel inequality in the world of people living with HIV and AIDS. Before the advent of triple therapy, the disease had united people living with HIV in the north and the south. Now it divided them. HIV-positive Africans who had attended international conferences since the 1980s now returned from these conferences feeling distraught and abandoned. Their life-and-death battles with the disease remained unchanged, but many of their former comrades had left the struggle. Northern activists now seemed preoccupied with adjusting to the challenge of unexpected longevity.

In general, the international AIDS fraternity had been slow to embrace the ethical challenge presented by the success of the new therapy.[238] Major organisations and donor groups continued to promote HIV prevention as the preferred goal. The cost of the drugs was only the first hurdle, they argued. Such a complex therapy also required a good health infrastructure and person-power, yet many health facilities in AIDS-affected countries lacked basic testing equipment, and sometimes even electricity and refrigeration. Then there was the cost and expertise required for the ongoing monitoring of what was a highly toxic drug regimen. For now, prevention and palliative care would have to do.

For HIV-positive people in low-income countries, their only hope was inclusion in a drugs trial, or in one of the tiny donor or NGO programmes piloting antiretroviral therapy in resource-poor settings.

The stark injustice of this new situation galvanised a small but vocal fraction of northern activists. They targeted the high price of drugs, and lost no opportunity to protest and lobby the industry. By 1998 they had made an impact on the international agencies that defined AIDS orthodoxy.

In 1998, the Twelfth International AIDS Conference[239] in Geneva represented something of a watershed in this debate. For the first time, the desirability of treatment for the poor was placed on the mainstream agenda.

The conference slogan 'Bridging the gap' referred to the widening gulf between the life-chances of rich and poor people living with HIV. At this conference, the high cost of drugs and the connection to pharmaceutical industry practices were flagged by participants from the UN agencies and academia as well as by the activists. A letter in *The Lancet*, for example, commented on the irony that the pharmaceutical industry supported the bi-annual conference financially, while not supporting its aims. 'Industry remains the only part of the AIDS community left unaccountable for its policies and priorities. The failure to call them to account is nothing less than a betrayal of those in the developing world.'

Activists from the north and south took to the streets, united in a new campaign to bring life-saving drugs to the poor. Their slogan was 'Pills cost pennies, drugs cost lives.'

South Africa was their first target.

They broke our hearts

This then was the climate in which the South African health minister would have to assess the Glaxo offer of discounted AZT.

On the one hand there was the pressure of the Big Pharma's legal challenge, which made the offer difficult to accept.

On the other hand, though, the infant death toll was clearly mounting and the growing band of disaffected activists, within and outside of the country, would seem to stop at nothing to get their way.[240]

By now the issue of AIDS was so politicised that anybody in the health minister's shoes would have struggled to negotiate this treacherous terrain. Zuma's relationship with the activists had been so damaged by the *Sarafina* and Virodene controversies that she did not seem predisposed to listen to their views.[241] The social contract between government and civil society, as described in the original National AIDS Plan, lay in tatters. At best, the activists and civil society organisations engaged in AIDS were tolerated by the government. At worst, they were dismissed as complicit in the conspiracy of forces opposing political transformation. Their demand for conventional pharmaceutical drugs, in preference to Virodene, seemed to confirm that view.

There were also broader economic considerations. The cost of the mother-to-child programme, including the discount on AZT, had been estimated at R80 million a year. This did not sit well with the government's new-look conservative macro-economic policy. Since 1996, economic growth, foreign investment and export earnings had been prioritised over social spending. A health budget expanded to mitigate the impact of a terminal disease was out of kilter with this goal of fiscal restraint. Beefing up the 'behavioural' prevention programme seemed like the better way to go.

Thus it was that in October 1998 the government renewed its commitment to HIV prevention as the basis of its AIDS programme. This was defined as prevention of sexual transmission between adults. They allocated a budget of R80 million — the exact price tag of the rejected mother-to-child programme.

This new strategy, The Partnership against AIDS[242], was intended to unite government departments and civil society organisations — from the health sector to the education sector, from business to religious leaders — in a powerful new AIDS response. This was an early attempt at mainstreaming AIDS, an innovative forerunner of what is now textbook UNAIDS strategy.

The initiative had been given much advance publicity, and President Mandela was scheduled to make a television address. It was anticipated by those in the know as a watershed event, the first time Madiba would talk to the nation about HIV and AIDS. Apart from the fact that this broadcast was scheduled not for prime time television but for midday on a Friday, it was a significant moment in the history of the government AIDS response.

There was a big build-up to this event. Government leaders urged all South Africans to stop what they were doing and listen to the broadcast. 'Invest ten minutes for the life of the nation on October 9,' was the call. Mandela even ordered that, on the day, the national flags be flown at half mast on all government buildings and foreign missions in memory of those who had died of AIDS.

A few days before the event, it was announced that the president was overtired and taking an unscheduled holiday in Mozambique. Deputy President Mbeki would deliver the Declaration of Partnership against AIDS in his stead.

Mbeki told the nation that HIV and AIDS were a threat to everyone. 'It walks among us. It travels everywhere we go.'

Young people were urged to delay their first experience of sex, and if not, to use a condom. Men and women were urged to be faithful to their partners, and if not, to use a condom. 'For too long we have closed our eyes as a nation, hoping the truth was not so real,' Mbeki said.

The Declaration was a wholehearted government dedication to reinvigorate the AIDS response, ending with the words 'Together as partners against HIV/AIDS we can and shall win.'

The health minister chose the occasion of the gala launch of the Partnership against AIDS in Pretoria to announce her decision on the mother-to-child programme. She told the media that the AZT programme was too expensive to be rolled out after all.[243]

'It is not cost-effective,' she said, 'because we do not have the money.' Zuma said that the government would be better off focusing on prevention programmes and public awareness. Additional money would also be put into vaccine research. She also expressed scepticism about the value of a programme where such large numbers of women would have to be treated to make a difference to so few babies. Of every 100 women who would receive the treatment, she said, only 15 babies would be saved from HIV.

'If you take all that into account and compare it to the benefit you would get from prevention, then we really have to deal with prevention.'

Sponsorship for the 18 pilot mother-to-child sites agreed to earlier in the year was withdrawn and all programmes were to cease forthwith. However, the minister did urge the public to join with her to put pressure on the pharmaceutical companies to bring down drug prices.

For the paediatricians, the researchers and the activists, this was a terrible blow. Dr Peter Cooper, who headed the department of paediatrics in Johannesburg General Hospital, recalls 'It was awful because the AIDS burden on the wards was just rocketing at the time, and not doing anything about it was just crazy.'

Public health facilities were not prevented from supplying the drug, but they would have to find their own sources of funding. Even for the Johannesburg General Hospital, one of the largest and best-resourced teaching hospitals in the country, this was a challenge.

'The drug itself was quite expensive at the time,' says Cooper. 'We couldn't just write it up and get it dispensed by the hospital, because it was expensive and it wasn't approved and it was not health department policy to do so.'

For the women attending antenatal clinics across the country, this was a tragedy beyond measure. At Chris Hani-Baragwanath, the support group had been praying regularly for the advent of the treatment that would prevent them from passing the virus on to their unborn children. Now, instead of praying, they wept.

'The new government let us down,' said Florence Ngobeni. 'They have broken our hearts.'[244]

Nkosi

It is a weekday morning in May 1997 and eight-year-old Nkosi[245] *is in the kitchen of his Johannesburg suburban home, feeding his fat grey cat.*

'I've made no allowance for his illness,' says foster mum Gail Johnson. 'It's not an issue in our house. He has his duties to do on a daily basis because he has got to be involved with life. If I allowed him to just sit on his little bum and say "I'm sick," he would not be with us today. So it's a balanced diet; it's normality – punishment when punishment is due, and… life.'

So far, 1997 has been a challenging year for Nkosi. He almost failed to gain admission to the local school because teachers and parents were not comfortable with his HIV status. The provincial health and education authorities then intervened with educational workshops at the school. Once parents and teachers knew more about the disease, they relented and Nkosi was admitted into Grade One. A few months into the school year Nkosi has made friends and is doing well. But a few parents have remained unhappy. They seem to demand a much higher degree of protection from risk of HIV than they do from other dangers that might befall a child at school.

Mindful of these feelings, Gail has taught Nkosi a basic drill which he is keen to demonstrate. It involves covering a wound with a tissue and going to the sick room. 'I personally believe that we should assume we are associating with infected people all the time,' says Gail. 'Have latex gloves in the classroom and don't discriminate. Any child falls, put gloves on and deal with it.'

Nkosi's experience at primary school has already had far-reaching consequences. Schools across the country are now obliged to draw up new regulations and in the future no child living with HIV will be discriminated against.

Xolani Nkosi was born in an East Rand township where he lived with his mother until he was two years old. Then, feeling unable to care for an HIV-positive child, his mother placed him in a children's home. Some months later the facility closed and one of the volunteer workers, Gail Johnson, took Nkosi home.

By the time he was 11 years old, Nkosi had become a spokesperson for children living with HIV and AIDS. In July 2000 he took the platform at the International AIDS Conference in Durban to tell a global audience:

'I want people to understand about AIDS… You can't get AIDS if you touch, hug, kiss, hold hands with someone who is infected. Care for us and accept us — we are all human beings. We are normal. We have hands. We have feet. We can walk, we can talk. Don't be afraid of us, we are all the same!'[246]

Nkosi died in 2001.

Chapter Eleven

A state of denial

The cutting edge

On any summer's day in the late 1990s, the wards of Murchison Hospital[247] on the south coast of KwaZulu-Natal are full to bursting. Many patients at this small community hospital are sleeping on mattresses on the floor. Others are stretched out on the green grass outside, sunning themselves in the bright light. Nobody is turned away.

The health services in the province are witnessing a dramatic increase in AIDS-related illness. 'I think the tidal wave is only really just hitting us now,' says Murchison's Dr Bill Hardy. 'I see ever-increasing numbers of ill people. I know that, given the time-lag in this epidemic, we are treating patients from five years ago.' Hardy fears what is to come.

The hospital operates on a strict budget that cannot accommodate the increasing numbers coming through the doors. And it's not just the numbers. AIDS-related illnesses are complicated to treat, patients stay for longer, and return more often than people with other diseases do. Without further resources, patients will be left to die, untreated.

Health professionals like Hardy feel that they have become gatekeepers for the health system's financial problems. There are drugs to treat the opportunistic diseases of AIDS, like thrush and tuberculosis, but they are expensive. It's a constant juggling act. 'We decide who gets the treatment and who doesn't. Every day you look at patients and you say, "Do I give this patient this drug, Diflucan, or don't I?"' says Hardy. 'This is something that goes against the grain, goes against all my own ethical values regarding medical treatment, and it's really painful to me because many of these patients, once treated, can be expected to recover and have a significant quality of life.'

In these difficult times the health authorities seem unable, or unwilling, to meet the challenge of this disease. But ordinary people in communities are faring little better. One of the greatest tragedies of AIDS is the barriers it creates: the social stigma, the sense of shame and sexual guilt.

This compounds the problems of those who are ill. 'We have become more and more aware that most people in our community who die of AIDS, die of starvation,' says Hardy, 'and they die alone, because they are rejected by their families.'

To alleviate this problem, the hospital and the local hospice train community health workers who in turn teach family members how to treat and care for the sick. One of their patients, a young man who will not be named, tells how his uncle (and only living relative) abused him and confronted the hospice team. 'He looked them straight in the eyes and said they should take me away. He said there was nobody even to feed me. He told them to take me to the government.'

Now he lives alone in a backyard room. Wheelchair-bound, he depends on the community health workers who visit regularly to dress his open wounds. They alone will care for him in his dying days.

AIDS, 'THE NEW STRUGGLE'

Alongside the political scandals of *Sarafina* and Virodene, and the conflict over the mother-to-child programme, HIV prevalence continued to soar. In 1997, the annual survey showed that HIV prevalence had risen to 17 per cent among pregnant women across the land. By 1998, it had reached 23 per cent. And as the epidemic of HIV entered its second decade, the epidemic of illness and death was beginning in earnest.

But despite the rising HIV statistics and the growing death toll, South Africans were still failing to get to grips with the crisis. Opinion-makers and ordinary people seemed to be in denial, and concern for the issue was largely left to a small group of activists, health professionals and health department politicians.

President Mandela, for example, had been strangely silent about HIV and AIDS. He had waited until February 1997 before making a major presidential speech on AIDS, and then it was to international leaders and masters of the global economy. He told the World Economic Forum[248] in Davos, Switzerland, that the disease was causing enormous suffering for individuals and families, and impacting on the efforts of the new democracy to achieve its goals of reconstruction and development. Mandela estimated that the epidemic would cost South Africa 1 per cent of its GDP by 2005, when up to three quarters of the health budget would be consumed in direct costs relating to HIV and AIDS.

Because of this, he said, South Africa's National AIDS directorate had made the call for 'a new struggle'. Using the language of the liberation movement, he promised to put the effort to combat AIDS on a higher plane. 'Future generations will judge us on the adequacy of our response,' he said.

South Africans who heard the speech waited for the president to kick-start a new national awareness campaign. But when Madiba returned home, he kept his own counsel.

For the health department's directorate for HIV and AIDS, it had indeed been a struggle. They had worked hard to try to turn the epidemic around, but their attempts had been overshadowed by political conflicts and controversies around the AIDS programme. In the wake of the *Sarafina* saga, director Quarraisha Abdool Karim had resigned and had been replaced by Rose Smart.[249] Under Smart's leadership a revitalised multi-media campaign, dubbed Beyond Awareness, was devised. This engaged several NGOs in creating educational materials that were distributed free to organisations across the county. The campaign promoted social action and the de-stigmatising of HIV — there were exhibitions and publications featuring the lives of people living with HIV, local artists worked together on murals in seven cities, and a national telephone helpline was launched. The international symbol of HIV and AIDS, the red ribbon, was formally adopted. It was a big campaign, with a wide reach. 'Our model was really getting stuff out to people who could use it, rather than a centralised approach,' says one of the architects, Dr Warren Parker.

But although the directorate had good leadership, new policies and competent and motivated staff, the national programme was faltering.[250] The team had insufficient capacity to spend the huge budget[251], and the independence of the provinces meant that they struggled to push their new programmes through.

Smart and her team also had the challenge of repairing the damaged relationship between the health department and the

NGO sector, which was still delivering the bulk of AIDS services in the country. A proposal to review[252] the National AIDS Plan provided a good opportunity to mend fences and renew the contract between government and civil society that had been made, in such good faith, in 1992.

Teams went out to every province to take stock of the AIDS response — to understand where it was best succeeding, and when, and why it failed. One day in August 1997, 600 AIDS activists and experts gathered in the Carlton Hotel in Johannesburg for a report-back and planning session. But when Minister Zuma spoke, she announced the decision to make AIDS a notifiable disease.

Once again, her approach proved too hard to bear. Many in the audience were enraged and stormed from the room. Smart and her co-workers were devastated. The renewal of the social contract between government and NGOs was again a distant dream.

This particular conflict had been simmering for some time, with government and AIDS experts in open opposition. One of the hallmarks of the original National AIDS Plan was a commitment to confidentiality and the rights of people living with HIV. Preserving confidentiality was not only a human rights issue but central to creating an environment in which people felt comfortable to come forward for testing.

The minister, on the other hand, had argued that the confidentiality principle was feeding into the vicious circle of stigma, secrecy, ignorance and denial. For several years she had been hinting at new legislation that would bring HIV into the open.

The AIDS fraternity did agree on the need to break the circle, though, and behind the scenes there were fertile discussions about 'shared confidentiality' and other ways this could be done. But legislation around notifiability was seen as a blunt instrument — it was not the way to go.

This, and many other conflicts, past and still to come, derived from the ideological differences between the AIDS fraternity and the government.

The AIDS orthodoxy had been shaped by the lessons learned in the northern gay epidemic of the 1980s; in South Africa many of the AIDS organisations were still led by white, gay men. On the other hand, the government was committed to an African perspective, an indigenous solution to the crisis, which they believed would yield better results.

Then there was the deeper layer of discord that derived from the clash of political culture between exile and 'inzile' politics, a clash that would haunt the land for years to come.

Those who stayed behind to listen to the report on that cold August day heard what they, in any case, already knew. The National AIDS Plan was being implemented slowly and imperfectly, if at all. In some instances it had become just another 'dusty book on the shelf'. The report also confirmed the suspicions that, outside of the Department of Health, there was little commitment to the government's AIDS programme, and little coordination between the many government players who ought to be engaged. Among the recommendations were that political leadership for the AIDS response be located in the deputy president's office, and that new structures be formed to strengthen and coordinate work across different sectors and government departments.

It was these recommendations that led to the Partnership on AIDS, which Minister Zuma launched in the midst of the mother-to-child controversy. They also led to the establishment of an inter-ministerial committee on AIDS. But as we have seen, by the time these reforms came into effect the AIDS debate had moved onto entirely new terrain.

Life skills

There was one section of the original National AIDS Plan that was slowly stuttering into life. This was a schools-based programme that was designed to raise awareness of sexuality, sexual health and HIV. It went beyond simple health messages, aiming to build skills that would help pupils to survive in a dangerous and challenging world. Negotiating gender relations and safer sex were included in the many topics.

Life skills, as it came to be known, was a compulsory programme intended to reach all eight million school pupils in the country. Age-appropriate multi-media materials were produced, and teachers were trained in what was to become the largest programme of its kind on the continent.

It was ambitious, and from its early days in 1996 there were problems. Although life skills had been a fundamental component of the National AIDS Plan, it took several years to get off the ground. Proponents battled to overcome the major obstacle posed by widespread moral qualms. Although all the research shows that sexuality education helps young people make good choices and delay sexual debut, there were still fears to the contrary — teachers and parents feared that the new knowledge would encourage young people to experiment.

Training the teachers was one of the biggest challenges. Many had no such education themselves and were mortified at the prospect of speaking to their pupils about subjects like STIs, contraception, masturbation and sex.

During training it was common for teachers to refuse to participate, for example, in the exercise where they were required to pin labels on diagrams of male and female reproductive anatomy. As Aloma Foster[253], one of the trainers from the Planned Parenthood Association explained, 'Their main fear is that they don't know enough. The virus has been around a long time, but they don't know the facts. Some say "In all my 40 years I didn't know that."' It soon became clear that the training was benefiting teachers as much as pupils. 'I recall one of the evaluation forms where a woman said this was the first training that she had had since she left college — this was a woman in her fifties,' says Dr Kenau Swart, one of the architects of the programme in the department of education. 'I realised that the training had a spill-over effect on their families and developing their own lives. That wasn't what the money was for, but that's what happened.'

The institutional arrangements were also complex. Because the programme required close cooperation between the departments of health and education, this was the first real test of the 'multi-sectorality' of the AIDS response.

At the time, the department of education was undergoing major restructuring and teachers were being retrained to meet the needs of a new national curriculum. This placed a huge strain on the system, and some managers were reluctant to allow space for another new programme. 'It was a difficult time in the country,' says Swart. 'We had major changes in the education system and you had the teachers all of a sudden going off for training.'

Once teachers were trained, they were often deployed elsewhere. Then there was more restructuring, and new batches of teachers had to be trained, all over again.

By the end of 1998 nearly 10 000 teachers had been trained

and were plying their new skills in classrooms across the country. But evaluations showed that some teachers still struggled to deal comprehensively with the subject. 'There's one thing I never started. Whenever I think of the topic my heart starts beating very fast...', one teacher told an evaluation team. 'That was demonstrating how to use a condom... I do not feel confident to go through with it.'

In the end, the life skills programme was mainly implemented by schools that had the capacity and supportive management. Coverage was patchy at best. An evaluation of over 100 secondary schools in 2000 found that the programme was fully operational in less than a third of schools, and more than half had no teaching materials.

For Mary Crewe, who chaired the committee that put together the programme, there were hard lessons to be learned. The experience challenged her notion of what life skills meant in a context of AIDS.

'Everybody sees it merely in terms of getting AIDS literate, but I don't think that's what it's about,' says Crewe. 'My sense is that... if you are in a country with one of the worst epidemics in the world, the whole way of teaching must change. And you need to understand how kids learn conceptually... because clearly, traumatised children are not going to learn in the same way as non-traumatised children do. So for me, life skills is absolutely fascinating because unless you have teachers actually thinking about how to change the way they teach, you are not going to confront this epidemic and how it is affecting education.'

THE MATERIALITY OF EVERYDAY SEX

The internationally endorsed HIV-prevention paradigm, with its emphasis on individual behaviour change, AIDS awareness and safer sex, was the basis of the South African government's AIDS response. But this paradigm is not without its flaws, and is regarded by some as a denial of the realities of HIV and AIDS. This is because the focus on behavioural change and prevention deflects attention from the deep structural problems that have rendered some communities so vulnerable to HIV.

In the early days of the epidemic, the apartheid system, with its dependence on enforced migratory labour, provided fertile ground for HIV to seed itself across the land. Then, during the dying years of the regime, new and complex phenomena like chaotic urbanisation, gender-based violence and martial rape had allowed the virus to flourish. While it might be hoped that the social ills nurtured by these violent times would diminish in the new South Africa, this was never going to be an automatic process.

In the mid 1990s, massive state energy and resources were devoted to healing the flagrant wounds of political violence, in the form of the Truth and Reconciliation Commission. But the more profound legacy of psychological wounding festered on, creating social problems that enhanced risk and vulnerability to HIV. One manifestation of this was a new epidemic of child rape that came to public attention in the late 1990s. Much of this rape was committed by young men whose violent actions fitted no Western definitions of paedophilia.

Researchers have speculated on what it was about the post-apartheid period that gave rise to such distorted masculinities. Writing about young men in the township of Sebokeng, sociologist Pule Zwane[254] suggested that the rise in rape was linked to the decline in political organisation in the early 1990s. Interviews with young men revealed that they felt displaced by the return of their senior comrades from prison and exile. As a result the young people, who had previously been 'struggle leaders', turned to violent crime. One group even formed a gang called the South African Rapists Association (SARA). A gang member explained why he joined:

'I was a comrade before joining this organisation. I joined it because we were no longer given political tasks. Most of the tasks were given to senior people. I felt that we have been used by these senior comrades, because I do not understand why they dumped us like this. Myself and a group of six guys decided to form our own organisation that will keep these senior comrades busy all the time. That is why we formed SARA. We rape women who need to be disciplined (those women who behave like snobs), they just do not want to talk to most people, they think they know better than most of us and when we struggle, they simply do not want to join us.'

Not only were the psycho-social legacies of the apartheid era lingering, but there were new problems in the making. The economic reforms of the late 1990s were contributing to rising unemployment and social inequality across the country. This twin crisis created new conditions of vulnerability to the epidemic, particularly for women.

In a textured and insightful piece of research, sociologist Dr Mark Hunter explored this dynamic in the squatter settlements of a high HIV-prevalence area of northern KwaZulu-Natal.[255] During the late apartheid years, black women had been increasingly drawn into the 'women's industries' — the garment and textile factories — of the area. For many, this was their first taste of financial independence, and their lives and relationships with men had changed, they thought, forever. But when the trade liberalisation of the new era opened South Africa to a flood of cheap clothing imports, these industries suffered, and with them went womens' jobs.

In this bleak environment women sought boyfriends who could help them maintain their former levels of prosperity. For some this meant rent and food on the table; for others, perfume and smart clothes. To accomplish this, more than one partner was usually required. Hunter relates a typical conversation between his research assistant and a local woman:

NONHLANHLA: How many boyfriends do you have?
THANDI: Three.
NONHLANHLA: Why do you have three boyfriends?
THANDI: Because I have many needs.
NONHLANHLA: What needs?
THANDI: To dress, I don't work, a cell phone… doing my hair so that I am beautiful for my boyfriends, they won't love an ugly person.
NONHLANHLA: What do they give you?
THANDI: One, money… another, Checkers groceries… another buys me clothes.
NOHLANHLA: Does your mother know where the groceries come from?
THANDI: She knows, but she doesn't say anything because of the situation of hunger at home.
NONHLANHLA: Do other people know that you have many boyfriends?
THANDI: Yes, they know. My neighbours, they criticise me, but not in front of me. They gossip about me, they say I am *isifebe* (prostitute) but my friends understand the situation, they say nothing…

NONHLANHLA: Do you use condoms?
THANDI: With one, but two don't agree. These two say that they want flesh to flesh sex, they don't want to eat a sweet still in its wrapper.
NOHLANHLA: What do your friends think about the future?
THANDI: They wish... like me one day, I wish to get the right person who is going to love me and do everything for me and we marry.

For their part, the men were acting out of a new sense of masculinity in which having multiple partners was the norm. Though this idea of masculinity was rooted in traditional concepts of polygamy, it had been shaped by the changing times; in the modern era, marriage was increasingly unaffordable, and casual sexual relationships were condoned.

Hunter spent six months living with and talking to the people of the shacks. What his work revealed was a dynamic reciprocity between sexual culture, socio-economic realities and traditional mores that led to the kinds of relationships that allowed the virus to flourish. Hunter argues for an historical understanding of this conundrum, and against fixed notions of culture and tradition.

Many researchers, before and since, have sought to document this type of 'gift relationship', which has become increasingly common across the continent.[256] A 2004 study in Soweto, for example, sought to quantify the link between transactional sex and vulnerability to HIV.[257] Interviews with women seeking care at community-based antenatal clinics confirmed the theory. Women receiving food, money and other gifts from multiple partners were much more likely to be HIV positive than those who did not.

Transactional sex is increasingly understood as a response to modernity and to economic stress, and as a boost for HIV transmission. HIV, gender and transactional sex are linked in many ways: dependent women have less say in safer sex and are less able to insist on condom use; richer men are usually older men, and older men are more likely to be infected with HIV.

The culture of transactional sex, and the sexual networks that result, is central to understanding why some communities are so susceptible to HIV. Recent research[258] suggests that it is not the number of sexual partners, nor the amount of sexual contact that creates vulnerability to HIV, but the fact of concurrent sexual relationships.

Mathematical models show that when people have concurrent partners, dense sexual networks are formed and these promote the rapid spread of HIV. This is in contrast with sexual cultures, such as those common in the north, where serial monogamy (with or without occasional extramarital encounters) has become the norm.

These new ideas debunk old myths about promiscuity and HIV. They also challenge simplistic notions of the relationship between poverty and HIV, for it is often poor women in wealthier societies who are most at risk.[259] It seems that inequality rather than poverty is at the root of the HIV crisis in many countries.

An understanding of 'the materiality of everyday sex' is crucial to the development of strategies to curb the spread of HIV. To be successful, these strategies must go beyond behavioural interventions to interrogate the ground beneath. But the prevailing orthodoxy has preferred to stick with the old prescription: a safe mix of behavioural and technological interventions to prevent HIV.[260] For Dr Liz Floyd, who has headed the Gauteng AIDS directorate for many years, it is this inappropriate model that has underwritten the failure of South Africa's AIDS response. In her experience, condom distribution and safe sex messages do not hold the key to stemming the epidemic. 'We have to reinvent prevention and move away from the biomedical model,' she says. 'If you look at the Western model you are really looking at individual behavioural change... and the assumptions are that you have the conditions and the ability to control your own sexual behaviour — which even in a middle-class environment has not been so successful. The psychosocial determinants of risky behaviour have not received enough resources.

'Sometimes I say, if you are trying to tell me that sex is a medical event then I don't know how to talk to you, I give up.'

The lessons are clear: whether they be concurrent relationships in the squatter camps of KwaZulu-Natal, sex work in the brothels of Bangkok, or anonymous sex in the baths of San Francisco, it is the materiality of everyday sex and the nature of sexual networks that determine people's vulnerability to HIV. Unless and until this is understood, AIDS prevention programmes are bound to fail.

An epidemic of AIDS hysteria

Of the many failures to respond to the AIDS crisis in these times, that of the mass media[261] was probably the most significant. By 1998, the newspapers and television channels were still neglecting to come to terms with the gravity of the issue. Instead of headlines about the soaring HIV rate and its implications, HIV and AIDS coverage revolved around the political scandals and intrigues of the day.

People living with HIV found this particularly difficult to understand. Interviewed in 1998, Peter Busse (who by now was national director of Napwa) said that 'The media have been extremely irresponsible. They have focused on the most sensational and shallow stories like Virodene and *Sarafina*... It is the greatest human tragedy. It is the closing story of the millennium, and the newspapers, the television, are just not seeing it.'

For their part, editors argued that to be faithful to their shareholders they had to cover stories the nation wants to read. 'News is all about controversy. It's not admirable, but that's the way it works,' said Dave Robbins, a senior health writer for *The Star*. 'How do you say to your press you have a moral responsibility to cover this subject? Their original responsibility is to their shareholders. The only other way is for there to be state control of the media.'

There was also a dearth of journalists who were trained to deal with complex health stories. The media had already burned their fingers with their triumphalistic reporting of the Virodene 'cure', and were unwilling to risk their reputations any further. 'Young journalists are asked to write about AIDS and they don't understand the issues,' says Robbins. 'They may not even understand what a virus is. There is no specialisation, and health is very low on the list of priorities for our media.'

The absence of in-depth debate in the broadsheets was linked in both cause and effect to the fractured nature of AIDS discourse in civil society. Outside of the AIDS fraternity, left-wing intellectuals, activists and civil society organisations avoided the subject. AIDS did, after all, represent a threat to all their plans. Busse, who at the time ran educational workshops for non-AIDS NGOs, found that they too were struggling to take the epidemic on board.

'Even the NGO sector, traditional ally of the poor and marginalised, has failed to relate to the epidemic constructively,' he said. 'The idea was that NGOs in various fields like education and rural development have a unique advantage in working against HIV because of their contacts in the community. But integrating the HIV message has not been easy. Most NGOs cannot see the links and impact on their work. And even if they do, they do not have the conceptual ability to address them.'

Even Cosatu seemed to be dragging its heels on this one issue that represented the greatest threat to their membership. For example, in 1997, the September Commission which reported on the broader forces shaping the trade union movement, failed to factor HIV into their scenarios for 2005.

There were many shades and shapes of denial of the AIDS crisis in late twentieth century South Africa: from the politicians who played down the seriousness of the crisis to the ordinary people who denied their own risk and vulnerability; from the mass media, which dodged difficult and meaningful debate, to the teachers who refused to talk about safer sex. It is not surprising then, that this national state of benign denial created the space for a more malignant version to emerge.

In the late 1980s the AIDS dissidents, or denialists, who rejected the orthodox view that HIV leads to AIDS, had created controversy in the international AIDS fraternity. But by the early 1990s the matter had been largely laid to rest and few publications continued to promote their views. However, their core supporters had remained true to the cause and were finding new opportunities to promote their ideas in the unregulated intellectual atmosphere of the world wide web. The influential UK-based news magazine *New African*[262], which was widely read in South Africa, also continued its mission to debunk conventional ideas about AIDS. In its pages the African origins of HIV, the epidemiology and aetiology of the virus, were all under attack. These articles were clearly Africanist in their ideological outlook and their critique of the AIDS orthodoxy was a radical one.

In 1998, *The Citizen* — a newspaper that was neither Africanist nor radical, having been started as a propaganda tool of the apartheid government in the 1980s — took up the dissident cause. In September it published an article entitled 'The epidemic of AIDS hysteria' by Charles Geshekter, a professor of African history in California.[263] He spelled out the denialist argument that the AIDS epidemic was an artificial construct, and that immune deficiency in Africa was a product of poverty diseases such as parasite infection, malnutrition and tuberculosis. Geshekter argued that the symptoms of these diseases and the symptoms of 'so-called AIDS' were one and the same.

One of the dissidents' favoured strategies has been to raise the most perplexing characteristics of the virus as evidence for its non-existence. For example, in this article Geshekter asks: 'How can one virus cause 29 different "AIDS" diseases almost entirely among males in Europe and America, but afflict African men and women in nearly equal numbers?'

To the uninformed, the fact that the virus has never caused a major heterosexual epidemic outside of Africa may seem to be proof of its non-existence. In a later article in *New African*, journalist Baffour Ankomah took up the refrain, asking how HIV could be transmitted by different methods in different regions — heterosexual sex in sub-Saharan Africa, homosexual sex in Australia, injecting drug use in Eastern Europe.[264]

'Interesting, isn't it?' he wrote, 'one virus, one "disease", deciding on different modes of transport (Concorde, Fokker, canoe, bicycle, etc) as it travels around the world. But that is AIDS for you.'

Precisely. That is AIDS for you. But in the absence of any in-depth discussion of the subject, it was difficult for an unsuspecting audience to differentiate between mischievous denialist sophistry and scientific questions.

By and large, the educational materials produced by the AIDS orthodoxy steered clear of these perplexing questions, restricting their content to simple prescriptive messages. All you needed to know to be safe was as simple as ABC: abstain, be faithful or wear a condom. For most people — black and white, north and south, intellectual and other — AIDS literacy was so basic that it amounted to little more than blind faith in the chosen orthodoxy.

And as *The Citizen* correctly guessed, in that spring of 1998, the theories of the Africanist denialists were exactly what many South Africans wanted to hear. Geshekter spelt it out. The virus is a hoax. 'The best predictors for "AIDS" anywhere in Africa are economic deprivation, malnutrition, poor sanitation and parasitic infections,' he wrote, 'not extraordinary sexual behaviour or antibodies for a virus that has proved difficult to isolate directly.'

Internationally, however, there was growing concern about the rapid escalation of the epidemic in the region. President Clinton's 1998 visit had put the South African epidemic squarely on the international agenda. By the end of the year, UNAIDS was calling the southern African epidemic an 'unprecedented emergency'.

On the eve of World AIDS Day, the Executive Director Peter Piot[265], speaking at a press conference in Johannesburg, confirmed that AIDS was nothing short of a development disaster. He said that life expectancy in the world's worst-affected countries, which were all African, would be reduced by 17 years. And in those that were hardest hit — Botswana, Namibia, Swaziland and Zimbabwe — more than one-fifth of all adults were infected.

'Whether measured against the yardstick of falling life expectancy, deteriorating household income, overburdened health systems, child deaths, orphanhood, or bottom-line losses to business,' he said, 'AIDS has never posed a bigger threat to development.'

The report released by UNAIDS the following day showed that South Africa had the fastest-growing epidemic in the world.

PART THREE

REASON ON TRIAL
1998 TO 2003

By the end of the 1990s an unusual alignment of forces had placed the South African AIDS response at serious risk.

Efforts to contain the virus were not succeeding, and the government and the AIDS fraternity were at loggerheads over how to deal with it. The advent of successful antiretroviral therapies had given HIV-positive activists new heart, and their demands for anti-AIDS drugs were growing increasingly strident. But government policy favoured prevention over treatment as the more cost-effective approach.

This formed the backdrop for the government's ongoing legal battle with the powerful pharmaceutical industry over the right to manufacture and import affordable drugs for all diseases. And while AIDS activists supported the government in this particular contest, their participation in the dispute concealed deepening antagonisms.

For the government these were impossible contradictions. Something had to give — and it did. By the turn of the new millennium, key government leaders had begun to question the fundamentals of scientific thought on HIV and AIDS....

Lucky

Lucky Mazibuko lived with his secret diagnosis for several years before deciding to make his HIV status known. But he was not content with disclosing to his family and friends.

'I had this burning desire to reach out to people,' he says. 'So one day I called Dr Aggrey Klaaste, who was an icon of nation-building in the country, a very respected leader, not only in his capacity of editor-in-chief of the Sowetan, but as a member of his community.'

Lucky's boldness earned him the invitation to write some trial pieces for the newspaper, and on the strength of these, he was commissioned to write a regular column.

At first there was some suspicion from Sowetan journalists. 'Everyone was very warm and accommodating, but... one of the first things I learnt was that most of them did not believe I was HIV positive because I looked so well and I was a happy-go-lucky type of guy.'

Perhaps this was the reason that his new employers asked him to go for a confirmatory HIV test. 'I was not forced, but I think now I know exactly what they were doing... they were thinking what if this guy is lying, so it was suggested in a polite way — let's go to Prof Reuben Sher. So I went there and I was diagnosed HIV positive.'

His column, Just call me Lucky, has been appearing in the Sowetan every week since March 1999. It has been enormously popular with people living with HIV, who until then had had so little public acknowledgement or understanding. Many wrote under strict conditions of anonymity, but Lucky often found a way to include their stories in his column.

Despite the success of the column, it took its toll on the writer, especially in the early years. 'It was just more than I bargained for,' says Lucky. 'I became a first-hand witness to the pain and trauma and anguish... to, really, sometimes the worst that humanity can dish up: the worst forms of discrimination, the worst forms of prejudice, by people of their own. Whereas with apartheid it was one race against the other, now I found the discrimination is perpetrated by people against their own.'

Chapter Twelve

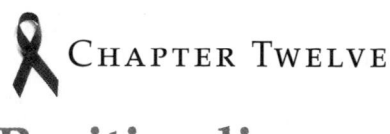

Positive lives

Death by stoning

On World AIDS Day 1998, a young woman from the township of KwaMashu in KwaZulu-Natal went public with her HIV-positive status on national television. Two weeks later she was stoned to death in the street by an angry crowd.

In the days following her disclosure, Gugu Dlamini and her family had received many threats from people who accused her of denigrating the neighbourhood. On separate occasions a group of women and a mob of armed youths visited the house demanding to know where Dlamini was.

Mandisa, Dlamini's 15-year-old daughter, told the press about the terror the whole family experienced during the days before her mother was killed. 'It was horrible and we were living in fear,' she said. 'Everybody had turned against us, even the neighbours whom we thought were family friends. People in the area, including some of my friends, stopped talking to me, and many said, since my mother had the virus, I too had AIDS.'

On the evening of her murder, Dlamini was assaulted by a young man. She contacted the police saying she feared for her life. A friend took her to see a nurse who tended to her wounds. On their way home, the pair stopped at a shebeen for a drink. There Dlamini was attacked by another man, who beat her to the floor and continued to kick her while she lay bleeding. Then she was dragged from the shebeen. Later, according to the neighbours, a group of young men came to the house and shouted at her saying 'How many people have you infected with this virus, you prostitute?'

They stoned and beat her to death and demolished the house. Dlamini died[266] in hospital the following day.

A few weeks later, four youths were arrested, then released into the custody of their parents. They were between 18 and 27 years of age.

Dlamini's murder, and the subsequent arrests, created huge divisions in the community, and her friends and supporters began to live in fear. Musa Njokwe, who was living openly with HIV, received an anonymous call from a man promising that she would follow Dlamini to the grave if she did not stop encouraging people to be open about their status. She was HIV positive, he said, because she was a prostitute and slept around with many men.

By the end of January 1999 the 'positive' camp began to retaliate. The *Sunday Times* reported that witnesses to the murder were fleeing the area. One resident said it was because Dlamini's friends were rumoured to be planning revenge. Pat Hlongwane, a spokesperson for the National Association of People Living with AIDS (Napwa), told the press, 'It is very tense in the area… We have received reports from a number of witnesses who say they have moved out because of intimidation. We have also heard that the alleged perpetrators are also leaving, not because of the police, but because of allegations that people living with AIDS wanted to retaliate.'

Despite the arrests and the plethora of witnesses, there were rumours that the charges were going to be dropped. People claimed this was because the investigating officer was a boyfriend of the shebeen owner, and that he knew the chief accused.

The AIDS Law Project took up the case and sent an attorney to meet the deputy director-general of public prosecutions. Apparently the docket failed to link Dlamini's death with her HIV status.

In response to this meeting, the police promised to see justice done, and appointed an eight-person investigative team. Nevertheless, charges were dropped in August due to insufficient evidence. According to the detective in charge of the team, the chief accused was missing from his home and work. The detective said there were no witnesses and the State's evidence was clumsy.

The AIDS Law Project and the AIDS Consortium continued to put pressure on the authorities. An inquest date was set, but the police failed to turn up. At the next date — two years after the murder — the sitting was postponed as the prosecutor was still interviewing witnesses.

The first hearing of the inquest was eventually held on January 12, 2001. AIDS Law Project spokesperson Jennifer Joni told the press that the family was too afraid to participate in the inquest and that key witnesses had since died. In addition, a new prosecutor had been appointed and the inquest was postponed yet again.

The inquest finally began in July 2001, and again witnesses described the events that had taken place three years before. But the inquest failed to reach a conclusion.

At the time of the murder, local and international activists spoke out against the stigma that provoked such violent consequences. Even Deputy President Mbeki invoked the tragedy when he was launching a new AIDS prevention campaign, soon after the events. Mbeki told listeners that 'the killing of brave KwaZulu-Natal activist Gugu Dlamini after she revealed her HIV-positive status must encourage the rest of us to support and protect those who speak out against AIDS. Women are particularly vulnerable to this disease and to society's reaction,' he said. 'We need to stand up and support their fight.'

The campaign they were launching was an 'AIDS train' that was to criss-cross the country, highlighting the gender dimension of HIV and AIDS.[267]

Both Mbeki and the minister of health used the occasion to ram home the lesson of Dlamini's death. Mbeki challenged men to become more involved in the struggle against AIDS, and Zuma called on rural women to lobby their male-dominated communities for better sexual health and rights.

'We need to demystify the taboos, expose the violence and propagate the hard facts about the impact of HIV and AIDS on women and children,' she said.

Gugu Dlamini became known as South Africa's 'first AIDS martyr' — a legend in the annals of the fight against AIDS, a tale of courage in the face of stigma and discrimination. In 2000 the Durban city council erected a sculpture of a red ribbon and dedicated a central park to her memory. But few know the shabby truth. During the many delays and postponements of the inquest proceedings, the police, the news media, the activists and the struggle lawyers all tired of the whole affair, and the case simply petered out. Despite the fact that her killers were named and identified, nobody was ever brought to justice for her murder.

Dlamini was buried in a quiet cemetery on the northern edge of Durban. Decorated with a red stone ribbon, the gravesite is still the destination of many international AIDS pilgrims to the country. The message on her tombstone reads: 'Let us all ensure that her brave endeavour to combat the conspiracy of silence that surrounds the disease will not be in vain.'

A visit to the Gugu Dlamini memorial park, in December 2005, challenges the optimism of those words. Located in a busy part of central Durban, the park plays generous host to hawkers and shoppers, travellers and office workers who pass through, or stop there to rest, eat, or meet their friends. That Christmas, the council had set up a toy train that had Santa and his dwarves whizzing round in dizzying technicolour. Children surf up and down the giant mosaic AIDS ribbon, but when questioned, few parents have heard of Gugu, though the park is clearly named for her. One of Santa's colourful rail stops even bears the sign 'Gugu Dlamini Park Station'. At last, it is a pair of youthful security guards who nod in recognition of the name. 'Yes,' they say, 'she was the girl who was gang-raped for having AIDS.'

TREATMENT ACTION

Back in late 1998, the harsh message of Dlamini's death was a wake-up call for people living with HIV.

Their organisation, Napwa, was still struggling to find its feet in a hostile world, and the murder of one of its spokespeople was a threat to its existence.

'The prime aim of Napwa was to be the voice for people living with HIV and AIDS,' says Peter Busse, who was Napwa's national director at the time. 'At that stage it was a fledgling organisation and the focus was building organisational capacity and dealing with a broad range of issues like disclosure, public speaking, making one's voice heard.' Dlamini's murder was testimony to how far they still had to go.

A fortnight earlier, HIV-positive activists had lost another fighting hero. Simon Nkoli, the first black gay man to be open about his HIV status, had been fighting AIDS-related illnesses for years now, and his hospital visits had become increasingly frequent. On November 30, his frail body could stand no more. Nkoli's death was a serious blow to Busse and others in the world of HIV as well as gay and lesbian activism who had known, loved and been inspired by Nkoli for more than a decade.

Nkoli and Dlamini's deaths made an impact on people living with HIV and AIDS. Judge Edwin Cameron, who had been living with HIV for more than a decade, was prompted to make a public disclosure of his HIV status. He was the first senior official to do so, and his courage earned him and the cause of HIV-positive people support and encouragement.

The two deaths also galvanised strategic thinking about HIV activism.

'Both deaths meant that it was time to start some sort of treatment advocacy,' says Mark Heywood, director of the AIDS Law Project at the University of the Witwatersrand. 'Not only treatment advocacy, but to take the AIDS movement out of the hands of NGO specialists and try to stimulate a movement of affected people that would reflect the demographics and the class base of South Africa.'

Since the advent of antiretroviral therapy in 1996, South African health professionals and HIV activists had discussed and debated the need to expand access to treatment. Throughout 1998, the growing international treatment campaign had intensified these debates. And Heath Minister Zuma's refusal to embrace a programme to prevent transmission of HIV from mother to child had lent urgency to the cause.

At the centre of these discussions was Zackie Achmat.

Achmat, who had disclosed his HIV status in July 1998, was a former director of the AIDS Law Project and a leader of the lesbian and gay movement. He had also been a youth activist during the township uprisings of the 1980s. Achmat now focused his political expertise on the AIDS treatment crisis.

In a later interview Achmat said, 'I had been thinking about treatment for a while and was asking how we could stand by and do nothing while people kept dying.'[268] His convictions sharpened when he became ill with a serious bout of thrush in his mouth and throat.

'I thought I was going to die. I couldn't swallow anything. Eventually I was prescribed fluconazole, a very expensive drug. My friends helped me pay for it and still it nearly bankrupted me… On top of Simon's death that was just the last straw.'

Achmat and Heywood, his long-time friend and comrade, approached Napwa about working together on a treatment advocacy campaign, and Napwa agreed. The time was ripe. Achmat gave force to the campaign by a public commitment to delay his own much-needed therapy until the drugs were available free in the public health system.

At Nkoli's funeral, Achmat called for people to join him and other Napwa members in a day-long fast on the steps of St Georges Cathedral in Cape Town. This would be the launch of a new treatment action campaign. On December 10, 1998, 15 people protested outside the cathedral, calling upon the government to provide treatment for people living with HIV. Their first demand was for a national programme to prevent the transmission of the virus from mother to child.

Passers-by were surprised: few knew that there was any treatment for HIV. By the end of the day they had collected more than 1 000 signatures.

One of the protesters was former human rights commissioner Rhoda Kadalie[269], who told journalists: 'Giving AZT to pregnant women to prevent them passing an HIV infection to their babies is a human rights issue, and women's rights are a priority.' She gave voice to the thoughts of many, by contrasting the reluctance of the government to fund the prevention of vertical transmission with their energetic budgetary allowance for beefing up the military. 'I'm tired of generalised notions of human rights,' she said. 'We have concrete ways to attend to issues that affect people with HIV and I don't see why we're spending billions on arms.'

The genius of this new campaign was that it could advocate strongly for treatment, without being the exclusive domain of HIV-positive people. This enabled supporters to challenge the stigma surrounding HIV without putting their lives at risk.

The strategy was given a human face by the T-shirt designed by Achmat for the formal launch of the campaign. On one side was a portrait of the slain activist Dlamini, with the words 'Never again'; on the other side, in bold purple letters, were the words 'HIV positive'.

The T-shirt was both a declaration and an advocacy statement that could be worn by HIV-positive and HIV-negative activists alike. Even President Mandela donned the shirt when he eventually began speaking about HIV in later years.

In the weeks that followed the first public event, members of the Treatment Action Campaign (TAC), as it became known, visited train stations in the Western Cape, speaking to commuters about mother-to-child transmission and collecting more signatures. A group of 100 TAC activists even managed to meet Finance Minister Trevor Manuel when the AIDS train arrived at Cape Town station. They handed over a statement calling on Manuel and Zuma to meet them to discuss an affordable treatment plan.

The Treatment Action Campaign was canny in its use of struggle language, strategy and tactics. It chose the familiar language of street politics for its slogans, and launched their campaigns on days of historical significance. Achmat and Heywood had cut their political teeth in the struggle years — with the former being in and out of jail during the student uprisings of the 1970s. Heywood, who was of British-Nigerian descent, had met Achmat in Oxford in the mid 1980s, when both were involved in the political underground.

The campaign for mother-to-child prevention was formally launched on Human Rights Day, March 21, 1999, with fasts and rallies across the country. Protesters wearing 'HIV positive' T-shirts collected signatures and handed out pamphlets. In Soweto, more than 500 people representing trade unions and religious bodies, and even government supporters from the ANC and SA Communist Party, gathered outside the Chris Hani-Baragwanath Hospital. After the speeches, the protesters lay down in the street and refused to move.

Florence Ngobeni, who was a counsellor in the Perinatal HIV Research Unit at the hospital, remembers being called from her work by excited colleagues to say that there were people toyi-toying outside for access to drugs. 'I was told there are people outside, the media is outside, doctors are outside advocating… come,' she says. 'So I went with some of the pregnant women from the support group. The exciting thing was that the doctors were there.

'It was just a blossoming excitement. It was a new day, a new era. It was… "Come, let's go, let's fight together." For the first time I saw the unity between health care workers and civil society. We were outside and they were handing out T-shirts. There were loudspeakers. There was a lot of media. You could feel the spirit. People's spirit.'

Three days after this protest, Achmat had an opportunity to exchange views with Minister Zuma at an ANC branch meeting. Achmat was able to assure her of his loyalty to the party, before questioning her on her rejection of the mother-to-child campaign. At this meeting, Zuma spelled out her objection to the programme — it was purely the cost of the drugs. 'If you want to fight for affordable treatment,' she said, 'I will be with you all the way.'[270]

TAC took her at her word. They immediately began lobbying Glaxo Wellcome to reduce the price of AZT, the drug used in the mother-to-child regimen. They asked for information about the manufacturing costs and on the nature of the discount deal previously offered by the company. A few days later, 100 TAC members demonstrated outside Glaxo headquarters in Gauteng.[271]

Glaxo's South African chief executive officer, Dr Bill Collier, told the press they were committed to making AZT more accessible. 'There is a moral imperative for all of those involved in treating HIV and AIDS to meet around one table — in the spirit of the government's Partnership Against AIDS programme — to work out solutions,' he said. A company spokesperson also pointed out that they had been negotiating drug prices with the government for the past two years. At this point they were offering an unconditional 70 per cent discount.

But apparently the 70 per cent discount had been insufficient. Mbeki had told the press that he too hoped that the protests would force the pharmaceutical companies to bring drug prices down. 'It is incumbent on the pharmaceutical companies to reduce the cost and price of AZT,' he said. 'As long as it is only available at exorbitant prices, it is impossible for the government to make it available to ordinary people.'[272]

Thus it was, in a spirit of construction and cooperation, that on April 30, 1999, Napwa and TAC members held their first formal meeting with Zuma about mother-to-child transmission. The minister assured them that she would issue a response to the drug discount offer by mid June that same year.[273]

After the meeting, they released a joint statement calling on all sectors of civil society to pressurise Glaxo and other pharmaceutical companies to 'unconditionally lower the price of all HIV and AIDS medications to an affordable price for poor people and countries'.

While the activists were hoping for an even greater discount from the company, health professionals were wondering what price range the government considered affordable.

The response of the national press to this development was interesting. While some newspapers gave a factual report, others read into the statement a further hardening of attitudes, running the story under headlines like 'Zuma rejects cheap drugs'[274], 'Ministry refuses anti-HIV drug discount'.[275] The *Mail & Guardian's* story led with an unsubstantiated allegation that the minister was waiting for proof that AZT was effective.

While Zuma had not reversed her October rejection of the discount, she certainly had not renewed it.

BROEDERTWIS

Despite the united front presented to Zuma at the meeting, there was a deep and growing rift between Napwa and TAC. Ostensibly this was about the relative importance of treatment in the Napwa programme. Busse remembers that there was a lot of criticism from TAC of Napwa for continuing to work on soft issues like disclosure and public speaking, which were considered a waste of time.

'I still don't agree to this day,' says Busse. 'Looking at the countries where treatment is available, there are still big issues around stigma and disclosure. They are barriers to treatment.'

Initially, however, Napwa had been happy to accommodate the TAC programme and had provided office space and financial support. But soon TAC's demands grew. 'What I particularly remember,' says Busse, 'was being called to a meeting with Zackie, Mark Heywood and Morna (Cornell of the AIDS Consortium), and being told that they thought it was a good idea that Napwa reneged on all its contractual obligations with its funders and gave all of its money to TAC.'

Mercy Makhalemele, who was Napwa regional coordinator for KwaZulu-Natal, felt that a false dichotomy was being posed. 'You couldn't change Napwa to become a campaigning organisation, that was just out of the question, and that was what Zackie was proposing,' she says. 'But you could have Napwa, and have a treatment action campaign, as a campaign leading off Napwa. But Zackie was not happy, so the division came. And there started the politics among people who were HIV positive.'

Rumours and conflicting stories were circulating about the conflict.[276] Some, like Shaun Mellors, were under the incorrect impression that Napwa had refused to get involved in treatment issues. 'As I understand it the idea of the TAC was first presented to Napwa to do something on treatment and they said no,' says Mellors. 'I was surprised because I think it was, in hindsight, the incorrect decision.'

There were other rumours concerning mismanagement and even misappropriation of funds by Napwa staff. Then there were allegations that white, gay men were getting priority treatment in the organisation.

There was clearly a lot of malign energy focused on Busse, despite the fact that he was extremely ill at this time. He had been living with HIV for 14 years, and was experiencing his first major episode of AIDS-related illness. With severe hepatitis, he was losing kilograms every day and his life was hanging by a slender thread.

Lucky Mazibuko, who had just begun writing his column in the *Sowetan*, became involved in the issue. He felt that, as an outsider, he could play a constructive role in the conflict. Mazibuko went to visit Busse in the Braamfontein office. 'He came across as a very polite person and it was a cordial kind of meeting,' says Mazibuko. 'He was very upright and honest and said that probably one of the reasons why he was being victimised was because he was not black and he was not straight and that he was not a populist.'

Mazibuko felt that it would be impossible for Busse to stay on. 'I thought he had no chance, in terms of the allegations that had been made, and the seriousness and the ferocity — and the severity of the hatred. You could cut it with a knife. It was not a conducive environment for him anyway,' he says. 'It was almost as if the plan was there for him to be kicked out, and of course racism was used against him which was a battle he couldn't win anyway.'

For their part the TAC activists felt that Napwa was a weak organisation and failing in its duties to mobilise people for the TAC protests and campaigns. Writing later, Heywood remarked 'Tensions emerged over Napwa's leadership's failure to mobilise people for demonstrations on 21 March, to demand a national mother-to-child HIV prevention programme and to monitor the police investigation into the murder of Gugu Dlamini. This led to a war of words and shortly after to a physical parting of ways…'[277]

After some weeks of rumours and allegations Achmat asked to address a Napwa board meeting[278], which was held at the Johannesburg airport. Friends warned Busse that Achmat had said he was going to 'bring Napwa down'.

Busse broke down in the meeting and said he could not go on. After tendering his resignation he collapsed and had to be taken home.

Achmat made serious allegations about the role and conduct of Napwa, and the legitimacy of its board and its membership. He believed that Napwa members were being 'wheeled out' to give a face to AIDS, and that people living with HIV were being manipulated by 'patronising whites'.

'It really destroyed me,' says Busse, 'I had been working in the field for a long, long time. I always thought I had been working for the greater good, and suddenly to be cast as the worst thing that ever walked the planet... I went off and I just laid low.'

'I have never forgiven them,' says Makhalemele. 'I felt nobody deserved to be treated in this way. If only people knew what the difficulties were when we started Napwa. The way they described Napwa, it became a low-level thing.'

This episode was enough to drive Makhalemele out of AIDS politics altogether. She resigned and went to live on a remote mission station in the mountains for several months. With the benefit of hindsight, Makhalemele attributes the conflict to the recent nature of Achmat's HIV disclosure.

'This is a typical thing,' she says. 'Once you have disclosed your status you have a sense of emergency, you want everything to change right now, and nothing else matters. Whereas we had disclosed our HIV status a long time ago and we knew the best way to do things was to work with everybody.'

For Mazibuko too, it was a formative experience. 'It was a very sad episode in my introduction to the AIDS world to see how those who were being discriminated against could actually mete out such cruelty and brutality and coldness to one of their own.'

Mellors, who had been engaged in HIV politics from the start, has another take. 'The challenge of the movement is that we are all so diverse,' he says, 'and we come from fairly marginalised communities and we have had to fight for our place as individuals first... If there is one group that has power struggles and personalities and in-fighting, it is people with HIV.'

Busse's departure was to have serious consequences for Napwa. In the words of Mazibuko, 'the people who ultimately replaced him ensured that Napwa died a very slow death.'

In the years to come Napwa became increasingly identified with the government's position, and openly hostile to TAC. TAC continued to make allegations of financial irregularity and by 2004 their relationship had broken down to a point where Napwa members were disrupting joint meetings and calling for Heywood's removal.

The great debate that wasn't

The intensity with which the treatment activists fought their corner was understandable; for them it was a matter of life and death. But the moralistic fervour with which the campaign was fought meant that it was difficult to have any rational debate over the complex issues that it entailed.

Even Busse, who was dying of an AIDS-related disease and had impeccable credentials in the world of HIV and AIDS, was not permitted to question the single focus of the campaign.

However, for a health minister still battling with the legacy of apartheid's inequalities, the challenges of providing antiretroviral treatment in the public health sector were unprecedented, and demanded serious consideration. Even if drug prices were slashed, the health infrastructure of the country was not well equipped for such a task. Within and without government, there were quiet voices questioning the wisdom, and the justice, of focusing so much of the health budget on such an expensive treatment for the benefit of so few. An even greater concern was the possibility that use of the drugs, with insufficient monitoring, could lead to resistant strains of HIV that would hamper all future treatment efforts. Then there was the concern over the sustainability of the programme. As more people stayed alive, thanks to the drugs, HIV prevalence in the country would increase, and without a successful prevention campaign, escalating costs would make the programme unsustainable.

For a health minister of a country with a massive HIV burden, the answer seemed clear: free treatment for all who needed it was an impossible dream. Even to concede on the cheaper mother-to-child programme would leave the government open to further attack by activists who would rightly be able to ask, why save the lives of babies only to have them orphaned? By October 1998 the health minister had done the maths and opted for a reinvigorated prevention programme instead.

But she was out of step with the times. The growing global 'access to treatment' movement had changed the terms of the debate, and treatment was no longer something to be easily denied.

The ethical and practical challenges implied by the demand for universal access to AIDS treatment could have been resolved by a rigorous national debate, but this was not to be.

For their part the government had lost faith in the organisations of civil society, from whom they had previously gained their strength. The controversies over Virodene and *Sarafina* had set them on opposing paths, which were unlikely to converge on this new emotive issue.

And behind the scenes, the lawsuit over the Medicines Act festered, providing a strong disincentive for any strategy with pharmaceuticals at its heart. Although the lawsuit was a matter of public record, the treatment activists were still largely innocent of its significance, or that their demand for drugs was pushing them ever further from the government's trust.

Busi

Busi Maqungo gave birth to her second child in April 1999. When Nomazizi was just one month old she became mortally ill with pneumonia and chronic diarrhoea. The hospital doctor suggested an HIV test and Busi readily agreed. 'I wanted to know what was wrong with my baby,' she says. 'I wanted the doctors to know exactly what they were dealing with.'

Busi and her partner had to wait three days for the result, which confirmed that their daughter was HIV positive. Although Busi didn't know much about HIV, she knew that Nomazizi could only have got it from her. There was no other explanation.

'Now all of a sudden you have to deal with this thing — you are living with HIV, and so is your partner. But the worst was the baby.

'Right at that moment I just didn't know what to think, I just didn't know what to do... Normally when people are told that they are HIV positive they think that they are going to die, they have a picture of a person who has AIDS. But the first thing that came into my mind was that I have infected my baby. I felt so sorry for her, I felt so guilty. Ja, I think that was the feeling at that moment. Everything was about her. She looked so innocent and I thought I don't know what I am going to do about this.'

On top of the guilt and the pain of infecting her baby, Busi also had to deal with her partner, who was going off the rails.

He had always been abusive, but after his diagnosis their relationship deteriorated, along with his health.

'He started doing drugs badly, this pill, Mandrax; he was drinking and became very abusive to me... and I was the only person who was working. I would keep money for the baby and he would steal it and go and buy drugs. The last money we had. He would sell my stuff.'

Believing that the situation would bring them closer together, Busi stayed with her boyfriend. But their relationship did not improve. Worse was the deterioration in the baby's health. Nomazizi was never well. She died in January the following year, after having spent most of her short life in hospital.

Chapter Thirteen

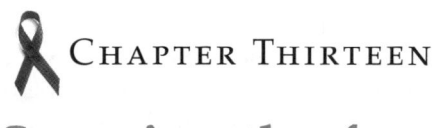

Securing the future

Watching out

April 30, 1999 was the day that Minister Zuma and the treatment activists released a joint statement pledging to bring down the price of AIDS drugs. It was also the day that the US Trade Representative published the annual Watch List, a list that identified countries breaking US trade rules. And like the previous year, South Africa featured on that list.

This time, however, the US Trade Representative's 301 Watch List Report highlighted the 1998 ruckus in the World Health Assembly as one of the reasons for South Africa's listing. 'During the year,' it read, 'South African representatives have led a faction of nations in the World Health Organisation in calling for a reduction in the level of protection provided for pharmaceuticals in TRIPS.'[279]

Already, the US government was withholding a previously agreed tariff deal on certain South African exports. Some were wondering if official US sanctions would be far behind.

April 30, 1999 also saw the promulgation of the new medicines legislation, written to replace the now-frozen Medicines Act. The legislation, written and debated during the previous year, had initially been welcomed by the pharmaceutical industry as an opportunity to start afresh. It hoped that some sort of compromise could be reached, which would allow it to drop its court interdict. But the South African government had chosen not to rewrite the contentious part of the law to please its foes. (Section 15C had been removed from the new legislation, not rewritten, and was to be reincorporated once the lawsuit was over.) And now that the law had actually been promulgated there was little hope of a negotiated settlement.

During the previous two years there had been little reporting about either the pharmaceutical companies' challenge to South Africa's new drug law, or the debate around intellectual property rights and pharmaceuticals in the World Health Assembly. But this year's placement of South Africa on the Watch List had provoked some interest in the US.

Consumer activists, such as Ralph Nader and James Love, saw opportunities to gain publicity for their cause. Love was the director of the Nader-founded NGO, Consumer Project on Technology[280], which had been campaigning around issues to do with intellectual property rights and access to medicines. It had a special focus on compulsory licensing.

The complexity of the issues and the lack of in-depth reporting had meant that there were few people able to see the big picture, or understand the connection between the two controversies running in parallel: the South African Medicines Act lawsuit and the international row over intellectual property rights/patents.

And though it may have been in the minds of some key players, neither of the controversies had been directly connected to the need to treat the growing number of South Africans who were dying of AIDS-related disease.

But times they were a-changing. The treatment advocacy movement at home and abroad had cast a spotlight on the high price of antiretroviral therapy, and by early 1999, AIDS drugs and intellectual property rights were being seen in public together for the first time. In March that year, representatives of 60 organisations — including activist groups, NGOs, governments, academics and trade organisations — gathered in Geneva[281] to discuss access to essential medicines.

Activists and health advocates argued that poor countries should be allowed to pass laws enabling them to make and import cheap generic drugs. The big breakthrough came when the World Trade Organisation (WTO) representatives agreed with this interpretation. There were clear provisions in the TRIPS agreement, they said, that would permit compulsory licensing and parallel importation under certain controlled situations. This was precisely the issue around which Big Pharma was taking the South African government to court.

Despite the WTO position, a representative of the US government's patents office told the meeting that his government remained opposed to compulsory licensing and parallel importation.

'We continue to regard the TRIPS agreement as an agreement that establishes minimum standards for protection,' he said. 'In certain situations, we may, and often do, ask for commitments that go beyond those found in the TRIPS agreement.'

This open admission shocked many of the participants. One of these was Eric Sawyer[282], a veteran US activist from ACT UP/New York, who got into an argument with Big Pharma. When Sawyer voiced his anger over the fact that his peers in the south were still dying for want of AIDS drugs, the industry representative replied that the activists' protests were threatening profits. If they continued with their tactics, he said, the industry's research and development programme would probably dry up. Sawyer was riled. Speaking later to a journalist he interpreted this as meaning 'Shut up, or we're not going to develop new drugs and we'll let you die.'[283]

This meeting was an important moment in the TRIPS/AIDS drug dispute. The legal position was clarified, making it clear that both the pharmaceutical industry and the US government were seeking greater intellectual property rights than those prescribed in the TRIPS agreement. (These have now been dubbed 'TRIPS-Plus' agreements.)

The Geneva meeting also provided the missing link in the activist chain, connecting those dealing with patent and trade issues with health professionals and AIDS activists. This new coalition of like-minded individuals agreed to build a joint advocacy strategy that would last into the coming years.

Less than a fortnight after the meeting, *Reuters* news agency ran the first major US story on the South African Medicines Act dispute. Under the heading 'Group says US hurts world access to AIDS drugs'[284], the article gave a platform to the views of activist organisations such as Médecins sans Frontières (MSF) and the Consumer Project on Technology. The opening sentence declared that the 'US government, on behalf of drug companies, is bullying developing countries into abandoning a trade remedy that could help them fight the escalating AIDS epidemic'. The article spelled out how compulsory licensing could allow poor countries to make cheaper generic drugs, and how Big Pharma's insistence on patent rights was ensuring that this would never happen.

For the first time, access to AIDS treatment was directly

linked to intellectual property rights in the popular imagination. The logic was undeniable and the emotions potent: a simple trade remedy would save millions from the agony of AIDS. At last there was a formula to repackage the complex issues of intellectual property rights in a way that journalists could understand and activists could use.

The charm offensive

This identification of the AIDS tragedy in Africa with drug access and patents spelled the beginning of the end for Big Pharma's AIDS drugs strategy.

But it was not ready to give it up just yet. For several years, pharmaceutical industry executives had been working on a range of drug discount and social responsibility campaigns. Some may have hoped that these would defuse the demand for reforming the drug patent rules.

The Bristol-Myers-Squibb (BMS) programme, Secure the Future[285], was one such example. After toying with the idea of offering drug discounts to poor countries, BMS eventually settled on a $100-million charitable initiative. Secure the Future aimed to provide funding for AIDS programmes in five southern African countries.[286] Though the company employed credible African-American and black South African consultants to draw up the scheme, it did not consult too widely with the governments concerned.

In April 1999, just one month before the programme was to be announced, BMS vice chairman Kenneth Weg and former congressman Ronald Dellums went to visit Health Minister Zuma with their proposals. It's not clear if they were innocent of the dispute between Big Pharma and the minister, or of her anger and frustration about the situation, but they seemed to expect a favourable hearing.

According to the *Washington Post*, Weg and Dellums handed Zuma a brochure that detailed their plans to fund medical research, educational projects and community-based programmes. They told Zuma and her staff that South Africa would become a full partner in implementing the initiative, despite the fact that some programmes had already been developed without her participation. One of these was an exchange programme to send African doctors to study in the US.

Zuma outlined a series of objections to the programme and told the pair that, without changes, South Africa could not endorse the initiative. Later, the new AIDS directorate chief Nono Simelela [287], who was also present at the meeting, told the journalist: 'This is our country. If Bristol-Myers-Squibb wants to be our partner they should act like a partner. They should not think they can simply come in here and tell us what is best for our people.'

Despite the rejection from the South African government, BMS went ahead and launched the programme — one month later — in Johannesburg and Washington. BMS chairman Charles Heimbold told his Washington audience: 'As one of the world's greatest pharmaceutical companies and a major developer and manufacturer of medicines for the treatment of HIV and AIDS, we feel a moral obligation to take action. One hundred million dollars over five years is our company's commitment to opening the door tomorrow for the millions of African women and children.'

At the Johannesburg event, UNAIDS director Dr Peter Piot described the initiative as 'a significant development in the global fight against AIDS'. Health ministers from four of the five participating countries were present. Minister Zuma did not attend.

But alongside the charm offensive, Big Pharma continued to pursue its opposition to the Medicines Act. The US PhRMA chair welcomed the listing of South Africa on the annual Watch List saying that the country 'fully deserves to be designated... South Africa could provide one of the first test cases for interpreting the scope of the protection provided by TRIPS to all fields of technology and thus has broad significance.' [288]

It was clear that patents were of paramount importance to the industry. While it was prepared to give away some of their profits in the form of charity, its intellectual property was what had made it one of the world's most lucrative industries, and would continue to do so.

But critical mass was steadily building against Big Pharma's stranglehold on patents. On May 24, 1999, the Fifty-Second World Health Assembly unanimously approved [289] the resolution on drug access that had caused such controversy the previous year. The redrafted Revised Drug Strategy asked member states to ensure that 'public health interests are paramount in pharmaceutical and health policies', and mandated the WHO to monitor and analyse the implications of trade agreements for public health.

After the meeting, Dr Ian Roberts, Minister Zuma's special adviser, told the press that 'the main importance of the new resolution is that health now has a role in all international trade and finance agreements... We will be collaborating closely with the WHO to ensure that we get affordable medicine to our people.'

GORE'S GREED AND THE FED-UP QUEERS

In the US, veteran activists who had fought and won their own cause for AIDS therapies, had been revitalised by the challenge of getting affordable medicines to the south. Sawyer and supporters from ACT UP and other organisations began the fight for cheap AIDS drugs in low-income countries. The South African Medicines Act was their primary focus. Sawyer told a journalist at the time: 'When you are no longer burying your friends, you have the luxury of time to try to save people in more remote areas.'[290]

For Sawyer this was much more than a political game. 'There is a tremendous sense of survivor guilt, which gives us inspiration to fight harder,' he said.

Working with ACT UP was James Love, economist and researcher from the Consumer Project on Technology. Part of their ammunition was an intriguing story that the research team had ferreted out, concerning PhRMA's relationship to the Clinton administration.

According to Love, Clinton's chief of staff was the brother (and former business partner) of a top public relations manager who represented PhRMA.[291] Other staff shifts suggested that there was something of a swing-door between the pharmaceutical industry and the current US government.

Then there were the stories about the generous donations made by the US pharmaceutical giants to the Democratic Party.

In the light of the forthcoming election, Vice President Al Gore was an obvious target. The activists also suspected that he was personally involved in the pressure on the SA government, and that he had threatened Mbeki with full-on sanctions during the February SA/US Bi-National Trade Commission.

Sawyer was quoted as saying: 'Gore has been carrying out the dirty work of the pharmaceuticals companies. He's putting a higher priority on trade than public health.'[292] And another activist claimed that 'If Gore blocked AIDS drugs in the US he'd be denounced as a genocidal despot. Instead, he's the Democratic Party frontrunner for president.'[293]

On the morning of Wednesday, June 16, 1999, Gore stood on the steps of the Smith County Courthouse in Carthage, Tennessee, to announce his candidacy for president. As he spoke, a group of 'supporters' stripped off their 'Students for Gore' T-shirts to reveal another slogan: 'Gore's greed kills'.

Before anyone could stop them, 15 protesters began blowing air horns and chanting 'Gore is killing Africans — AIDS drugs now.' The protest was captured by a news crew and the piece played on virtually every television broadcast that night.

This was the first of many demonstrations organised by Sawyer, Love and co. Protesters, some ACT UP and some paid members of a New York direction action group called the Fed-Up Queers, vowed to follow Gore's campaign across the land.

They were as good as their word. The following day, five protesters managed to get themselves seated behind Gore at a meeting where he was addressing 300 people in Manchester, New Hampshire. After he began speaking, they popped up with a banner reading 'Gore kills. AIDS drugs for Africa', and began chanting.[294] For his next stop, Wall Street, on the same day, a similar disturbance had been arranged. And so it continued throughout July and August 1999.[295] And in October, the protesters turned their attention to the US Trade Representative offices and the White House.

The US and international media were riveted by these displays, and the South African trade dispute made its way onto the front pages of many US newspapers, where it was sympathetically treated. An editorial in the influential *New York Times*, for example, said that Washington should stop pressurising South Africa.[296] Others commented that the trade dispute was beginning to tarnish Gore's reputation with his core liberal supporters.[297]

Gore's defenders claimed that he had been unjustly targeted by the activists, and insiders claimed that the vice president had personally opposed trade sanctions in the light of South Africa's health crisis. Gore, they said, had been making a concerted attempt to find a new framework that would allow the South

African government to get cheaper drugs.

Writing in *Business Day* in August, Simon Barber claimed that this framework involved a written bilateral agreement that South Africa would be able to purchase drugs outside of patent-holder marketing channels, as long as this was done in a way that was TRIPS-consistent.[298]

This deal would be sufficient to get South Africa dropped from the sanctions list, but it was unlikely to satisfy the needs of Big Pharma, which had relied on the US government to press for TRIPS-plus provisions. In other words, the implication was that Gore was responsible for driving a wedge, albeit a tiny sliver of a wedge, between the industry and the government. Whether this was humanitarian goodwill or a panicked response to activist pressure was beside the point.

Washington-based South African journalist Rich Mkhondo concluded: 'Gore's political rivals have deliberately manipulated the facts for political expediency in a more complicated debate. AIDS activists are either ignoring facts or have been hired by Gore's enemies. This is a debate with no easy solutions.'[299]

DRAMA WITH SAMMDRA

By now, the government back home was dealing with a whole new headache: the South African Medicines and Medical Devices Regulatory Act (SAMMDRA). This was the new Act designed to replace the frozen Medicines Act. It was almost identical to the old Act, but had been written and pushed through much too quickly.

In its haste to get the new legislation going, the inexperienced drafting team had neglected to draw up any regulations or drug schedules to accompany the new Act. This meant, among other things, that there were no longer any controls over medicine sales.

Pharmacologist Dr Andy Gray was one of the few keeping up with these complicated developments. 'If the regulations are not available at the time that the Act is brought into effect there is real chaos because you can't interpret the Act,' says Gray. 'The SAMMDRA Act repealed the existing schedules and... there was no effective control of medicines from that moment onwards. It was immediately obvious that you could go and buy things like morphine over the counter. Journalists went to pharmacists to buy it, but pharmacists told them to push off.'[300]

By July, newspapers were reporting that scores of drug dealers were escaping conviction because there were no schedules prohibiting the sale of hard drugs.[301] One leading Johannesburg lawyer said that he had clients escaping prosecution every week because the drug ecstasy was no longer illegal. The South African Narcotics Bureau estimated that at least 200 accused had their cases thrown out of court since the 30 April promulgation of the law.

This undesirable state of affairs brought the health minister and the Pharmaceutical Manufacturers' Association into a curious new alliance. They approached the court together with an appeal for the promulgation notice to be set aside. And they were refused — on legal grounds.[302] A series of complex legal actions followed, involving the High Court and the Constitutional Court, and President Mandela (who had signed the Act into law), and the whole saga took until February 2000 to get sorted out.

AID FOR AFRICA

The ACT UP Zaps, as the US protests were called, were taking their toll on the American vice president. Gore responded by re-affirming his government's resolve to address the AIDS crisis in Africa. During July 1999, in a highly publicised speech alongside Archbishop Desmond Tutu, he announced the largest US budget increase for AIDS funding abroad: a new investment of $100 million.[303] Gore also unveiled a new report that assessed the extent of the AIDS crisis in Africa. The report, from which he quoted, said 'AIDS is the worst infectious disease catastrophe in the history of modern medicine. More than 20 million people are now infected and nearly 500 more become infected each hour. We hope that this initiative will not only provide much-needed relief but will inspire decisive action by other countries and institutions — and bring hope to the millions of children and families trapped in this horror.'

Whether or not this was a cynical attempt to save face, as many activists believed, it represented a turning point in the US government's engagement with the global AIDS epidemic, which would last into successive administrations.

And this new engagement had massive spin-off effects — boosting the growing international awareness of the AIDS crisis in Africa. Within five months, HIV and AIDS was on the UN Security Council agenda for the first time, and within two years, a special session of the UN General Assembly was devoted solely to HIV and AIDS.

By now it was clear that the US government's active support for Big Pharma, and for TRIPS-Plus patent protection, had diminished. After lengthy negotiations, an agreement was announced on September 17 that led to the removal of South Africa from the 301 Watch List.[304] This was widely misinterpreted as South Africa backing down on the Medicines Act, but the South African government maintained that it had simply reiterated its intention to abide by the World Trade Organisation's TRIPS rules. The pharmaceutical companies were also responsive to this new environment, and temporarily suspended their lawsuit against the Medicines Act.

On World AIDS Day 1999, President Clinton announced that the office of the US government was committed to a cooperative approach[305] on health-related intellectual property matters, one that was consistent with the goal of helping poor countries to gain access to affordable medicines. The announcement stressed that the TRIPS agreement allowed countries the flexibility to respond to public health crises and urged other partners to improve access to essential medicines.

In less than two years since the first fiery debates about the Revised Drug Strategy in the World Health Assembly, the environment for access to AIDS drugs in low-income countries had changed forever. But although it was Minister Zuma's determined struggle for the right to affordable medicine that had broken the logjam, it would be many years before South Africans living with HIV would benefit.

Lucky

From the day his first column was published, Lucky Mazibuko began receiving letters and telephone calls from young people keen to talk about the difficulty of living with HIV in South Africa. This contact has given Lucky some unique insights.

'The social dynamics are too complex. It is too simplistic for us to say, "It is stigma and discrimination"... It is far too deep for that,' says Lucky. 'When you find communities that are poor and where there is a dog-eat-dog kind of scenario, you will find petty divisions in the household. Someone did not cook last week... really petty stuff that actually widens the divide, and then AIDS simply aggravates the problem. These are very common problems in the township; I don't know why our leaders are not talking about it.'

'On one of my shows I had a caller who made all kinds of allegations about how her family had kicked her out of home... Then one of her sisters phoned in and said that it was nonsense. She said, "No, we never reacted against her. She was the one who caused all of this, because when things were rosy for her (apparently she was married to a foreigner who had money, flashy cars, a big house in the suburbs), she never cared for anyone else. We asked for assistance and she refused, and now that she is sick her husband has kicked her out she came back to us, but we couldn't help her."

'HIV is not a problem for me. The problem is the family structure. There is no harmony, there is no peace. There is a lot of discomfort and lies and secrets. But when AIDS gets into the picture everything distorts, the story becomes AIDS. A lot of people I help will tell you — my biggest problem is not AIDS, it is my own family...

'Most of the children of my generation, including myself, were not properly fathered, and we grew up in broken homes. Most of us were brought up by our grandparents instead of our mothers, and some of us were fathered by different men... so the fabric of the family is shaky ground and when AIDS creeps in, it causes all these divisions. On my show young people call and say, "We can't speak to our father and our mothers." They can't even speak among themselves. As soon as you become 15, 16, you must find your own way.

'What we need now is a societal transformation that is not based on morals but simply seeks to set a new culture. We need a massive programme to demystify sex, you know that seeks to say: sleeping around is not trendy; if you sleep around you are a fool!

'We really need a societal revolution, to create a new mentality and identity among our people. A cleansing of some sort... a healing.'

Chapter Fourteen
Where the truth lies

WE CAN DO THIS!

By the time the US government had changed its position on the Medicines Act, important political changes had taken place within South Africa. In June 1999 Nelson Mandela retired from active politics and Thabo Mbeki became the new president. During the past few years as deputy, Mbeki had become increasingly engaged with AIDS issues, giving encouragement to those working in the field. In his first cabinet shuffle, Mbeki made Dr Manto Tshabalala-Msimang[306] his new minister of health, promoting Dr Zuma to the post of foreign minister.

Tshabalala-Msimang had gone into exile with Mbeki in the early 1960s, and had lived abroad for 28 years. A medical doctor, she had a convincing track record on HIV and AIDS. During the 1980s, Tshabalala-Msimang had been one of the exiles who had urged the ANC leadership to take HIV seriously, and on her return to South Africa had played an active part in the design of the National AIDS Plan. Later, during her chairing of the parliamentary health portfolio committee, she had opposed some of Minister Zuma's more controversial decisions. People living and working with HIV rejoiced at the prospect of having what, for them, might be viewed as a more supportive, and less combative, minister in the health portfolio.

Minister Tshabalala-Msimang began her term of office with an unexpectedly upbeat approach to the AIDS issue. Determined not to inherit Zuma's enemies along with her portfolio, she took immediate steps to appease them. 'She came in deliberately trying to mend fences that Zuma had broken,' says TAC activist and AIDS Law Project director, Mark Heywood. 'She called a meeting very soon after the election, of all civil society groups, and she and Ayanda Ntsaluba (the director-general of health) sat through a two-day meeting and listened to people's suggestions.'

Next, the minister hosted a three-day workshop with young people about sexuality and HIV, and confirmed her commitment to the faltering schools-based life skills programme.

Under Tshabalala-Msimang's new leadership there were also signs that the Medicines Act lawsuit might be over. Local industry representatives hinted that now that the 'hard liners' had left the building, there had been a change of heart. According to the US PhRMA, 'the industry immediately made multiple overtures to the new government for the purpose of reaching a mutually acceptable solution.'[307]

A while later the South African Pharmaceutical Manufacturers' Association said that they were temporarily suspending the litigation[308] to allow for a resolution to be reached.

Tshabalala-Msimang also announced that she was reconsidering her predecessor's position on the prevention of mother-to-child transmission of HIV. She told the press that curbing HIV infections was her 'number one priority for the year', and that she believed the time had come to review the decision not to supply AZT to HIV-positive pregnant women. This announcement came shortly after publicity around the success of new trials using the inexpensive drug nevirapine.[309]

To support this new optimism, the UK's department for international development offered to fund the minister and a group of colleagues on a fact-finding trip to Uganda, where they could learn firsthand, from African peers, about their successful HIV prevention programmes.[310] The party also planned to talk to researchers who were using nevirapine in their programme to prevent mother-to-child transmission.[311]

Tshabalala-Msimang was so inspired by what she saw in Uganda that after the first day she phoned a colleague in the hotel in the early hours of the morning, saying, 'We can do this. We can make it work.'

A NEW KIND OF POISON

The optimism created by Dr Tshabalala-Msimang's first 100 days as health minister was soon dashed by a turn of events stranger than fiction.

In the spring of 1999, during the new president's first

address[312] to the National Council of Provinces, he cast doubt on the safety of the drug AZT. His comments, which were supported by Tshabalala-Msimang, became the focus of intense media attention[313], and a whole new controversy around AIDS was born.

This controversy surpassed the antagonisms that dogged the previous minister, resulting in long-term and inestimable damage to both the government's AIDS response and its international reputation.

Mbeki's closing remarks on that fateful October day drew attention to the urgent need to address the society's twin scourges of HIV and rape. 'We must wipe out of our communities this scourge of violence and abuse of our people,' he said. 'One rape is a rape too many. Similarly, we are confronted with the scourge of HIV and AIDS, against which we must leave no stone unturned to save ourselves from the catastrophe which this disease poses.'

However, he urged caution about the current demand for AZT to be made available in the public health system.

'Two matters in this regard have been brought to our attention,' he said. 'One of these is that there are legal cases pending in this country, the United Kingdom and the United States against AZT, on the basis that this drug is harmful to health. There also exists a large volume of scientific literature alleging that, among other things, the toxicity of this drug is such that it is in fact a danger to health. These are matters of great concern to the government as it would be irresponsible for us not to heed the dire warnings which medical researchers have been making. I have therefore asked the minister of health, as a matter of urgency, to go into all these matters so that, to the extent that it is possible, we ourselves, including our country's medical authorities, are certain of where the truth lies.'

Mbeki also urged members of parliament to do their own research and access the huge volume of literature on this matter available on the Internet, so that they could all 'approach this issue from the same base of information'.

From the manner of delivery, these remarks — coming as they did at the end of a much longer address — did not seem to be the stuff of a major new announcement. However, they were interpreted as such by the mass media and the AIDS fraternity. In the press conference held immediately after Mbeki's parliamentary address, Tshabalala-Msimang was closely questioned on the issue. She confirmed that there was indeed a body of research that indicated that AZT was a dangerous drug and 'had not been designed for treatment of HIV and AIDS'.[314] Because it was unable to target only the virus, she said, it further weakened the immune system. There was also a danger that the drug might produce children with disabilities. In addition, there were no data proving that AZT was of any use to rape victims.

'We have to be very cautious, very sensitive,' she said. She told journalists that her ministry would not like to look back 10 or 15 years later and find it had exposed the vast majority of historically disadvantaged people in South Africa to a dangerous drug.

Members of the public were justifiably confused by this information, and many believed that there was new evidence about AZT toxicity. Researchers were taken aback, and the manufacturer, Glaxo Wellcome, pointed out that AZT had been registered in South Africa by the Medicines Control Council for the treatment of HIV for nearly a decade.

Glaxo's medical director also denied that there were any ongoing legal cases, anywhere in the world, concerning AZT toxicity.

At this stage, the situation did not seem irredeemable, but as in previous controversies about AIDS, a press campaign built and attitudes hardened. Insiders say that the final blow came when leading black AIDS researchers added their voices to the chorus of critical voices. Despite meeting with Glaxo the health minister continued to hold to her doubts on the drug.

Within days, the Medicines Control Council delivered a preliminary report summarising the research on AZT. There were known side effects, said new council chief Dr Helen Rees, but the potential benefits outweighed the risks. The minister was not satisfied by this superficial report, and asked for a more in-depth investigation that would set her mind at rest. In the face of mounting criticism from the media and the medical community, the president and the minister stuck to their position.

It must be remembered that the president and the health minister had their own good reasons to find fault with AZT. On top of the escalating demand for an expensive mother-to-child programme, Glaxo, which had been pressing the government to accept a discount on the drug, was one of the multinational pharmaceutical companies that had been holding the Medicines Act to ransom.

It soon emerged that the source of the president's information on AZT toxicity was Anthony Brink[315], a lawyer with no medical training.

Brink was preparing a court action for the widow of an HIV-positive friend who had allegedly died from a single month's course of AZT (taken over two months because the side effects were so serious). Glaxo stood accused of negligence for supplying the deceased man with a 'dangerous and defective drug'.

Brink says that he passed his dossier to the minister of health's special adviser, Dr Ian Roberts. Other sources claim that it was the Vissers of Virodene fame that alerted the president to Brink's work.[316]

In the course of preparing the case against Glaxo, Brink had written a lengthy treatise on AZT, and his views had been published in *The Citizen* in March 1999. What was interesting about Brink's article, apart from the emotive language in which it was written ('in the orgy of stupidity that characterises the AIDS age…', 'dying of AIDS on AZT is a racing certainty…', etc), was its selectiveness.

The article dealt with the early trials, which showed that AZT was ineffective as a single drug; with the possible side effects of the drug; and with its toxicity to liver and bone marrow, particularly at high doses — all aspects acknowledged by researchers in the field. But it failed to deal with AZT's part in the triple therapy breakthrough of 1996, which had led to dramatically reduced death rates of people with HIV in the US and other high-income countries. The article also failed to give even a hint of the history of active engagement of HIV-positive people in treatment issues, characterising them rather as passive victims of researchers who were in the pay of the pharmaceutical industry.

Brink's writing on AZT bore the hallmark of writers from the denialist school, whose proponents reject the fundamentals of AIDS science (ie that HIV is a virus and leads to AIDS). And indeed it was to these writers that Brink referred to back up many of his claims. Highly selective of the published science on the subject, and mixing detailed accounts of biological processes with subjective statements, Brink's article resembled sophistry rather than science.

The president had clearly been concerned about Brink's reference to legal cases 'against Glaxo Wellcome in England and the USA, arising out of the deaths of family members killed by their doctor's prescriptions of AZT'. But in fact the paper only mentioned its author's own case, which yet had to come to court — and indeed was dismissed without trial in 2001.[317]

But herein lies another tale....

This new controversy over AZT toxicity had a strong ring of déjà vu. As with the Virodene episode, new scientific evidence was presented in a political forum to an audience of laypeople, by the highest political authority in the land. And once again it seemed that the country's political leaders had been misled by medically unqualified researchers claiming to have bucked the scientific establishment. But now the stakes were very much higher. In the two years since the Virodene episode, access to AIDS drugs had become an inflamed political issue, and from this point there would be no going back.

On November 16, 1999, the health minister gave a comprehensive address[318] to parliament on the issue of treatment for HIV, in which she demonstrated a detailed knowledge of the current research. She identified many challenges of the mother-to-child programme, including the fact that breast-feeding HIV-positive mothers would have to be persuaded to use breast-milk substitutes. This would be a difficult task, and an additional expense to the State, she said. But in her costing she conflated the cheaper mother-to-child prevention programme with treatment for adults, estimating the price tag of a national programme at greater than the total health budget of the country.

Tshabalala-Msimang also repeated her concerns about the toxicity of AZT for babies. She drew attention to the small percentage of babies that would be saved by subjecting all pregnant HIV-positive mothers to what she felt was an untested therapy.

'Can we truly justify exposing 75 per cent of the healthy babies to toxic drugs in order to make sure that an extra 8 per cent overall do not run the risk of becoming infected when we have very little, or no idea, of what the long-term effects of the drugs on the babies/children will be?' she asked. 'We must remember that five years is the longest time that we have had so far to study the effects on children who were given AZT as babies.'

There was now the possibility of using the alternative nevirapine regimen, she said, which would cost R30 per mother and baby, in comparison with the AZT regimen, which came in at R400. The minister explained that she was waiting for the outcome of a South African study (the Saint trial)[319] that would assess its cost-effectiveness before making her decision.

As the months dragged by, it was clear that the mother-to-child prevention programme was again in stalemate. Now the Treatment Action Campaign began discussing a legal challenge to the government on the basis of the right to health guaranteed in the 1997 Constitution.

Gore's greed revisited

If the activists at home were dismayed by this new setback to the mother-to-child programme, their peers abroad were still working from an older script, the one that saw the South African government squaring up against Big Pharma for cheap AIDS drugs.

For the consumer activists, linking intellectual property rights with the AIDS crisis had been a major coup, and small glitches in the story were not going to get in their way. James Love of the Washington-based Consumer Project on Technology told a journalist: 'We were completely unsuccessful for five years on this thing. Now we're kicking ass.'[320]

Although the US government and the pharmaceutical industry had rested their case, events in late 1999 created the opportunity for a whole new rash of press articles on the subject. As international activists geared up to protest the World Trade Organisation meeting in Seattle, journalists searched for good stories about trade injustice. Despite the complicated domestic scenario, the international media remained enthralled by the image of the US Goliath crushing South Africa's brave freedom fighters at the AIDS barricades.

On December 19, under the headline 'How drug giants let millions die of AIDS', the UK's *Observer* reprised the story of the previous year: the close relationship between the Clinton administration and Big Pharma, and the vested interests that had led to the US government supporting the pharmaceutical industry in the South Africa case. The naming of Mandela as first respondent provided additional hype.

This choice, wrote journalist Ed Vulliamy, 'was brazenly defiant… it was some years since Mandela was faced with a legal charge.'

In this article, the pharmaceutical industry's challenge to the Medicines Act was seen as the sole obstacle to the South African government's brave fight against AIDS. The 'cabal' in the White House, it said, 'and their friends in the big drug companies' lobby, have put South Africa's desperate attempts to combat AIDS on hold, while millions stand to die'.

Anyone with even a passing acquaintance with the South African AIDS story might have been surprised by this interpretation, but it remained the dominant one in the international media and in the minds of the international activists for years to come.

'It was just bad reporting, sensational reporting,' says Mark Heywood of the AIDS Law Project. 'Journalists didn't properly understand what was going on in South Africa with AIDS and with the legislation, and wanted to see into the issue something that wasn't there. The Act could have had a specific purpose around AIDS drugs, but that wasn't the purpose of the South African government. That Act had a much broader purpose.'

While the international activists might have been deluded about the health minister's intention to roll out antiretroviral therapy, their suspicions about the pharmaceutical industry were not too far out.

Despite the new consensus that the manufacture and importation of generic drugs could be TRIPS-compliant, Big Pharma persisted in statements to the contrary. However, it must be said that the ambiguous wording[321] of the offending section 15C of the Medicines Act gave the case some credence. While the section could be read as permitting compulsory licensing and parallel importation within the rules of TRIPS, it could also be read as empowering the health minister to override patent rights at will.

As the year drew to a close, it was clear that the South African Pharmaceutical Manufacturers' Association was tiring of its attempts to get the government to rewrite the offending section 15C. The temporary suspension of the lawsuit was running out of time....

TALKING TO THE DENIALISTS

By early 2000 there was a rumour circulating that President Mbeki was questioning the premise that HIV was an infectious virus, or that it was the cause of AIDS. The president had a list of eight technical questions[322] about the current knowledge base of

HIV and AIDS, and he was asking the health minister and others to provide him with the answers.

The president's doubts were likely to have been raised by his reading of Brink's thesis on AZT toxicity; scouring the Internet to check on Brink's references would have led straight into the AIDS denialists' camp.

Brink later boasted about his role in these events. In his essay 'Just say Yes Mr President'[323], he approvingly repeats the words of a friend who has said that 'the story of how a lone radical activist lawyer had blocked the world's largest pharmaceutical corporation and turned South Africa's president and health minister adamantly and vocally against its popular drug' was worth telling in its own right.

As it turned out, the president and Brink were not the only South Africans rethinking the fundamentals of HIV and AIDS at this time. In December 1999, Dr Sam Mhlongo, who headed the family medicine department at Medusa medical school, hosted a seminar on 'Rethinking Core Concepts of AIDS'. To this he had invited prominent US AIDS denialist Prof Charles Geshekter, the author of the article 'An epidemic of AIDS hysteria' published in *The Citizen* the previous year.

Whilst he was in South Africa for this event, Geshekter had allegedly met with the health minister and the registrar of medicines of the Medicines Control Council, Dr Precious Matsoso.[324] They allegedly discussed, among other things, the effectiveness of AZT and other antiretroviral therapies, the reliability of HIV tests, and the interpretation of the annual HIV prevalence surveys. The fact that Geshekter was not a scientist of any sort, but a scholar of African history, seemed not to dent his credibility on these important matters. At the meeting with Geshekter, the minister had mentioned the idea of convening a panel in which global players in the field of HIV and AIDS could thrash out their views.

Soon after this meeting, President Mbeki made email contact with Geshekter and his close colleague and denialist Dr David Rasnick, at their base in California. According to Rasnick, Mbeki asked them to comment on his list of questions, and on Tshabalala-Msimang's replies. The following day the pair faxed a nine-page reply. They suggested that Mbeki add to the list some 'even more fundamental questions'. These were: 'Is AIDS contagious? Is AIDS sexually transmitted? Does HIV cause AIDS? Do the anti-

HIV drugs promote life and health? What is the justification for lumping together the well-known diseases and conditions of poverty, malnutrition, poor sanitation and parasitic diseases that Africans have been suffering from for generations and renaming them as AIDS?'

Much of their fax dwelt on many of the issues dear to the heart of denialists, including the claim that the HIV test is unreliable and that there is no proof that HIV-positive children live shorter lives. The drift of their logic inclined towards the inevitable denialist conclusion that HIV is not a harmful virus, nor sexually transmitted. On the other hand, they focused heavily on the link between poverty and ill-health. 'We suggest that the link to HIV is irrelevant,' they wrote, 'but the link between AIDS and socio-economic status is truly the underlying basis of AIDS in Africa. The HIV and AIDS establishment is blaming the consequences of poverty, malnutrition, poor sanitation, parasitic diseases, etc, on a harmless virus. There are billions of dollars available for AZT and condoms, but hardly a penny for food, schools, education, clean water and jobs.'

Describing the malnutrition and tuberculosis that he witnessed in a hospital in northern KwaZulu-Natal, Geshekter wrote authoritatively: 'Here's where all the slander about truck drivers, wandering male workers away from home seeking prostitutes... all fuses together to become the HIV and AIDS viral epidemic caused by sexual promiscuity'.

It is not difficult to see how these ideas would appeal to a president struggling to overcome the legacy of apartheid; sensitive about racist sexual stereotyping; at war with the pharmaceutical industry; and on the defensive against attacks by activists. This new explanation would soften the horrifying implications of an escalating epidemic of a fatal disease.

What is surprising, though, is that two US academics — qualified in their own fields, but not in HIV and AIDS research — could be more convincing than the host of African researchers working on the issue across the continent.

Even more perplexing is Mbeki's notion that the majority of thinking African people would be willing to collude in the invention of a new terminal disease, when old diseases and explanations would have done perfectly well.

It is known that Mbeki discussed these issues with trusted health professionals such as Professor William Makgoba, as well as his own ministers who were medical doctors. But whatever the outcome of these discussions, he continued to talk to the denialists. On January 21, Mbeki had a ten-minute telephone conversation with Rasnick, allegedly asking for support on his stand on AZT. The president then said that he was planning to write to President Clinton and other heads of state to ask them to join his efforts to bring about an international discussion on AIDS and the treatment thereof.

At this stage the denialists' influence seemed to be having the effect of deepening the president's views on AIDS. For example, in his opening address to parliament in February 2000, he commented: 'What seems to be clear, as of now, is that in addition to the work that is being done and which must be intensified, regarding the sexual behaviour of our people and the use of condoms, all possible interventions will have to be made to deal with the challenges of poverty and malnutrition, a whole range of well-known diseases such as tuberculosis, malaria, hepatitis and others, as well as the development of the required vaccines.'[325]

A few weeks later, however, the issue burst into the news in a way that was to colour all future debate. Roberts announced that the health minister was convening a panel to 'look into AIDS in Africa and the way forward'[326]. SAPA reported that the panel 'would surely re-appraise the scientific evidence that HIV leads to AIDS'. The panel, which would consist of about 30 experts, was aiming to include well-known denialists such as Californian molecular biologist Dr Peter Duesberg. The plan was that the panel would meet twice, and between the meetings participants would correspond on the Internet. The main aim of the panel was to come up with therapeutic interventions suitable for Africa.

On the face of it, it was difficult to see how a meeting of two groups with dissonant paradigms could be of benefit to anyone. The AIDS establishment was astonished. As far as its members were concerned, the denialist controversy had been laid to rest more than a decade previously. The Treatment Action Campaign immediately issued a challenge to the minister to distance herself from this statement.

Tshabalala-Msimang responded by elaborating on plans for the panel. She confirmed her belief in the existence and seriousness of AIDS, though refused to deny that dissidents had been invited to the panel. 'My personal view,' she said, 'is that those with more extreme views will be unwilling to participate because we are looking for a consensus view.'

But it seemed that the more extreme view was now coming from the office of the president himself. One newspaper reported how he wrote personally to a critic implying that the AIDS establishment's views were coloured by vested interests.[327]

'I am taken aback by the determination of many people in our country,' he wrote, 'to sacrifice all intellectual integrity to act as salespersons of the product of one pharmaceutical company' (presumably referring to the Glaxo/AZT debate).

On April 3, 2000, the diplomatic pouch to the US contained a hand-addressed letter to President Clinton from Mbeki.[328] It began by summarising the strategies adopted by his government to combat HIV and AIDS and the extent of the AIDS crisis in southern Africa, which differed from that in the west. The letter went on to criticise the 'orchestrated campaign of condemnation' against his search for specific targeted solutions to the problems in South Africa. His critics were demanding, he wrote, that he freeze discourse on the subject by quarantining those with alternative views on AIDS. This was 'intellectual terrorism', for which some agitate 'with a religious fervour born by a degree of fanaticism which is truly frightening'. 'The day may not be far off,' he wrote, 'when we will, once again, see books burnt and their authors immolated by fire by those who believe that they have a duty to conduct a holy crusade against the infidels.'

One of the most telling lines in the letter explained the president's insistence on his prerogative to espouse an alternative view. 'It may be that these comments are extravagant,' he wrote. 'If they are, it is because in the very recent past, we had to fix our own eyes on the very face of tyranny.'

Some US officials were allegedly so surprised by the tone of the letter that they felt obliged to check whether it was genuine.[329] The Clinton administration, as well as the office of UN Secretary General Kofi Annan and officials of other governments who received the letter, apparently decided to restrict its distribution in an effort to protect Mbeki's reputation. But as things happen in the world of politics, one unnamed US official passed the letter to the *Washington Post*.

The denialists were delighted by this turn of events, which boosted their faltering mission, and Mbeki soon became their new poster boy. Even today the opening page of their website, virusmyth.net, sports a pensive portrait of the president and a tagline asking 'Support President Mbeki to find out the truth about "AIDS".'

The news magazine *New African*, which had long espoused denialist views, opened its story with the words 'South Africa is coming alive with discussion and hopes for the government's "expert panel of inquiry".'[330] The article commented that the debate was rattling the foundations of the 'professional status and market penetration of medical and pharmaceutical establishments'.

The timing of this new controversy was disastrous for the government, which was gearing up to host the bi-annual international AIDS conference. This major event on the international AIDS calendar was being held in a southern country for the first time. Twelve thousand of the world's leading scientists, researchers and activists in the field of HIV were scheduled to convene in Durban to advance the knowledge base of HIV and AIDS. This conjunction of events focused world attention on the president's views and threatened to hijack that event. Soon there were rumours of a boycott.

The conference organisers, including leading AIDS researchers Drs Jerry Coovadia and Salim Abdool Karim, soon became embroiled in the deepening hostilities between the minister and the AIDS fraternity. 'I can't count the number of times (Tshabalala-Msimang) asked us to fly up to Pretoria and she had some angry response to us about something,' says Abdool Karim.

Tshabalala-Msimang got wind of a manifesto, called the Durban Declaration, in which established AIDS scientists declared their commitment to the orthodox AIDS paradigm. Though the organisers were signatories to the declaration they were not the originators of the document. 'She heard that we were going to pass a resolution at the conference condemning the government,' says Abdool Karim. 'We said this is not a political meeting — there is no resolution, scientific conferences do not have resolutions. But she saw it as a personal affront and felt that we were undermining her on this issue.'

These were tricky times and, as always, AIDS issues were easily tangled with the politics of the day. Matters came to a head when Abdool Karim and Covaadia told members of the Democratic Party, in what they thought was a private briefing, that they were critical of the government's response to the epidemic. What they did not know was that there was a journalist in their midst who would paste their words all over the national press. 'Both Jerry and I are well-known ANC supporters,' says Abdool Karim, 'and boy, all hell broke loose because now we were doing the unthinkable. It's not that we were attacking the party, because we were allowed to do that, but we were siding with Tony Leon (the DP leader). That was unthinkable... It did us a lot of harm.'

With each unfolding drama the battle lines became more sharply drawn. It is not difficult to see how party loyalties and political allegiance would shape the government's position. If the AIDS orthodoxy was in cahoots with the political opposition (and the pharmaceutical industry), perhaps it was the denialists, with their supportive demeanour and radical views, that represented a new, true direction for South Africa's AIDS response?

More poison

Throughout the early months of 2000 there was mounting pressure on the government to provide the drugs that would reduce HIV transmission from mother to child.

By now there was a choice of two drugs, AZT and nevirapine, both of which appeared to reduce transmission by 50 per cent, but the government was still prevaricating. Although Glaxo had finally agreed to meet the government's price on AZT, for the minister, the toxicity questions were now paramount. In February it was revealed that the minister had already rejected two reports from the Medicines Control Council that had confirmed its safety.[331]

Nevirapine was now the drug of choice, but the minister was still waiting on the outcome of the Saint trial, which would prove the new drug's efficacy. In the earlier discussions, the Treatment Action Campaign had agreed to mute their protests until the results of this trial were known, but their patience was wearing thin.

This, then, was the state of affairs when the minister of health received information that five women had died during a drug trial in Kalafong Hospital outside Pretoria. Although this study was not part of the Saint trial, and in fact did not include pregnant women, nevirapine was one of the drugs being tested. The report of the deaths seemed to confirm all the minister's worst fears about the toxicity of antiretroviral drugs.

The minister chose to report the deaths during an afternoon session in parliament.[332] To this alarming news she added a quote from a recent report by World Health Organisation that appeared to caution against the use of nevirapine in mother-to-child transmission on the grounds that it led to drug resistance.

The minister's statement provoked an angry debate in parliament, in which opposition speakers accused her of looking for ways of delaying the mother-to-child programme. Predictably, her supporters rejected the accusation, countering it with their own view that the opposition was but part of the pharmaceutical industry's conspiracy.

Outside the halls of parliament, activists and AIDS experts were puzzled and concerned. The medical establishment pointed out that toxicity had not yet been seen in mother-to-child transmission where nevirapine was given as a single dose.[333] Nevirapine's manufacturer, Boehringer Ingelheim, claimed that only two women had died on the trial, and the link between the deaths and nevirapine was, as yet, inconclusive.[334] The company spokesperson said he feared that the minister's statement could be a 'complicating factor' in the Medicines Control Council's decision to register nevirapine for use in preventing mother-to-child transmission.

As for the new fear of resistance, it seemed that the minister had misquoted the WHO report. Its concluding paragraph contained the words: 'Given the potential value of NVP (nevirapine) in reversing the dramatic trends of AIDS-related paediatric mortality in developing countries... the new information is not considered sufficient to interfere with plans to make NVP more widely available in pilot MTCT-prevention programmes or in research settings.'

The minister's pronouncements on the toxicity of antiretroviral drugs were to have a deep and lasting influence on her people. Florence Ngobeni was one of the health workers who witnessed the fallout from this every day. The hospital where she worked was involved in testing some of the new antiretroviral drug regimens, and when Ngobeni's immune system began to fail, she joined one of the clinical trials.

When Ngobeni experienced weight gain and skin pigmentation changes from the drugs, members of her support group became alarmed. 'They were discussing how Drs Gray and McIntyre had put black people on these ARV trials without letting them know they are dangerous,' says Ngobeni. She found out later that members of her support group were planning to take action on her behalf. 'They were saying I'm exploding,' says Ngobeni 'and I'm so dark it looks like I am going to die and they must do something about it.'

Then, and later, the minister's attitude prevented many from taking the drugs that would prolong their lives. 'The main questions people would ask were "If I start taking these drugs, what about side effects?" says Ngobeni. 'People were really, really, really afraid of side effects. I used to explain that side effects were something that just happens for six months or a year... Yes there were other side effects like gaining weight on different parts of your body. But I usually said, "What is better — to try and buy yourself a little time, or not to try at all?"'

Mercy

After a lengthy retreat at a mission station in the mountains of KwaZulu-Natal, Mercy Makhalemele returned to her work as an advocate for people living with HIV and AIDS.

It was the turn of the millennium, and the South African AIDS community was preparing for the international conference that would be held in Durban in July.

'You know everybody was thinking "The year 2000, what is going to happen..." and for me being HIV positive I was thinking I would probably die at that time.

'It was the conference, so I started writing all these things down and saying to my father — I was very, very close to my father — if ever I should be invited, and I die, you should go and speak for me. So I was doing all those things with my father.'

But a month before the conference, Mercy's father, jazz saxophonist Mike Makhalemele, died unexpectedly of a heart attack. Mercy was so devastated that she was unable to speak for eight days. 'For me it was one of those spiritual things, a feeling that says you can't predict your life. Nobody can say how long you are going to live.'

Despite her preparations, Mercy felt too fragile to play an active part in the conference, choosing instead to participate in a silent protest.

'We had actually written a letter to Nelson Mandela's office, asking him to call on people living with HIV and AIDS to join him on stage as he was giving the closing speech. We had hoped that would reflect the presence of the global community of people living with HIV — that would have had an impact. But there was no feedback from his office, so what we did was a silent protest.'

Mercy and a northern activist positioned themselves at the doorway of the conference hall.

'She had embroidered ARV tablets on her fancy evening gown and she was standing there with an umbrella, and I was on the floor in a black African outfit with red paint poured all over me,' says Mercy.

'What we were saying was "in the US people have this medicine and they can play around, but these African women do not have this medicine and they are dying". We were just at the exit that Nelson Mandela had to use, and he actually had to step over us. For me this was very symbolic.'

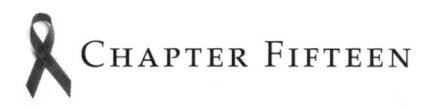

Chapter Fifteen
Behold a pale horse

WISE MEN AND FOOLS

One Friday evening in May 2000 found leading AIDS denialists nibbling canapés with world-renowned AIDS researchers at the Sheraton Hotel in Pretoria.

The next morning the nearly three dozen scientists[335] who represented the President's Advisory Panel on AIDS were seated around a conference table, ready to begin. Their mission: to inform and advise the government on the most appropriate course of action in dealing with its AIDS epidemic. They had been asked to come to a consensus position, to find an African solution.

From the start it was obvious that the denialists, who numbered about a third of the total, subscribed to a different paradigm from the orthodox scientists. They rejected the very notion that HIV was a harmful virus that could cause disease, or even that it had been seen or measured. It is unclear whether the president hoped that one side would convert the other, but the notion that two such groups could come to a consensus was far-fetched indeed.

The attendance of the orthodox scientists at this meeting was something of a duty call. Their commitment to the president and the AIDS response was such that they were prepared to spend two days debating the assumptions on which their life's work was based. They represented a global community of thousands of researchers who had been tussling with the complexities of the virus and its impacts for nearly two decades.

For the denialists, this meeting represented a unique opportunity to gain publicity for their views, which since the early 1990s had fallen into disrepute. This was the first time that any international figure of standing had given them any credence, a fact that they liked to attribute to the hegemonic power of the AIDS establishment. The denialists represented a vocal network of theorists, with a strong presence on the world wide web. None of them worked with people living with HIV and AIDS, and only one — an academic — was a black South African.

Several leading South African experts who had previously clashed with the government had been left off the invitation list for this first meeting. Unfortunate, too, was the absence of eminent African researchers who had identified the virus in the early days and whose ongoing population-based studies in rural Uganda, for example, have provided many of the insights into how the epidemic works. It was unclear why such a high-profile stab at an African solution to the AIDS epidemic would exclude many of the people who had been searching for the same thing.

Mbeki himself opened the proceedings, welcoming the participants with a reading of an Irish verse:

'Since the wise men have not spoken, I speak,
   but I am only a fool;
A fool that hath loved his folly...'[336]

Mbeki told the panel that there were times when he had asked himself whether his investigation into HIV and AIDS was one of folly or of grace.

It was because of the seriousness of the AIDS epidemic in South Africa, he said, that he had wanted to learn more about it himself, and to that end, had ploughed through a large amount of scientific material in a language that by his own admission, he did not understand.

As he spoke, the president revealed the question that neither his advisers nor his home-grown study course had managed to answer. Centrally it concerned the difference between the course of the epidemic in the US and Africa. Having read the early journal articles, he said, he understood that in the 1980s HIV was present only among homosexuals in South Africa, as it was in the north — though there were heterosexual cases in Central Africa. The articles had concluded that HIV was not endemic in Southern Africa.

'That was 1985,' he said, 'but clearly something changed here. In a period of maybe five, six, seven years after 1985, when it was said that such transmission in this region was not endemic in Southern Africa, there were high rates of heterosexual transmission. Now, as I was saying, being a fool I couldn't answer this question about what happened between 1985 and the early 1990s. The situation has not changed in the United States, up to today, nor in Western Europe with regard to homosexual transmission. But here it changed very radically in a short period of time… Why?'

It is not surprising that the president had not found easy answers to that question. The beginning of South Africa's second epidemic is a complex tale, about which there is scant primary research. This is not an accident: issues concerning vectors and vulnerable groups in the virus's journey across the continent to South Africa have been so fraught with sensitivities and ideological tensions that no agreed narrative has emerged (see Chapter Two).

'We were looking for answers because all of the information that has been communicated points to the reality that we are faced with a catastrophe…', said Mbeki. 'You have to respond to a catastrophe in a way that recognises that you are facing a catastrophe. And here we are talking about people — it is not death of animal stock or something like that, but people. Millions and millions of people.'

Perhaps it was the absence of answers in the literature of the AIDS orthodoxy that made the denialists' views so attractive. But when the president stumbled upon their school of thought, again, he found his advisers were of little help. 'I am embarrassed to say that I discovered that there had been a controversy around these matters for some time,' said Mbeki. 'I honestly didn't know. I was a bit comforted later when I checked with a number of our ministers and found that they were as ignorant as I, so I wasn't quite alone.'

The reaction to his interest in alternative theories about HIV, he said, had taken him completely by surprise. 'There was this very strong response saying: don't do this.'

But for Mbeki, this was tantamount to freezing debate and scientific discourse. And his motivation in calling together this panel was to get at deeper truths. He concluded:

'Indeed when eminent scientists said, "You have spoken out of turn," it was difficult not to think that one was indeed a fool. But I am no longer sure about that, given that so many people responded to the invitation of a fool to come to this important meeting.'

After this introduction, participants were given an opportunity to position themselves in relation to the issue of the day. Although the stated aim of the meeting was to advise the government on its AIDS response, according to a diary published anonymously in the *Mail & Guardian*, the invitation clearly asked 'What causes AIDS?' The first speaker lifted up the invitation, and simply said his name, and 'HIV'.

One by one, participants spoke.[337] Some argued for the introduction of antiretroviral medicines into Africa, others claimed that AIDS does not exist at all. Some wanted to focus on solutions, others argued that it was the drugs that killed, not HIV. The day seemed endless, discussions dragged on with no conclusion.

Afterwards the denialists gave interviews to the press. Austrian doctor Christian Fiala said 'They have nothing, just fairy tales about friends dying, architects dying, all these funerals…' Professor Peter Duesberg commented: 'The conventional view has not produced anything… It has not cured one single AIDS patient in 18 years.'

This of course was an accurate, but mischievous use of language. Proponents of antiretroviral therapy have never claimed a cure, but the drugs have been shown to prolong the lives of the majority of people who use them. Many who began the drug regimen at death's door are still alive today.

For the orthodoxy, the discussion was complicated by the fact that within the dissident camp there were contradictory views. Professor Alan Whiteside describes it like this: 'When you sat down and tried to analyse what they were thinking, there were a number of distinct groups. There were those that believed there was no such thing as HIV. There were those that believed that there was a virus, HIV, but it was harmless. There were those that believed that there was HIV and it caused AIDS but the whole thinking was designed to make money for the drug companies… and then there were those that you never understood what they did believe. They were not united by any means. They were just enjoying their moment in the sun.'

On the second day, talks broke down altogether and the two groups separated, with predictable results. The denialists' conclusions were that HIV does not cause AIDS, AIDS is not infectious, antiretroviral drugs are poisonous, and that it is important to treat the opportunistic infections.

The orthodoxy recommended that the government step up efforts to reduce blood-borne infections, vertical transmission and sexual transmission, and to provide antiretroviral treatment.

At the end of the day a four-person team (two from each camp) was appointed to review the scientific data and construct experiments that would deal with as-yet-unanswered questions. The health minister also requested that the discussion be continued on the Internet until a second meeting in July, when conclusions would be drawn and recommendations made. Both the Internet panel and the second meeting were to be opened up to a greater number of participants, including some of the previously uninvited South African scientists.

Despite the lack of consensus, the denialists hailed the whole event as a great triumph. 'In 14 years of AIDS journalism,' wrote Celia Farber in the *New York Press*, 'I've never seen the AIDS leadership writhing in the kind of agony they now find themselves in daily. The prospect of having to debate, defend or quantify their paradigm is melting them down.'

'It felt like the period around the time of the Velvet Revolution when former authoritarian socialists suddenly started talking about the importance of "socialism with a human face".'

Acting out

The Internet discussion that followed the first panel was dominated by the denialists, and failed to reach any fresh conclusions. The orthodox group had apparently decided not to debate each point, but to prepare broad responses to the questions posed by the president. Writing in *The Village Voice*, journalist Mark Schoofs reported that this upset Health Minister Tshabalala-Msimang, who felt betrayed by South African scientists for discouraging foreign panellists from joining the debate.[338]

Whiteside, who entered the panel at the time of the Internet debate, was one of those that came to regret his participation. 'Being a good protestant I thought it would be rude to ignore it,' says Whiteside. 'But there was no logic, and in my opinion my colleagues who didn't participate made the right decision. I just didn't realise because I hadn't met the people, just to what extent they were flat-earthers.'

After the first panel meeting, leading scientists decided to publish a statement outlining their position on the debate. The Durban Declaration, which was signed by 5 000[339], refuted revisionist theories about HIV and AIDS. 'HIV causes AIDS,' it read. 'It is unfortunate that a few vocal people continue to deny the evidence. This position will cost countless lives.'

Word of the declaration had got out before it was published, and the health minister and her colleagues were outraged. The president's spokesman, Parks Mankahlana, who died (officially from anaemia) three months later, aged 36 years, told SAPA that the declaration belonged in the dustbin. 'People can't… circulate a petition all over the world condemning the president,' he said.[340]

The panel reconvened in early July, in the slipstream of the publicity created by the Durban Declaration. By now relations between the government and the orthodox AIDS scientists were at a low ebb. The orthodoxy found that their first speaker, Professor Jerry Coovadia — convenor of the International AIDS Conference and a signatory to the Durban Declaration — had been disallowed, and they were forced to choose a substitute.

The second panel got no further than the first.

During this meeting, the denialists made complex scientific and theoretical arguments to support their position. Their starting point was that the virus had never been properly seen, isolated or imaged. One of the proponents of this view was an eminent electron microscopist, who repudiated the images that orthodox scientists claimed to have made of the virus.

'To some extent that is not totally untrue,' says virologist Professor Barry Shoub, who heads South Africa's National Institute of Virology. 'Because HIV is an enveloped virus it is totally impossible to get pure virus, because you always get some membrane components. That doesn't mean that you can't visualise them and you can't study them…' says Schoub. 'All the biochemical, biophysical and virological studies have been done and HIV has been extremely well characterised.'

But Schoub, who was present at the second panel meeting, was unable to make his views heard.

There was also a protracted discussion about the reliability of the HIV test, which the denialists claim is notorious for producing false positives. The orthodox scientists agreed that there had been a problem in the early days when the tests were less sensitive, but they provided contemporary data showing that the HIV tests commonly used in South Africa were reliable. This evidence too was dismissed. Dr David Rasnick went so far as to strongly motivate for all HIV testing to be stopped. This, he said, would bring an immediate end to the AIDS epidemic.

Similarly tautological discussions ensued around other aspects of HIV. For example, when scientists put up a graph that illustrated rising death rates in the younger age group, the denialists argued that this was a reflection of poor record-keeping and medical care in the bad old days of apartheid — though why the youth should be differentially affected was not explained.

Professor Mhlongo expounded at length on the theory that diseases of poverty were responsible for what scientists had misunderstood as AIDS deaths. According to the official report of the panel, Mhlongo 'spoke of the preoccupation with biomedicine in an attempt to be scientific, even at the expense of the wider distressing situation of poverty, poor housing, lack of sanitation and a multitude of diseases associated with the deprivation and urban squalor that characterise the reality of the majority of black South Africans'.

So the days went on ... The denialists repeated their theories, and the orthodoxy rebutted them, as before. This time, however, the commitment to good behaviour had diminished, and tempers flared. Schoofs, who was one of several invited journalists, described a serious row about paediatric HIV.

Researchers at Chris Hani-Baragwanath and the US Centers for Disease Control (CDC) had produced a large amount of material that showed that babies with HIV have a higher death rate than those without. 'And so holding the CDC data in his hand, Duesberg asked (the CDC's Dr Helene) Gayle whether the babies with HIV had received AZT,' wrote Schoufs. 'Gayle started to answer but (denialist Harvey) Bialy cut in saying yes, the babies had received the drug. Duesberg then shouted that that was probably what had killed the babies, and as Gayle kept trying to answer his original question, Duesberg stormed out of the room. Eventually Gayle explained that some of the babies had received the drug while others hadn't and that the CDC was preparing a breakdown for the dissidents to analyse.'

With the reliability of the HIV test in question, and the death statistics disputed, the denialists had book-ended the subject in a way that seemed to render all discussion futile. 'It's like engaging with fundamentalists on an issue of faith,' says Whiteside. 'If it's your faith you are going to believe it and I can't argue with you logically about it.'

For Schoub, who had worked on HIV since its arrival in the country in the early 1980s, the whole thing was a circus.

'The humorous thing was that the dissidents were quarrelling amongst themselves as well as with the scientists,' he says. 'At one stage one of them stormed out of the meeting over the extent of denial — whether the virus exists at all or whether it was a harmless virus. They were just a querulous lot. The actual discussion was not a scientific discussion or debate, it was just a shouting match.'

When Shoub found himself seated next to Rasnick he challenged him to a test. 'I said to him well, will you inject it (HIV) into yourself, and he said he would, provided that I would, instead, take AZT.'

But Schoub withdrew because he thought it unethical. 'It would have been an interesting experiment,' he says, 'cos AZT is toxic, it is true, but I would have taken AZT and I would have stopped. But he would be infected.'

While this may have seemed like fun and games for idle minds, for those who had spent the past decade working in public health facilities trying to treat the exponentially rising numbers of young people with inadequate drugs, it was an outrage. They did not need elaborate theoretical arguments to prove what they had painfully discovered for themselves, and the denialists' sophistry was hard to take.

'They would have these 1 200 references and it would look really impressive, and it would say that this paper shows that, and then they would take half the sentence and insert it so the less you know about this, the more authoritative the documents look,' says paediatrician Dr James McIntyre, who attended the second panel.

'The more you know about it, the more useless it is to try and rebut everything, because each rebuttal leads to another 500 references taken out of context… It was not so easy for the politicians to see. The politicians argued that "they are scared to debate or they won't debate" or whatever. But in reality it was not possible.'

The official panel report[341] lists a large research agenda proposed by denialist scientists: to investigate HIV causality, the reliability of the HIV test[342] and other disputed aspects. The work was to be performed within a year — using government funding. Schoub was involved in the first experiment, which showed that South African laboratories provided accurate HIV tests. But he believes that since then the whole idea was abandoned. 'These experiments, and having to go to these meetings, are very, very time-consuming and very energy-consuming. And that is wasteful energy, particularly in a country like South Africa,' says Schoub.

Much of the terrain the denialists hoped to cover had, in any case, been traversed by the orthodox scientists for years. For example, papers showing the correlation between viral load and health, or comparative rates of heterosexual transmission at different viral loads, or the relationship between HIV infection and infant mortality were readily available in the large peer-reviewed scientific literature — a literature that the denialists had clearly not deigned to read.

The fate of this research is still not clear. In December 2005, the health minister confirmed that the work was ongoing.[234] In February 2007, Bialy made an Internet posting about his research at Medunsa University, which purports to discredit the HIV test.[344] However, results have yet to appear in a peer-reviewed journal.

Breaking the silence

A few days after the conclusion of the second panel, the 13th International AIDS Conference began in Durban. This year the conference theme was 'Breaking the silence' about HIV and AIDS.

For the government, the environment could hardly have been more toxic. The Durban Declaration was headlined in all the newspapers, and the health minister was engaged in daily verbal fisticuffs with querulous reporters. The president's office commented that they hoped the conference would not turn into a 'Mbeki-bashing bazaar'.[345]

Not only was there fallout from the panel, but legions of international activists had descended on the steamy sub-tropical city of Durban to strut their stuff. The Treatment Action Campaign and US activists from ACT UP and Health Gap had organised a Global March for Treatment[346], to take place just before the grand opening ceremony of the conference.

Protesters representing over 230 organisations from 33 countries congregated in front of the Durban city hall, where they were addressed by political and religious leaders. 'One dissident, one bullet' was the chant, and banners to that effect were draped over statues in the central city park. The protesters then marched to the conference, where they presented the health minister and conference organisers with a petition calling for affordable drugs, and a national programme to prevent mother-to-child transmission.

Inside the conference venue on that opening Sunday night, 1 400 AIDS experts — and the world press — were waiting to hear what the president had decided about the truth of HIV. Perhaps he had not had a chance to view the video tapes of his advisory panel, but instead of making a clear statement on his conclusions about the relationship between HIV and AIDS, he chose to dwell at length on the enormous burden of ill-health on the African continent, and its roots in poverty. He quoted from a 1995 World Health Organisation report.

'The world's biggest killer and the greatest cause of ill-health and suffering across the globe,' he said, 'is listed almost at the end of the International Classification of Diseases. It is given the code Z59.5: extreme poverty.'[347]

Mbeki then went on to tell the world's leading academics, health professionals, counsellors and activists that he did not believe that one virus could be responsible for the collapse of the immune systems of young people on the continent. He ended by assuring the audience of his government's commitment to fight HIV and AIDS and outlined some of the elements of the government's HIV control programme.

Mbeki's speech infuriated a large segment of his audience. Hundreds walked out as he spoke, and local activists had difficulty controlling their international comrades.

'They wanted to invade the platform and shout at Mbeki,' says Mark Heywood. 'We had to explain that it's not about satisfying your own consciences by saying that you shouted at Thabo Mbeki. For us it is about building a movement. People in this country would not understand or sympathise with that type of action — the very type of people who we need to mobilise in the long term.'

The next to take the podium was 11-year-old Nkosi Johnson, who spoke about being a child living with HIV. 'I hate having AIDS', he said, 'because I get very sick and I get very sad when I think of all the other children and babies that are sick with AIDS.' Johnson pleaded with the government to make treatment available. 'I just wish that the government can start giving AZT to pregnant HIV mothers to help stop the virus being passed on to their babies,' he said. 'Babies are dying very quickly and I know one little abandoned baby who came to stay with us and his name was Micky. He couldn't breathe, he couldn't eat and he was so sick and mommy Gail had to phone welfare to have him admitted to a hospital and he died. But he was such a cute little baby and I think the government must start doing it, because I don't want babies to die.'

But the tiny boy's personal plea fell on an empty seat — Mbeki had already left the arena for his next engagement.

So the conference proceeded as usual, with its reports and discussions and display stands hawking this treatment and that prevention programme. This year the denialists had a greater presence than on previous occasions, and in the margins of the conference there were assorted shenanigans. Anthony Brink, of AZT-bashing fame, found himself festooned by a bowl of curry and rice from an angry HIV-positive activist. For their part, denialists spread the rumour that ACT UP was financed by the drug company Merck.

Dissident South African journalist Anita Allen, writing in *The Citizen*, claimed that this year conference participants were better informed about HIV and AIDS, 'thanks to the ever more vigorous debate here and abroad raised by the African leader and his chosen ones who want the scientist in Africans to wake up.'[348]

THE JA-NEE PRESIDENT

Former President Mandela had been invited to make the closing speech of the conference. This was his first major public utterance on the subject of HIV and AIDS since his 1997 address to the World Economic Forum in Switzerland. He defended Mbeki's right to question the cause of AIDS, but said the dispute was distracting from real life-and-death issues.

'The ordinary people of the continent and the world… would, if anybody cared to ask their opinions, wish that the dispute about the primacy of politics or science be put on the backburner, and that we proceed to address the needs and concerns of those suffering and dying,' he said.

Predictably, the denialists interpreted Mandela's support for Mbeki as a major victory, and as tacit support for their position. On the other hand, the orthodoxy read into it a mild rebuke for the president — instructing him to cast aside his doubts and get on with the job. They knew that, traditionally, African politicians do not criticise each other in public, and Mandela would never have done so on a global platform.

The fact that this occurred under the gaze of the world media led to widespread speculation and debate across the globe. The world waited for Mbeki's next move, to see if the elder statesman's words had hit home. When it came, it was a shock. On 11 September, 2000, *Time* magazine (with a global circulation of 1.5 million) published an interview with Mbeki[349] in which he reiterated his original position on HIV and AIDS, and the role of poverty in disease.

TIME: You've been criticised for playing down the link between HIV and AIDS. Where do you now stand on this very controversial issue?
MBEKI: Clearly there is such a thing as acquired immune deficiency. The question you have to ask is what produces this deficiency. A whole variety of things can cause the immune system to collapse. Now it is perfectly possible that among those things is a particular virus. But the notion that immune deficiency is only acquired from a single virus cannot be sustained. Once you say immune deficiency is acquired from that virus your response will be antiviral drugs. But if you accept that there can be a variety of reasons, including poverty and the many diseases that afflict Africans, then you can have a more comprehensive treatment response.

Again Mbeki was conflating AIDS with all immune deficiency and, predictably, it was widely seen by the media as a confirmation of Mbeki's denialist position. What it did confirm, certainly, was the president's antipathy towards antiretroviral drugs. But it was the next section of the interview that was most widely quoted.

TIME: Are you prepared to acknowledge that there is a link between HIV and AIDS?
MBEKI: No, I am saying that you cannot attribute immune deficiency solely and exclusively to a virus.

South Africans who have seen the transcript of that interview say Mbeki did not say 'No', but used the phrase 'Yes-no', a peculiarly South African expression indicating equivocation.

The health minister also found herself in the same 'Ja-nee' hot water — being unable to contradict the president she held in such esteem in public, but reluctant to identify herself with the denialist views. The week before Mbeki's interview, she and *Radio 702* presenter John Robbie had fallen out over the issue. The interview ended with Tshabalala-Msimang castigating Robbie for calling her by her first name, and Robbie telling her to stop talking rubbish and 'go away'.

ROBBIE: You have said that the policy of the ministry is well known. Do you accept that HIV causes AIDS?
TSHABALALA-MSIMANG: Why do you ask me that question today? I have answered that question umpteen times.
ROBBIE: Yes, and the answer is?
TSHABALALA-MSIMANG: Umpteen times I have answered that question. My whole track record of having worked at the area of HIV and AIDS for the last 20 years is testimony. Why should you ask me that question today?
ROBBIE: You haven't answered the question, Manto.
TSHABALALA-MSIMANG: Why should you ask me that question?
ROBBIE: To avoid confusion.
TSHABALALA-MSIMANG: I have never said anything contrary to what you want me to say today.
ROBBIE: So, therefore, you accept that HIV causes AIDS.
TSHABALALA-MSIMANG: You are not going to put words into my mouth.
ROBBIE: I am not putting words into your mouth. I am asking you a question.
TSHABALALA-MSIMANG: Yes you are.
ROBBIE: I am asking you a straight — now hold on a second — I am asking you a straight question, the minister of health of South Africa, I am asking you a question: does HIV cause AIDS?
TSHABALALA-MSIMANG: I have been party to developing a strategic framework and that strategy testifies what my policy understandings of the HIV epidemic are. If you haven't read that, please go and read it. And then you will understand where I depart from.
ROBBIE: Manto, Manto. A simple yes or no is the answer I am looking for.
TSHABALALA-MSIMANG: You will not force me into a corner, into saying yes or no.

Around this time Tshabalala-Msimang's office also distributed a document that suggested that HIV had been developed as part of a conspiracy to reduce world population. A photocopied chapter from the book *Behold a Pale Horse* by American writer William Cooper had been placed on desks of key officials across the country. The covering letter attached to the photocopy was addressed to 'all African health ministers', and warned that the virus could be in any vaccine bought by or donated to any African country. This was just one of Cooper's conspiracy theories, which included ideas about UFOs and alien abduction.

The appearance of HIV, a new and lethal virus that appeared to favour gay men and Africans, had given rise to an abundance of conspiracy theories in the past. These included theories that the virus had been engineered in the US (CIA/Pentagon) for biological warfare/genocide campaigns and that it had been distributed (accident/design) in vaccination programmes. Conspiracy theories now seemed to be gaining ground among African leaders like Namibian president Sam Nujoma[350], who had made a public statement to this effect at an International Labour Organisation conference in Geneva earlier in the year.

This new interest in the subject on the part of the health minister sent chills through the AIDS establishment. However, Patricia Lambert, Tshabalala-Msimang's spokesperson, reassured them that this was just one of many documents that had landed on the minister's desk, and that she did not necessarily endorse it.

'There's nothing unusual at all in this case, said Lambert 'because it's part of stuff she routinely sends to the provinces so they can be aware of the kind of stuff that's coming into her office.'

All these events, clustered in the first two weeks of September 2000, brought the political temperature of the AIDS debate to a new high. Despite the speculation and rumour, nobody actually knew what was happening behind the scenes. Neither the president nor the health minister had actually denied the denialists, but nor had they come out in clear support of orthodox scientific views on HIV and AIDS. Even Mbeki's admirers were flummoxed by these goings on.

For example, reporters at the *Sowetan* newspaper gave up hours to do a forensic review of their archive. 'We put a whole team together to look into the president's speeches,' says Lucky Mazibuko, 'to see whether we can find somewhere where he said

HIV does not cause AIDS. We couldn't.'

For Mazibuko and his peers, the president had been deliberately misconstrued. 'There is that mentality in the AIDS world that says it's either "A" — or nothing. But I also think he victimised himself by not spelling out clearly what he means.'

As with the *Sarafina* saga of 1996, the media's response to this episode was revealing. 'It was interesting that the media seemed so hell-bent on criticising Mbeki, instead of using it as an opportunity to do some in-depth reporting about HIV and AIDS,' says Mary Crewe. 'Mbeki asked important questions — how does HIV lead to AIDS years later; and what about "African AIDS" and its relationship with poverty. But he was mocked and treated like a Third World character. The media painted him as a stupid geek that surfed the Internet. Why weren't they more subtle? They sent us into a spiral.'

But there were also many within the ANC who were not willing to give the president the benefit of the doubt, and the AIDS question was becoming politically divisive. The ANC's two major political allies, the Congress of South African Trade Unions and the South African Communist Party called on the government to end its scientific speculation about the causes of AIDS and concentrate on providing affordable treatment to people infected with HIV. And in a confidential document, members of ANC's own health committee called on Tshabalala-Msimang and Mbeki to unequivocally reject the denialists' views.

On September 15, the government took the unprecedented step of placing half-page advertisements in the country's newspapers to clarify its position. The advertisements clearly stated that neither the president nor his cabinet colleagues had ever denied the link between HIV and AIDS. A few days later the president confirmed this in parliament.

Losing their grip

Although the president had clarified his stance in public, there were still many doubters in the central and provincial government. By now this had become an essentially political dispute, and it would have devastating and long-term consequences for the rollout of AIDS programmes in the provinces. While some provincial leaders used all their powers to advance AIDS prevention efforts, others were less enthusiastic.

The health minister of Mpumalanga province, Sibongile Manana, was one of the latter. She mounted a lengthy campaign to oust an NGO that was providing care and counselling to rape survivors[351] in one of the provincial hospitals.

This story has its roots in the furious row between the president and the leader of the official opposition party over rape and its remedies — and that in turn, had its roots in the earlier dispute over the toxicity and efficacy of AZT.

This is how it happened.

From November 1999, when Minister Tshabalala-Msimang had told the press that there was no evidence that AZT was an effective HIV prophylactic for rape survivors, there had been fierce disagreement. Many members of the medical establishment, as well as rape survivors, were asking that post-exposure prophylaxis be made available in the public health system. With the discount offered by the manufacturer, the treatment would be affordable, costing around R200 per person.

In July 2000, Democratic Alliance leader Tony Leon challenged President Mbeki in parliament[352] over the issue. Subsequently they exchanged letters, and this emotionally charged correspondence was later published in the press. What began as a disagreement with a factual basis soon escalated into an acrimonious personal exchange. Insults were traded on both sides, and over all sorts of extraneous subjects — including the Zimbabwe land crisis, the rule of law, racism and the motives of the pharmaceutical companies.

Essentially Leon argued, correctly, that there was a strong body of medical opinion that supported the efficacy of post-exposure prophylaxis with AZT, and that it was inexpensive enough to be made available in the public health system. On the other hand Mbeki argued, also correctly, that AZT was not licensed for this purpose — either in South Africa or in the US. Mbeki also made the point that if post-exposure prophylaxis was a reliable form of prevention, it would be as good as a vaccine, and would be widely used. He concluded that to prescribe AZT for this purpose was not legal.

This fevered debate simply inflamed the passions on both sides, and it was a small NGO that worked with rape survivors that took the heat.

Since May 2000, the Greater Nelspruit Rape Counselling

Programme (Grip)[353] had been providing post exposure prophylaxis to rape survivors, along with other support and counselling services. But in early October, Manana ordered them to stop, summonsing 14 Grip staff members to tell them they were contravening government policies. She told them that AZT was a dangerous drug, and as Grip had no permission to be on hospital premises, they deserved to be charged and jailed. She allegedly accused them of being part of a plot to undermine the president.[354]

Manana then evicted project workers from the hospital, saying that they were 'illegal squatters' who had never been given permission to operate there. She told the press that 'the government can therefore not allow itself to be blackmailed by organisations masquerading as good Samaritans, while the truth is (that) they have a clear agenda to undermine the present government.'

'This route is followed,' she said, 'in order to safeguard the country and Mpumalanga province from being a mirror of a banana republic.' She then accused Grip of abusing the hospital and their staff with their 'unethical research', and of preventing the hospital from doing its work.

At the time the Mpumalanga health department had failed to spend more than 80 per cent of its AIDS budget, and there were no services in Mpumalanga's 23 hospitals for rape survivors.

Later Manana fired several of the hospital's officials for having allowed the project to operate within its walls. Others were charged with misconduct. She went on to ban AZT from all government facilities in the province, forbidding hospital doctors from writing prescriptions for the drug.

Although Manana was eventually forced to allow Grip back into the hospital, she continued exploring all legal means against them. Over the next two years she pursued Grip through the courts, running up bills of R140 000 before she abandoned her quest.

Towards the end of September 2000, in a closed meeting of around 200 ANC members and cabinet ministers, Mbeki revealed his personal views on the subject for the first time.[355] According to reports leaked to the press, he told them that he believed that the CIA was working covertly with American drug companies to discredit him, because he was threatening their profits by questioning the link between HIV and AIDS. He alleged that the

Treatment Action Campaign was part of this conspiracy, as they received funding from the drug companies and had 'infiltrated' the trade unions to spread the call for the government to provide treatment for people with HIV.

Mbeki also raged against members of his own cabinet saying that they should join him in fighting off attempts to undermine him, instead of becoming the unwitting tools of powerful international forces ranged against him. He allegedly told them that it was their duty to inform themselves so that they could counter the propaganda offensive that was being mounted to say that HIV causes AIDS.

According to writer William Gumede[356], there was stunned silence in the room, and his audience was so deeply shocked by the virulence of his attack that they did not challenge anything Mbeki said.

A fortnight later Mbeki's spokesperson announced that the president was 'scaling down his direct involvement' in the AIDS question, and was passing the baton to his health minister, who would continue to liaise with the advisory panel and receive and process their final report.[357]

Thus it was that South Africa's second democratically elected president abdicated from leadership on AIDS, and from the defining crisis of his administration.

Busi

After her diagnosis, Busi Maqungo began attending a support group for people living with HIV. One day a doctor who was also a member of the Treatment Action Campaign came to the hospital to talk to them about the organisation. 'I was sitting there thinking to myself maybe this is what I have been looking for,' *says Busi.* 'I needed a place to belong as an HIV-positive person. I wanted to go and join these people.'

The doctor invited her to accompany a TAC delegation to the Parliamentary Health Portfolio Committee hearings on AIDS and treatment access.

When they arrived, the room was full of parliamentarians, journalists and television crews. Although Busi had never disclosed her HIV status, she decided that she wanted to participate.

'I had never spoken about HIV, or me being HIV positive to anyone apart from the support group and the doctor,' *she says.* 'Now I am going to speak to parliament people, hmmm... it felt strange, but I was not afraid. After my baby's death I felt that I needed to do something. Because it felt like, all this time I had been covering up for HIV, and now that it had killed my baby I wanted to expose it and not cover it anymore.

'So I spoke about the unavailability of PMTCT (prevention of mother-to-child transmission) and how I lost a child to HIV. I told them it felt like my baby had been robbed of her life. If this miracle AZT was saving the kids from getting HIV, why wasn't I given that to save her?'

'Afterwards I felt proud... fulfilled, that's the word I am looking for.

'That's how the whole thing started, and I've never stopped. I've been with the TAC ever since. I've toyi-toyied with the TAC, I've been to night vigils, I've been to courts with the TAC, suing governments, suing pharmaceutical companies, and ja, and I've also been a role model in my community as a person living with HIV.'

Chapter Sixteen

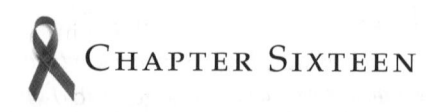

In the court of public opinion

Defiance!

When TAC leader Zackie Achmat heard that the president had accused them of involvement in a Big Pharma conspiracy, he reacted with surprise. 'We are the ones calling for the manufacture and importation of generic drugs that would reduce their profits. Does this sound like an organisation in the pay of drug companies?' he asked. 'We challenge the president to provide a shred of evidence to back up his claims.'[358]

Shortly after this, TAC officially launched a new campaign — the defiance campaign[359] against drug company profiteering. Using the terminology and tactics of the African National Congress resistance of the 1950s, TAC committed to defying unjust laws. The first action: smuggling.

On October 18, 2000, Achmat flew in to Cape Town airport from Thailand with 5 000 capsules of a generic anti-fungal drug hidden in his luggage. Busi Maqungo was in the crowd of TAC supporters that met him at the airport. 'It was so wonderful; it really felt that he had brought life into the country,' she said, 'because fluconazole[360] wasn't available at the public hospitals. And if you went to the chemist to buy it, it was too expensive. One pill cost about R80 and that is too much, especially for a poor person from the shacks.'[361]

The drug, manufactured by Pfizer, is used in the treatment of thrush and cryptococcal meningitis, both crippling opportunistic diseases of AIDS. People suffering from these diseases need to take the medication for an extended period, and thus free access to the drug is literally a matter of life and death. But because of the cost of the branded drug, it was seldom available in the public health system.

Achmat told reporters that he had bought the generic drug for R1,78 a capsule: his smuggling operation had netted a saving of nearly R400 000. This was the first time that the high cost of branded drugs had been so clearly demonstrated, and there was an immediate outcry against the manufacturer.

In fact TAC's campaign had begun earlier in the year when activists had challenged Pfizer to reduce the cost of this same drug. Pfizer had responded by offering a free supply to the South African government. But when TAC heard that the offer was limited to the treatment of meningitis, and available only until the patent expired — two years down the line — they had reacted angrily, accusing the company of 'fraud to protect profits'.[362]

Despite the anger of the activists, or perhaps because of it, Minister Tshabalala-Msimang had accepted the offer. But months later the drug was still not available. Thus fluconazole became the first target of the campaign against Big Pharma. TAC organised marches and pickets in front of Pfizer offices, in which they were joined by Cosatu.

TAC's smuggling operation was welcomed by many in the South African medical community. Although the smuggled drugs were confiscated and charges were laid against Achmat[363], eventually the generic version was legalised, on condition that it was prescribed by qualified health professionals. Pfizer objected to the breaking of its patent rights, but took no further action. It took until March 2001 before Pfizer's first donated drug became available at public health clinics.

Behind the headlines of TAC's campaign were very many quieter acts of defiance against the medicine's status quo. Friends, NGOs and activists smuggled life-saving generic antiretrovirals through airports and over borders. Many doctors participated in such schemes, feeling that their Hippocratic Oath was compromised by their inability to supply these drugs. One public sector hospital in Johannesburg had even found a way of fiddling the accounts to purchase unauthorised drugs to reduce the transmission of HIV from mother to child.

But even these life-saving ventures were constantly thwarted by the impact of the president's controversial views on HIV and AIDS. At Chris Hani-Baragwanath Hospital, where drugs to reduce mother-to-child prevention were available (from research trials), many pregnant women were afraid of taking them. In October 2000, a Reuters journalist interviewed women in the queue for antenatal care and heard a common refrain: 'I don't believe HIV causes AIDS. I don't believe AIDS exists. Mr Mbeki told us.'[364]

Counsellor Florence Ngobeni was in despair. 'My job got harder when the government began questioning the link between HIV and AIDS,' she said. 'I have to find ways to convince (patients) that HIV exists and that it does cause AIDS... I feel exhausted.'

BIG PHARMA VS MANDELA

In the months since September 1999, when the Pharmaceutical Manufacturers' Association (PMA) suspended the court challenge to the Medicines Act, there had been little said about the matter. According to industry insiders, there was yet a hope that the South African government would rewrite the offending law; the PMA was therefore holding out for a negotiated settlement.

In the meantime, the industry had pursued a vigorous and visible strategy of donations and discount offers on AIDS drugs, which had bought it new friends across the globe. For example, in May 2000, just before the 13th International AIDS Conference in Durban, five leading drug manufacturers had announced an initiative[365] in which AIDS drug discounts could be negotiated on a company-by-company, country-by-country basis. The South African government had rejected this UNAIDS-approved programme, saying that they would prefer to maintain independence by exploring the local manufacture of pharmaceuticals.

Indeed Big Pharma's social responsibility campaigns had failed to impress the South African health minister, who had rejected several offers, including five years' free supply of nevirapine, the drug used to prevent mother-to-child transmission. Pfizer was the only company whose charitable offer had been accepted — perhaps because they had stayed out of the Medicines Act lawsuit, or perhaps because fluconazole was not an antiretroviral drug.

Every rejected offer garnered the health minister fresh criticism and insults, but the South African government was holding out for rights rather than charity. As they saw it, the TRIPS agreement gave them the right to import and/or manufacture affordable drugs for the public sector. This was what had been envisaged by the Medicines Act, and this was what they were determined to do.

In the years since the PMA interdict, Big Pharma's chances of a court victory had declined precipitously. A series of events had transformed the court action from a test case for intellectual property rights into a gigantic public relations disaster for the pharmaceutical industry.

Firstly, the fevered debates in the World Health Assembly, and the passage of the Revised Drug Strategy, had reshaped the normative environment for drug patents. Next, the linking of the lawsuit with the rising death toll from AIDS had cast the industry as the clear villain of the piece. The publicity campaign of the activists had even cost the industry the support of the US government.

The dramatic entry of the generic drug manufacturers into the mix had been the final blow. In September 2000, Cipla [366] — an Indian generic drug manufacturer — had announced that it could provide the triple drug cocktail for $800 a year, in comparison with the branded drug price of $9 080. By February 2001, Cipla's price was down to $350 per person per year.

In making this offer, Cipla had not only removed the first serious barrier to AIDS treatment, but more importantly had indicated the true cost of manufacturing these drugs. Cipla's offer exposed the huge profit margins of the research-based industry. After the Cipla announcement, the price of patented AIDS drugs began a steady tumble. [367] By early March 2001, Glaxo, Merck and Bristol Meyers Squibb announced discounts of up to 90 per cent for drugs in low-income countries.

In this new environment, the South African government's attitude to the Medicines Act lawsuit hardened. [368] According to the US industry group PhRMA, it was now the South African government that was responsible for ending the suspension of the litigation. In an official document in November 2000, they said that 'the minister's legal advisers have insisted that petitioners continue litigation on the existing law — refusing to allow the continued and logical suspension of the case... PhRMA members would ultimately prefer a negotiated settlement and the forging of a partnership that immediately seeks to address the AIDS pandemic in South Africa'.

Thus it was that the long years of wrangling about the wording of a little-known law came to an end, and the court date was set down for March 5, 2001.[369]

In the run-up to the court case, TAC and its allies abroad embarked on a massive campaign in support of the government. Despite all their disagreements with the minister and the spat with the president, TAC made common cause with the government on this issue and applied to become a friend of the court (*amicus curiae*). This would enable them to use the court case to examine the broader issues surrounding the case, which for TAC were the high price of patented drugs in an era of HIV and AIDS. TAC's intervention was the final turn of the screw. From a dry legal contest over intellectual property rights and public health, the court case had been transformed into a personal battle between Big Pharma and AIDS activists who were fighting for their lives.

Protest groups across the world worked hard to create adverse publicity for the Pharma action, which soon became synonymous with AIDS deaths. London's *Guardian*, for example, ran a series of articles[370] with emotive headlines that could not have been bettered by the activists themselves: 'Drug giants sue to cut HIV lifeline', 'The profits that kill', and 'Evil triumphs in a sick society'. They even gave crime fiction writer John le Carré column space to describe the background research for his latest thriller[371], in which innocents die in bogus drug trials and whistleblowers are murdered. While effective as propaganda, this coverage resulted in some lingering confusion between fact and fiction.

Interestingly, Big Pharma did little to ward off the battering it was getting in the media. In South Africa its CEO and spokesperson, Mirryena Deeb, made infrequent but abrasive press statements[372], which failed to gain the sympathy even of financial journalists. Writing in *Business Day* at the time of the court case, for example, Pat Sidley commented: 'For many journalists of my vintage, the activists were manna from heaven… They were always available to teach and explain. Pharmaceutical companies, evasive and secretive at the best of times, retreated further into their shells.'[373]

While all of this spelt doom for Big Pharma's lawsuit, it was not entirely to the South African government's liking. Their intention had never been to use the law to get cheap AIDS drugs, and they had consistently rejected demands for antiretrovirals to be made available in the public health system. The events of 2000 — the controversy around the president's panel and the Durban Declaration—had only served to sharpen their antipathy towards the drugs, which they seemed to truly believe were too toxic for routine use. Heywood confirms that the minister and her allies disapproved of the TAC's campaign. 'They were uncomfortable because we used the PMA case to focus on the pricing of ARVs,' he says. 'They weren't trying to encourage interest in that kind of treatment because by that time Thabo Mbeki's denialism had become entrenched in the ANC and the presidency. Although its full extent was probably not understood in the society, it was understood in the Department of Health.'

According to Heywood, 'Although the press were generally unable to grasp the point, the minister of health understood that the *amicus* intervention was but a stage in TAC's campaign for treatment access, which would lay the foundations for intensified criticism of the government's policies'.

If this was the minister's perception at the time, she certainly did nothing to dampen the media campaign, which served her interests so well.

US consumer activists represented another set of interests in the case. For James Love of the Nader-established Consumer Project on Technology, the South African Medicines case chimed with his organisation's interest in intellectual property policy and practice. They had long-standing concerns about the practices of the transnational pharmaceutical industry that restricted access to medicines. For them, the South African case represented a chance to set a precedent for parallel importation and compulsory licensing under the TRIPS agreement.

Although the health of ordinary people was at stake, over time the Medicines Act court case had become the plaything of powerful, cross-cutting vested interests.

The case that wasn't

The case opened on March 5, 2001 amid widespread protests. TAC had called a global day of action against drug company profiteering, and supporters around the world were out on the streets. 5 000 activists marched past the US Embassy in Pretoria, ending outside the High Court building.

'It was very exciting. It was the beginning of a movement,' says Heywood. 'South Africa suddenly became the centre of the universe for a few days and everybody from CNN to the Australian Broadcasting Corporation was there.'

The courtroom was packed with ANC, trade union and TAC supporters wearing 'HIV Positive' T-shirts. International observers from organisations like Oxfam and Médecins sans Frontières were also present. Within a day, the case was adjourned to allow the industry's legal representatives more time to study the TAC's submission. The judge directed the PMA lawyers to address the TAC's allegations in a point-by-point reply.

During the six weeks that followed, pressure mounted on Big Pharma to drop the lawsuit.[374] Amnesic of their earlier support, several European ministers spoke out against the case, and UK Chancellor Gordon Brown urged the pharmaceutical companies to 'accept their share of responsibility'. When Nelson Mandela added his voice to the chorus of disapproval, his words were published around the world. 'I think the pharmaceutical companies are exploiting the situation that exists in countries like South Africa and in the developing world,' he said, 'because they charge exorbitant prices which are beyond the capacity of the ordinary HIV/AIDS person. That is completely wrong and must be condemned.'

Soon there was talk of a split within the industry group — with Merck and Glaxo pushing for a strategic retreat. The London *Observer* reported that when senior industry lawyers in New York and London saw the TAC's papers for the first time, they were forced to rapidly reassess their chances of success. Buried in the large mound of documents was an affidavit that challenged the basic tenets of their case. They had long argued that patent protection was necessary to create the profits they needed to research and develop new life-saving drugs. But James Love's affidavit[375] detailed his investigation into the development of new drugs in the USA, including the importance of academic research and government funding to their success.

'After we were admitted as *amicus curiae* they had to respond to the allegations in our founding affidavit,' says Heywood, 'and the allegations concerned profiteering, concerned price margins and concerned the actual cost of research and development. So if they had decided to continue with the case, then they would have had to reveal some of that — or explain why they couldn't, which would have been bad for them.'

Soon UN Secretary General Kofi Annan was brought on board to broker a compromise. He allegedly told representatives of the five leading pharmaceutical companies that their position on the court case was indefensible. He also telephoned President Mbeki in an attempt to facilitate a new round of negotiations.

When the case reopened on Wednesday April 17, PMA's South African lawyers were complemented by a second, slicker international team. Rumours abounded that a deal had been struck. A smiling health minister hinted at this when she told a barrage of local and international reporters that if the judge had any indication that the different parties would not reach a settlement, he would have thrown them out of court.

By Thursday it was all over. Big Pharma had withdrawn its case. The scenes inside the courtroom were as joyful as any political victory in bygone days. Government supporters danced on the wooden benches, popping open bottles of champagne. Outside, activists toyi-toyied and punched the air with their fists. There was jubilation and dancing in the streets. David had whacked Goliath, and lives would be saved.[376]

The health minister told the waiting press: 'Obviously this is a victory for us all.' She thanked everyone who had played a part. Tshabalala-Msimang confirmed that the deal had not forced the government to renege on any part of the legislation, but promised to seek pharmaceutical industry involvement when drawing up the regulations for the once-contested law. 'The government reiterates its commitment to honour its international obligations, including TRIPS,' she said.[377]

In question time the minister worked hard to correct the mistaken assumptions about drugs for HIV and AIDS. While there was no policy *not* to use antiretrovirals, she said, there were key issues that had to be sorted out before such drugs could be made available in the public health system. These were the same old issues of affordability and safety.

The director-general of health, Dr Ayanda Ntsaluba, followed this up with the confirmation that 'As of now, there is no offer on the table that puts antiretrovirals in the ambit of affordability for the South African public'. He also dismissed the prospect of offering post-exposure prophylaxis for rape survivors in the public sector.

For TAC leaders this was no surprise. But they had hoped, at least, for some acknowledgment for the role that they had played, expecting thanks, if not an olive branch. 'It was just the most unbelievable slap in the face,' says TAC spokesperson Nathan Geffen. 'Her callous statement that ART would not be implemented, and her failure to recognise TAC's role, was unbelievably rude, thoughtless and callous,' he says. 'That was the turning point in my mind. After that day things steadily went downhill with the government and Manto in particular.'

So after a brilliant and successful campaign, South Africa's 4,7 million HIV-positive people were no nearer to receiving life-saving drugs. For activists, it was an empty feeling. 'We weren't in this heady atmosphere that people were going to get access to treatment,' says Heywood, 'because we understood well enough that there was a very deep political resistance to HIV in South Africa.'

There were other reasons to be less than pleased with the outcome. The withdrawal of the case meant that there was no binding legal precedent on which future cases could draw. Furthermore, the government's defence of the law had indicated that they were not intending to use the law to allow local manufacturers to make cheaper generic alternatives to branded drugs (compulsory licensing). Although this had been one of the initial goals of the government's campaign, observers feared that it had been quietly negotiated away. What the government was really holding out for was the right to shop around abroad for branded drugs at the cheapest prices (parallel importation).

However, the case had thrown a spotlight on pharmaceutical industry practices and the world had pronounced judgement on the conflict between intellectual property rights and public health. This was to have immediate and long-term consequences. In November a new discussion opened at the World Trade Organisation around the interpretation of the TRIPS agreement. This resulted in the Doha Declaration on the TRIPS agreement and public health, which confirmed (in paragraph 4) that 'the TRIPS agreement does not, and should not, prevent members from taking measures to protect public health. Accordingly, while reiterating our commitment to the TRIPS agreement, we affirm that the agreement can and should be interpreted and implemented in a manner supportive of WTO members' right to protect public health and, in particular, to promote access to medicines for all. WTO members have the right to grant compulsory licences.'

This development removed the first and most obvious barrier to expanded access to antiretroviral treatment in poor countries. It paved the way for the WHO campaign to treat three million people by 2005, and the subsequent global pledge to universal access to AIDS treatment.

The irony of this tale is that it was the South African government — from its gutsy Medicines Act to the revolt in the World Health Assembly — that had been pivotal in removing obstacles to antiretroviral treatment in low-income countries across the world. But South Africans living with HIV and AIDS would continue to die for the want of these drugs for many years.

In the wake of its public relations debacle, Big Pharma worked hard to regain respect. AIDS drug prices continued to tumble. In South Africa the price of antiretrovirals in the private sector dropped to one-third of its former price. Even though the drugs were not available in the public sector, increasing numbers of wealthier people could now afford to pay for their own treatment.

Even for the TAC it was not all gloom. In its court papers the government had stated that affordability was the sole barrier to the use of antiretrovirals in the public sector. Writing later, Heywood commented that 'these unambiguous admissions have laid the foundations for the next stage of the TAC's mobilisation as well as for further litigation'.[378]

'Dr No'

If there had ever been any hopes for a détente between the TAC activists and the health minister, these were swiftly dispelled by their first joint meeting[379] after the court case. In early June, representatives of TAC, the trade unions and other organisations went to Pretoria to discuss the endless postponements of the promised programme to prevent mother-to-child transmission of HIV.

By now, none of the government's previous objections to the programme were valid. Not only were drug prices at a new low, but clinical trials had demonstrated the safety and effectiveness of nevirapine and it had been licensed by the Medicines Control Council. With the final obstacles removed, it was difficult to understand the continued delays around a programme that was estimated to cost under R1,99[380] per person and had the potential to save around 14 000 small lives a year.

In the meeting, Tshabalala-Msimang allegedly berated Heywood and Achmat, calling them 'sell-outs' and criticising them for singling out the needs of people with HIV and ignoring broader health needs. She dwelt on the impact of poverty in South

Africa's epidemic and the need to direct state resources to fight it. Antiretroviral drugs, she said, were too complicated, too toxic and had too many side effects to use in Africa. The TAC leaders were offended and aggrieved: they had repeatedly campaigned for strengthening health systems and fighting poverty alongside their demands for AIDS treatment.

Now that the fragile truce between the government and the treatment activists was over, TAC leaders returned to their former idea of mounting a constitutional challenge over the mother-to-child programme.

In July 2001 the TAC sent a letter to the government asking for legally valid reasons why the government would not make nevirapine available in the public health sector. The letter went on to ask whether the government would undertake to 'put in place a programme which will enable all medical practitioners in the public sector to decide whether to prescribe NVP (nevirapine) for their pregnant patients, and to prescribe it where, in their professional opinion, this is medically indicated.'

The three-page letter was so carefully crafted that it had taken the TAC and its lawyer Geoffrey Budlender a month to get it perfect; the way it raised the issues and the manner of the response would determine the outcome of a future court case, and indeed the future of treatment programmes in the country.

When the minister's reply finally came, it acknowledged the ethical dilemma for health workers but concluded that 'at the same time we need to balance their desire to provide the best treatment that they can for their patients with the government's obligations to root our public policies in the practical realities of the daily life experiences of all our citizens equally'.

For the TAC this was a major concession. As Heywood wrote later, the letter was the first admission by the minister that she knew the policy was intruding on the ethical duties of doctors.

Despite the sympathetic tone of the letter, the answer to the second question was an unambiguous 'no': the government would not make nevirapine available outside of the current research sites.

Minister Tshabalala-Msimang's response earned widespread condemnation — and the nickname 'Dr No'.

For a member of the liberation government, this nickname was a huge affront, as it was shared not only with the Bond villain but with a former politician of the extreme right-wing.

While there were reasonable grounds to fear the challenge of rolling out a full treatment programme, the continued refusal to prevent mother-to-child transmission was difficult to understand. On the minister's part, it seemed to be rooted in the conviction that antiretroviral drugs were toxic, and a desire to support the president's lingering affection for the denialist school of thought.

On August 21, 2001, the TAC filed a constitutional claim against the liberation government that it had supported for so long. It asked the court to confirm that the current policy infringed the right to health as guaranteed in the South African Constitution. It also asked the court to order the government to make nevirapine available in the public health sector to HIV-positive pregnant women to reduce the risk of vertical transmission. A series of affidavits[381] set out the scientific, legal and moral reasons why such an order was justifiable and why the government's policy was unreasonable.

Toxic shock

News[382] in September 2001 suggested an alternative explanation for the health minister's reluctance to roll out the mother-to-child programme. Virodene, the president's love-child of 1997, was back in the picture. And in a big way.

The press unearthed an incredible story of dodgy dealings and intrigue that gave pause to wonder if Virodene was not perhaps still the government's drug of choice. Although the Virodene trials had been officially halted by the Medicines Control Council in December 1998, this had not brought an end to the work: it just went underground.

The story only came to light because Virodene manager Zigi Visser was arrested in Tanzania for immigration control offences. It turned out that he had been organising clinical trials of the drug, which had been running for at least a year. The drug was being tested on HIV-positive Tanzanian soldiers, apparently against the wishes of the Tanzanian National Institute for Medical Research (NIMR), which like its South African counterpart had rejected the trial methodology. Visser claimed that the Tanzanian health minister endorsed the trials, which in any case were exempt from the usual procedures as they were being conducted in a military clinic. Another set of trials was taking place in a private clinic owned by the Tanzanian inspector-general of police.

By September 14, 2001, Visser was back in South Africa telling the press that his deportation was part of a plot by global pharmaceutical companies who were afraid of the potential impact of Virodene. 'It is a smear,' he said. 'Our work is top secret so I can't say much, but large international pharmaceutical companies and elements of the media are afraid of Virodene.'

Visser claimed that they had had excellent results. He said that they were going to Phase Three trials within six months and would soon be ready for global registration. He also told reporters that he did not believe that HIV was sexually transmitted or that it led to AIDS. Visser was convinced that world-approved antiretroviral medicines were too toxic.

Apparently Visser and his colleague had also been arrested the previous year for illegally importing Virodene into Tanzania. Around the same time, Tanzanian inspectors had seized a consignment of a compound called Oxihumate K[383], which was marked as being imported by the Tanzanian chief of defence. It turned out that Oxihumate was a nutritional supplement manufactured by Enerkom, a company owned by the government's Central Energy Fund. And it was being fed to soldiers at the Lugalo military hospital in Tanzania, the site of the Virodene trials. Tanzanian NIMR chief, Dr Andrew Kitua, said that 'there seemed to be a connection' between Oxihumate and the Virodene research.

A later report by the Department of Minerals and Energy claimed that Oxihumate was effective in the management of HIV and would be marketed some time in 2001. However, a year later, Enerkom was auctioned off and the nutritional supplement disappeared into obscurity.

The press then began asking hard questions about where the Virodene team had got the funding for its ongoing research. It was known that part of the money had come from the drug's new owners — a black business consortium headed by Joshua Nxumalo, a former ANC guerrilla turned businessman. But the news of the Tanzanian operation made it clear that the company had received other large cash injections over the years.

Journalists uncovered a cash trail from a black empowerment consortium whose CEO, Max Maisela, had strong links to the ANC and was said to be close to the president.[384] The funding allegedly amounted to over R17 million between June 1999 and September 2001. Maisela denied that the money had come either from him personally or from the consortium. But he freely admitted to being the go-between for a secret donor, or donors. The *Mail & Guardian* claimed that ANC treasurer-general Mendi Msimang, who was also the health minister's husband, had played a lesser role in these transactions.

The extent to which the Virodene business may have influenced the government's approach to antiretroviral drugs will probably never be known. Certainly at the time of the health minister's response to the TAC legal letter, it was not entirely out of the frame. It was clear that the health minister and the president had been receiving regular letters from Olga Visser throughout the year. In August 2001, Tshabalala-Msimang had even accepted Visser's invitation to visit the Tanzanian clinic where they were testing the drug. Tshabalala-Msimang's spokesperson denied that the department had any involvement in the Tanzanian trials, saying that the minister had visited the clinic only as a matter of interest.

A lecture[385] Mbeki gave at the University of Fort Hare, in October 2001, revealed the huge toll that the accretions of controversy had taken on his world view. Speaking on the theme of the responsibilities of African intellectuals, he hit out at certain black intellectuals who, he claimed, were influenced by their higher education to unconsciously reflect colonial and racist ways of thought. In what can only be seen as a reference to those who supported scientific views on HIV and AIDS, he said:

'And thus does it happen that others who consider themselves to be our leaders take to the streets carrying their placards, to demand that because we are germ carriers, and human beings of a lower order that cannot subject its passions to reason, we must perforce adopt strange opinions, to save a depraved and diseased people from perishing from self-inflicted disease... Convinced that we are but natural-born, promiscuous carriers of germs, unique in the world, they proclaim that our continent is doomed to an inevitable mortal end because of our unconquerable devotion to the sin of lust.'

Lucky

Lucky Mazibuko's profile as an HIV-positive newspaper columnist and spokesperson earned him an invitation to participate in the government's AIDS programme. 'The first thing I did was to work on the funding committee, where we had to scrutinise the funding applications from NGOs and CBOs,' says Lucky. 'It was fun for me because I was doing exactly what I wanted to do — helping the government to assist organisations that were doing sterling work in the communities. There are hundreds and thousands of people on the ground who cannot put up a financial plan properly, so my presence there ensured that organisations that I knew were doing exceptional work in the townships and rural areas got funding.'

Later Lucky was invited to sit on the South African National AIDS Council (SANAC). This was the body that determined AIDS policy, and was headed by the deputy president, Jacob Zuma. 'It was a wasted two years. When it came to the core issues, such as the provision of treatment, SANAC was toothless. When it came to the issue of "Does HIV cause AIDS?", SANAC was a government spokesperson. There were really crucial issues where SANAC should have showed itself but it never did... That caused me a lot of aggravation. I was very, very embarrassed that I had fallen into this trap.'

Lucky became increasingly uneasy at the elitist nature of the job. He felt that politicians needed more contact with ordinary people who were bearing the brunt of the crisis. 'The reality is, as soon as they become prominent leaders they live in a different world, they have bodyguards, they have chauffeurs, so their lives are such that they almost lose touch. So we need to remind them constantly of what is going on.'

Despite his frustrations with SANAC, Lucky feels that the government programme has been poorly served by journalists who lack an in-depth understanding of the complex issues around HIV, particularly antiretroviral therapy. 'You can't give it (ART) to everybody. What do they do in the meantime? You are not supposed to ask those questions, the president is not supposed to ask those questions. The minister, when she talks about garlic and beetroot, is being ridiculed by medical doctors... But you can pick up any form of medicine and the label says "Shake well, eat before you drink". But these people are saying "give antiretrovirals" irrespective of whether this person has eaten or not. And when the minister says "Eat beetroot and garlic" she is called Dr Beetroot, and all sorts of disrespectful names.'

Chapter Seventeen

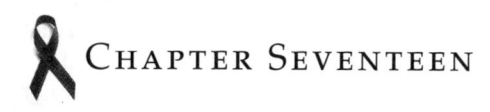

Little white crosses

The mother-to-child story so far...

Back in December of 1998, the founding mission of the Treatment Action Campaign had been to lobby for a programme to reduce the risk of mother-to-child transmission of HIV. At that time, the high cost of the drug AZT had been a major obstacle to implementing this programme across the country. Although the manufacturer offered a substantial discount, Health Minister Zuma had decided that a national programme was still unaffordable. After some months of conflict, TAC activists and Zuma pledged to work together to bring down the price of the drug. The manufacturer offered the named price, but by then the heat over the Medicines Act lawsuit had made the deal unacceptable to the government.

By early 1999 there was a new drug on the scene, which was both cheaper and easier to administer than AZT. Research (called the Saint trial) to confirm its efficacy was underway at Chris Hani-Baragwanath hospital and other sites around the country. The nevirapine regimen required only a single dose to both mother and child around the time of birth, at a total cost of about R25.[386] The new health minister, Dr Manto Tshabalala-Msimang, had welcomed nevirapine and was placing some importance on the outcome of the research

The Treatment Action Campaign agreed to tone down their demands until the results of the research were out, and the new drug was registered for perinatal use by the Medicines Control Council. All was going according to plan, albeit at a much slower pace than many would have liked.

Into this scenario, with its cross-cutting interests and complex science, came the president's exploration of AIDS denialism. The denialists' literature cast doubts on the efficacy of antiretroviral drugs and raised issues around their toxicity. AZT and the issue of antiretroviral therapy for pregnant women were high on their hate list. In the climate of hostility towards Big Pharma created by the Medicines Act lawsuit, the denialist paradigm seemed to make some sense, if only to the president and the health minister.

Next came the news of deaths on a clinical trial for nevirapine.[387] Although the drug was not being tested for mother-to-child transmission, nevirapine's status as the drug of the future seemed to be over.

In this environment of scientific scepticism and political paranoia, the cost of the drugs was of diminishing importance. In July 2000, when Boehringer Ingelheim offered a five-year supply of nevirapine free to all low-income countries, Tshabalala-Msimang reacted with undisguised suspicion. She said to the press 'What's very strange is that we met with them last Friday and they did not for even one minute indicate that they were going to make such an announcement, yet they made it about us and did not involve us in it'.

She refused the offer, justifying her inaction with reference to a WHO report that she misquoted as 'recommending that it (NVP) should not be used on a wide scale'.[388]

The Saint trial reported at the 13th International AIDS Conference in Durban, amid the controversies around the President's Advisory Panel on AIDS.[389] By now relationships between the government and the AIDS research community were at an all-time low. The research showed that nevirapine reduced transmission of HIV from mother to child by about 50 per cent, and compared favourably to another more expensive regimen using two drugs. Though the twin obstacles of price and efficacy had been adequately met, the minister failed to act on the long-awaited research.

In August 2000, the head of the government's AIDS directorate, Dr Nono Simelela, told a meeting of provincial health ministers that it was ethically important to provide nevirapine to pregnant HIV-positive women. However, the meeting ignored her recommendations and came up with a plan for a pilot programme with two sites in every province.

Throughout this period the pending Medicines Act lawsuit continued to muddy the water for any programme based on antiretroviral drugs. But even after the court victory in April 2001, it was clear that nothing was going to change. Babies were continuing to die for want of a programme that the UNAIDS had declared as cost-effective as immunisation — and South Africans wanted to know why.

It took the TAC until August 2001 to make the radical step of challenging the government in court.[390] Just over a month later the government replied to the charge — with 1 000 pages of papers defending their decision. A new court battle was about to begin, and this time the activists and the government were on opposite sides.

Making a plan

Behind the headlines of court action and protest, medical professionals across the land had been quietly ignoring the rules and getting on with the business of saving babies' lives.

Since the first health minister's rejection of the mother-to-child programme in 1998, officials in the Western Cape health department had gone their own way.[391] In January 1999, they began dispensing AZT to HIV-positive pregnant women in Khayelitsha, outside Cape Town. This was enabled by a quirk in the national political landscape that had seen the ANC losing political control of the province. The Democratic Alliance provided a unique space for alternative AIDS policies, although ironically both the provincial health minister of the day, Ebrahim Rasool, and the prime mover of the programme, Dr Fareed Abdullah, were ANC members. 'Ordinarily a civil servant at my level had the authority to… start a new programme, as long as you had the budget to do it,' says Abdullah, who was chief director responsible for health services in Khayelitsha at the time. 'So I used my authority and went ahead. I was asked to go to Pretoria and present the AZT programme to Dr Zuma, and there was quite a bit of discussion about it. There was certainly quite a bit of room to talk and to disagree.'

The programme survived two changes of provincial government, gaining strength and expanding along the way. When Abdullah heard about the Boehringer offer, he accepted, and scaled up the programme from two sites in Khayelitsha with AZT to 300 sites with nevirapine. By August 2001, the Western Cape programme was reaching half of women who needed the drug.

'Programmatically we just continued. Of all the work this

was the one programme that was top priority in thought and in practice,' says Abdullah. 'I just couldn't stand the injustice of a child becoming infected when it didn't have to happen. It consumed me personally for years, and it still does.'

Both Abdullah and the provincial department came under fire from the Department of Health for their actions on several occasions.

Out of fear of repercussions, or party loyalty, the other provinces chose not to follow the Western Cape's example. Tricky politics aside, their higher HIV burden would have made it difficult for them to roll out the programme without central government support. In these areas it was up to individual health facilities to try to make their own plans. And they did.

Throughout the late 1990s hospital doctors went to extraordinary lengths to procure the drugs they needed. There were many different ways this could be done.

At Chris Hani-Baragwanath doctors started their programme with drugs left over from their research programme. 'We had some mechanism to give AZT to people who didn't want to go onto the study. We had a little stash,' says Dr James McIntyre. 'We were lucky because we had a legal way to do it, but we could not expand outside the hospital.'

Then when that supply ran out, the team raised funding from UNAIDS, but they had to wait for three months for government permission to accept the donation. At the time McIntyre's colleague Dr Glenda Gray told the press: 'It's a relief to know AZT will be available. We have been waiting since March and have been forced to turn away about 200 women a month.'

Their commitment to their work earned them the displeasure of the minister. 'We were often quoted as the salesmen for Glaxo,' says McIntyre. 'In some ways I feel really offended by this, because the record we have and the work we've done speaks for itself, in terms of finding better solutions. We have been and still are, in some studies, funded by the pharmaceutical industry… Does that mean we blindly advocated pharmaceuticals as solutions? No. I don't think so.'

On the other side of the city, paediatricians at Johannesburg's largest teaching hospital were also making a plan. Without making too much fuss they provided treatment to pregnant HIV-positive women with donations from a church group. 'At that time there was nothing that said you can't do it,' says Dr Peter Cooper, who was senior paediatrician at the Johannesburg General Hospital.

'There were no consequences. Even at provincial department level, if they had known about it they would have been happy.'

In KwaZulu-Natal, where the HIV load was highest, some hospital doctors were buying nevirapine with their own money. In the remote northern reaches of the province, one medical manager had bought a R743-supply of the drug, and his colleagues were waiting in line to pay their share. Almost a third of the patients attending the antenatal clinic were HIV positive, and they wanted the drug. Doctors were prepared to offend the government, they said. 'It costs only 86 cents for a baby and R7,67 for an adult. It's a small cost and it's so easy,' they said.

As the death toll in the paediatric wards rose, rumblings of dissent and discontent in the provinces grew louder. In September 2000 the Gauteng premier's committee on AIDS announced that it would be expanding its research on mother-to-child transmission.[392] By December 2001 there were 12 pilot sites in local hospitals and clinics across the province, instead of the two stipulated by national government. Premier Mbazima Shilowa had even been alleged to remark that he would have only one pilot site for the new programme — and that site would be the whole province of Gauteng.

BACK TO COURT

Despite open revolt in the provinces and disagreements within her own department, the health minister stood her ground. She even ignored a letter from the TAC inviting her to settle the matter out of court.

In the run-up to the court case, the TAC took the widespread discontent over government policy to the streets. But there was a new tone to these protests. 'The images were very different,' says Mark Heywood. 'I remember one of the marches where people left a pile of a few hundred white crosses on the steps of the Senate House Building in Pretoria. You know to lay that responsibility at someone's door is not something you do lightly, and to lay that responsibility at the door of a progressive government, and of a government that comes out of our history is particularly not something you do lightly.'

On the eve of the court hearing in late November, 600 TAC supporters held an all-night vigil in a tent near the court in Pretoria. The weight of the issues and the heaviness of the final break with government seemed to permeate the night air. 'It was very tense and quite harrowing,' says Heywood. 'There was a lot of emphasis on people talking about their own experiences, mothers of children who had HIV…'.

Busi Maqungo was one of those mothers. 'We were singing the whole night and in the morning we made the small white crosses,' she says, 'and each had to write the name of a child that had died, and I wrote the name of my baby… It had been a long time since she died but I still felt sad. Lots of people were crying…'.

Maqungo's testimony was also one of several appended to the TAC founding affidavit.[393] In it she told the story of Nomazizi's fight with the illness that took her life. It ended simply, with the words 'I gave birth to an HIV-positive baby who should have been saved. That was my experience, the sad one, and I will live with it until my last day.'

Other affidavits came from medical professionals who attested to the urgent need for the drugs to be available in the public health system, and economists who demonstrated the affordability and practicability of the nevirapine regimen.

The State opposed the programme on the grounds that it was unaffordable, that the safety and efficacy of nevirapine was not fully proven, and that its widespread use risked a public health catastrophe. Neither the national nor provincial health ministers appeared in court. (The case was left to Director-General Ntsaluba and AIDS Director Simelela to argue, the two government officials who were known to be least opposed to the programme.) The cost of providing a comprehensive programme, including counselling and testing and information about breastfeeding and breast-milk supplements, was an important part of their case.

The TAC's case was strengthened by the fact that nevirapine was already being widely used. Affidavits from paediatricians like Cooper were able to describe the use of the drug in private practice and in a general hospital. 'Basically it was an ethical argument,' says Cooper. 'It was an ethical responsibility. If you've got the drug available you should give it. And because it is so cheap it should be provided free.'

The TAC's lawyers also provided evidence that there was sufficient capacity to allow the programme in many parts of the country. Approximately 84 per cent of all South African women gave birth under medical supervision, and HIV testing and counselling was already available in many antenatal facilities.

The High Court judge was speedy in his assessment of the case. In just over a fortnight he found in favour of the TAC, saying that a countrywide PMTCT programme was an 'ineluctable obligation of the State'.

The activists greeted this news with enthusiasm tempered by the knowledge that this was just the first in a long line of battles. Heywood told the *Saturday Independent*, 'we pursued the issue and now children can get the medication, but they need parents.'[394] He said that the TAC would now intensify its campaign and call for a national treatment plan.

Dr No strikes back

The health minister was out of the country at the time of the ruling, but on her return her response indicated that there would indeed be a battle. And it was not what TAC was expecting. Tshabalala sought leave to appeal the judgement — and she took this directly to the Constitutional Court.

In response, the TAC's lawyers asked the court to order the government to act on the judgement while awaiting the appeal. This was granted. But the minister was determined to hold her ground. The TAC's lawyer Geoff Budlender describes the circus of attack and counterattack that then ensued.

'The judge ordered that his order would not be suspended, pending the outcome of the appeal. Then they appealed against the judge's order that his order was not suspended, and they said now his order that it is not suspended is also suspended, therefore the original order was suspended, and so we went back to court again for an order that is not suspended. It was sort of leap frogging... and the result was we were in court over and over again.'

Not only was the minister determined to fight tooth and nail in the courts, but she continued to reject the recommendations of her own advisors. In January 2002, a progress report on the pilot sites was presented to a meeting of provincial health ministers. The study, commissioned by the Department of Health, recommended that the pilot sites be expanded, and that ways be found to reach women not covered by these sites. In short, it found that there was no good reason for delaying a national rollout of the programme. Despite this, the meeting decided to wait until the pilot programmes had been running for one year before rolling out the programme. When Tshabalala-Msimang finally gave a detailed account of the report to parliament[395], she told them: 'I know that some members of this house are looking for a simple "yes or no" answer from me. And they will, for the present, be disappointed.'

Although the court case was tied up in ongoing actions, the judge's initial finding seemed to remove the remaining obstacles in the provinces. Within a short space of time the leaders of the KwaZulu-Natal, Gauteng and Eastern Cape provinces announced their intention to scale up the programme. Even the president appeared to be in favour of expansion, telling a television audience in early February that provinces should provide the therapy according to their respective capacities.

But Tshabalala-Msimang still said 'no'. She publicly rebuked the provincial leaders for breach of policy and continued to pursue her case through the courts. By now, former President Nelson Mandela[396] had become involved in the dispute. He presented a prestigious award to McIntyre and Gray for their pioneering work on preventing vertical transmission, saying that the worth of the programme was 'beyond argument or doubt'. He also requested a special meeting with senior ANC leaders to discuss government AIDS policy.

In March 2002 the judge allowed the TAC's execution order on the grounds that it could save ten young lives a day. The minister then opposed this judgement, telling the Constitutional Court that the programme had the real potential to cripple an already over-burdened healthcare system.[397]

Then came another unforeseen complication. Registration of nevirapine for mother-to-child transmission was withdrawn in the US on the grounds of irregularities in the documentation of the original Ugandan trial. Although this was unrelated to the efficacy of the drug[398], and the WHO and UNAIDS were still prepared to attest to its safety, the Medicines Control Council indicated that it was considering de-registering nevirapine. This was one more weapon in the minister's arsenal. She told the SABC: 'I think the court and the judiciary must also listen to the regulatory authority, both of this country and the regulatory authority of the US.' She threatened to disregard the court's judgement. When asked for confirmation she replied 'I say no. I am saying no.'

Although the justice minister contradicted her, the ANC Youth League came out in strong support, saying, 'We wonder why does the court reduce itself to become an agent to drug profit for multinational pharmaceutical companies whose only interest is to make money out of sick people.'[399]

The minister's next court application raised new information on the safety of nevirapine. But that too was unsuccessful.

It is worth noting that nevirapine was never the TAC drug of choice. Although its efficacy and safety was not in question, there were combined drug regimens that were thought to be superior to the task. The TAC action centred on nevirapine solely because it had been the government's drug of choice, and the most affordable. In all their court submissions, the TAC specified that the programme should employ the best possible regimen for efficacy and cost.

OF SHEEP AND GEESE...

Although their arguments were never raised directly in the court case, the dead hand of the denialists cast a shadow over the proceedings. 'The unspoken argument of the case is the denialist argument,' says Budlender. 'It was never raised in the case because the Medicines Control Council had registered the medicine and WHO had said it was safe. Denialism is the only way to explain their opposition rationally. They weren't against MTCT programmes, they were against antiretrovirals.'

Two of the denialists who had served on the president's advisory panel, Drs Roberto Giraldo and Sam Mhlongo, had sought to influence the government's case at various times. In a paper written in October 2001, 'to provide technical assistance to the lawyers of the ministry of health', Giraldo expanded on his theories about causes and cures.[400] This paper repeated the denialist claim that poverty and malnutrition were the root cause of AIDS in South Africa, and proposed good nutrition as a solution, and even as a means to prevent mother-to-child transmission. 'Scientific studies support the contention that the use of vitamins by themselves could be enough to avoid what is known as mother-to-child transmission of HIV...', he wrote. 'If this is the case, as many clinical trials and scientific papers contend, it would constitute a very inexpensive and non-toxic practice for South Africa and other countries.'

Nutritional supplements, including vitamins and minerals, were also suggested as therapy for AIDS-related illness. Giraldo claimed that these ideas were not widely accepted because of 'the propaganda spread by pharmaceutical companies to commercialise their toxic antiretroviral medications'.

Giraldo's views were clearly valued by the minister, who invited him to South Africa in early 2003 to 'tap his expertise in the field of nutrition'.[401]

There were other indications that the government was taking nutritional therapy for HIV extremely seriously.

Enerkom, a company falling under the government's Central Energy Fund, had allegedly received some R80 million for research into a 'nutritional supplement' called Oxihumate. This chemical, created by the oxidation of coal, was being openly tested on HIV-positive people at Kalafong Hospital, in a Phase One trial sanctioned by the Medicines Control Council.[402] Later, Enerkom officials told the press that they were running Phase Two trials with 350 HIV-positive people in a Tanzanian military hospital — the same hospital that Zigi Visser had chosen for his Virodene trials (see Chapter 15).

Events in March 2002 confirmed the suspicion that the denialists were still at work in the subtext of the government's AIDS response. Under the leadership of the charismatic former ANC Youth League leader, Peter Mokaba, the denialist camp regrouped and made a public comeback. Mokaba had allegedly been approached by denialist journalist Anita Allen, and with her encouragement began distributing denialist literature within ANC structures.[403] Towards the end of the month, an emergency meeting of the ANC's highest body, the National Executive Committee, was held to discuss the matter, and Mokaba was given the floor. Observers commented that it seemed as if Mokaba had the 'endorsement of the party leadership'. The *Mail & Guardian* alleged that the minister tried to bring in health professionals who were members of the ANC health secretariat, and was not allowed to do so.[404]

This was followed by the distribution of an 80-page document outlining the denialist position.[405] The essay entitled 'Castro Hlongwane, Caravans, Cats, Geese, Foot & Mouth and Statistics' was a bewildering mix of fact and fantasy, acuity and misunderstanding, logic and paranoia. Written in flowery language and quoting liberally from philosophers and writers — from Herbert Marcuse to Mark Twain to John Le Carré — the document acknowledged the problem of AIDS in South Africa but rejected most aspects of orthodox AIDS science. The central accusation of the document was that the AIDS orthodoxy — referred to as 'the omnipotent apparatus' — downplayed the relationship between poverty, HIV and AIDS in order 'to sustain a massive political-commercial campaign to promote anti-retroviral drugs'.

The second familiar theme was that the scientific paradigm of HIV and AIDS reflected deeply entrenched white racist beliefs and concepts about Africans and black people.

'The war to defeat AIDS,' it said, 'is also a war to defeat the humiliation and dehumanisation of the African people.'

Like the president in his Fort Hare speech, the document was deeply critical of Africans who went along with the AIDS orthodoxy, saying:

'They too shout the message that — yes indeed we are as you say we are!

Yes, we are sex-crazy! Yes we are diseased…

Yes, we the men abuse women and the girl-child with gay abandon! Yes, among us rape is endemic because of our culture!

Yes, we do believe that sleeping with young virgins will cure us of AIDS! Yes as a result of all this we are threatened with destruction by the HIV/AIDS pandemic!

Yes, what we need and cannot afford because we are poor, are condoms and anti-retroviral drugs!

Help!'

Mokaba later admitted to co-authorship of the document, giving a round of interviews to the local and international press. 'HIV? It doesn't exist,' he told the *New York Times* [406]. 'The kind of stories that they tell, that people are dying in droves? It's not true. It's not borne out by the facts.'

This episode raised the ire of many within the party. In particular Dr Saadiq Karrim, who chaired the ANC's National Health Committee. He said people who believed the document might as well believe that the moon is made of green cheese. In reply, Mokaba accused him of being an ill-disciplined party member. The document had after all been adopted and endorsed for release by the ANC's National Executive Committee and the president. 'I want to know why he (Karrim) is fighting for just one tablet?' Mokaba asked.

On March 20, the ANC released a statement confirming that its policy was based on the assumption that HIV causes AIDS[407], but rejected both the TAC demands and the court order on mother-to-child transmission. It also stated unequivocally that antiretrovirals would not be made available in the public health system.

And Mokaba? He died of pneumonia less than three months later. He was 43 years of age.

Florence

In 2002, Florence Ngobeni landed a job in the human resources department of a large parastatal company that was beginning to grapple with the impact of the epidemic. 'People were off sick, people were dying,' says Florence. 'People were coming in with opportunistic infections and they were not willing to talk to anyone about it.'

The company was planning to introduce antiretroviral therapy and wanted to get a picture of the extent of HIV in the workforce. But people were reluctant to come forward.

'I worked to try and convince people to take up VCT (voluntary counselling and testing). I had a very bad experience. Because there were about 38 000 employees, and among those, none was openly positive.'

By now Florence was an internationally recognised HIV-positive advocate, and had five years of counselling and community work behind her. But the corporate world was alien to her, and she to them.

'My direct executive was really questioning my existence,' she says. 'She came to me once and said, "Do you know, you are so lucky to be here. People who are in your position (because I was a consultant) have at least two degrees." So she would tell me off all the time, and remind me that I'm not equivalent to them. I was the only person known to be positive... It was just too hard.'

There was also an undercurrent of hostility to the programme on the part of the line managers, who were suspicious and resentful of the fact that she had been appointed by top executives. 'Some of them were very reluctant to involve me in their problems or give me time to talk to their employees. You had executives pushing for VCT uptake, but the line managers were not sure... they wouldn't respond to my emails, if I called a meeting they didn't take me seriously.'

Despite the offer of life-saving drugs, the workers had good reasons to avoid the programme.

'Everyone back then was afraid. I came at the time when they were retrenching a lot of staff,' says Florence, 'and stigma was a big thing. Most of management were white people and the relationship between them and the employees was very shaky. Some of them (workers) asked me how I did it, because they couldn't see themselves coming forward. I had an office where they could just walk in privately. But they never came. People sometimes called me at home, and I would see them at home, or in a restaurant. A lot of them did confide in me, but not as part of the workplace programme.'

'By the time I resigned they were starting to get a grip. But it was too hard, too stressful, too bad for my health.'

Chapter Eighteen

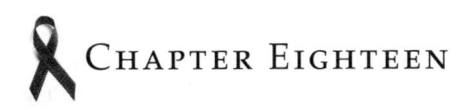

The moral economy

The turnabout

In early April 2002 the Constitutional Court made a decision on one of the many appeals that now comprised the tangled mother-to-child legal case. For the moment, at any rate, the government was obliged to implement the contested programme.[408]

Throughout all the wrangling, President Mbeki had kept his own counsel. But the day after the April court hearing he allowed his frustration with the activists to percolate through his weekly article[409] in the online journal *ANC Today*. In it he reiterated his views on the reciprocal relationship between poverty and ill-health. The president also lashed out at unnamed groups of people who he said were 'very determined to impose the view on all of us, that the only health matters that should concern especially the black people are HIV/AIDS, HIV, and complex anti-retroviral drugs, including nevirapine.'

'Some individuals engaged in politics and public health,' he wrote, 'seek to obtain public prominence on the basis of leading an extremely harmful and unacceptable campaign to deny our people all information and knowledge about the incidence of diseases of poverty in our country.'

Mbeki assured his readers that the government would not accept the harm caused, and the insult implied by these people. 'We will not be intimidated, terrorised, bludgeoned, manipulated, stampeded, or in any other way forced to adopt policies and programmes inimical to the health of our people,' he wrote. 'That we are poor and black does not mean that we cannot think for ourselves and determine what is good for us. Neither does it mean that we are available to be bought, whatever the price.'

But by now it was clear that there were serious differences within the party over the issue of AIDS and its treatment. The 'Castro Hlongwane' document and Peter Mokaba's outlandish statements about AIDS had created a whirlwind of adverse publicity for the government, and once again the country's international credibility was at stake. The health minister's battle with the highest courts in the land to avoid providing drugs for HIV-positive mothers added to the shame and confusion felt by many loyal ANC supporters.

The president, the health minister and several provincial premiers and party hotheads were ranged against a numerically stronger group of leaders who supported orthodox views on AIDS. Several of the latter group were themselves affected by the disease, and some were direct beneficiaries of the civil service medical aid scheme that paid for antiretroviral drugs. When the issue threatened to precipitate a major crisis, senior politicians acted swiftly to mitigate the damage, as they had done after the denialist controversy in 2000.

On April 17, 2002 an official cabinet statement confirmed the government's intention to abide by the temporary ruling of the Constitutional Court, and promised a national roll-out of the nevirapine programme. The statement included the first formal acknowledgement by the government that antiretroviral drugs could help improve the health of people living with HIV. It also reversed the ban on prophylaxis for rape victims and announced a new presidential task team on AIDS. The AIDS budget was to be almost doubled to R1,8 billion by the year 2004/5.[410]

But it was not all good news. The cabinet statement warned that antiretroviral drugs were still too expensive for universal access to treatment in the public health system. For TAC, and for people living with HIV, the struggle would go on.

BORN FREE

Despite the cabinet's acceptance of the nevirapine programme, the case had yet to make its final appearance in the Constitutional Court. It was an emotional day, even for the honourable judges. Justice Albie Sachs wrote this account:

'When we filed into court to deliver the judgment I saw that... it was packed with people — young and old, men and women, black and white, the nation — wearing T-shirts marked

"HIV Positive". There were also journalists from all over the world. The atmosphere was heavy as Arthur Chaskalson, the chief justice, in a magisterial voice read out a summary of our decision. The gist of our judgment was clear: since the drugs were available without cost and were deemed safe enough for use in the private sector and in the test sites, limiting their supply on the grounds that the government wanted to do further research on operational problems, was not reasonable. It had to be borne in mind that large numbers of children were unnecessarily going to be born with HIV in the meantime, and that doctors had said clearly that they wanted to prescribe the drugs but were prevented from doing so by directives from the ministry.

'... After the judgment was given, there was total silence. We filed out of the court and stood together for a moment in the passage behind. Then cheering erupted. And once more, I cried'.[411]

The TAC's Busi Maqungo, whose affidavit was one of several personal stories that had so moved the judge, was also elated at the news.

'I was really happy because I knew our kids were going to be born HIV free,' she says. 'It felt so good that I was part of the court case because I knew that my baby's death wouldn't have been in vain. Had she not died I would not have been involved in those struggles. But I had something pushing me from behind. I needed to do it.'

The outcome of the case galvanised the treatment programmes in the provinces. 'The impact of the court case was huge,' says Western Cape AIDS chief Fareed Abdullah. 'When there was national policy, that's all the provinces needed — a bit of room to go ahead. And they did. The court case was a turning point in AIDS history in this country.'

Health Minister Tshabalala-Msimang did not share in the elation of the moment. She was attending the Barcelona International AIDS Conference when the judgement was announced, and allegedly commented to a US journalist: 'The High Court has decided the Constitution says I must give my people a drug that isn't approved by the FDA. I must poison my people.'[412]

The judgement also had a wider significance. It confirmed that the social and economic rights outlined in the Constitution are legal rights that can be enforced by the courts.[413] 'The TAC case says... that the court will look at the reasonableness of the policy which is used to fulfil the rights in the Constitution, like the right of access to health care services,' says TAC attorney Geoff Budlender. 'It doesn't mean that the courts will say we are going to determine what best health policy is, but they will determine an envelope of what is reasonable and the department must bring itself within that frame of reasonableness.'

That frame did not require the government to implement the programme nationally with immediate effect, but instructed it to do so when and where it was appropriate and feasible. In this approach lay a threat to the government's long-stated arguments against a general treatment programme. By the same token, activists could now argue that parts of the public health system were ready, and able to provide antiretroviral therapy. It was a blow to the government's long-held argument about the unaffordability of treatment.

'The mother-to-child case was very deliberately chosen as the soft underbelly of the system, as the most compelling and obvious case: it was only one drug, very cheap and easily administered, and it was for children. And it was for prevention,' says Budlender. '(So) when it came to the question of a general treatment programme the government was on the back foot and they didn't know what arguments to put up.'

The activists immediately stepped up their campaign for a general treatment programme. Mother-to-child prevention was not enough, they said: babies need mothers, and HIV-positive mothers need drugs to prolong their lives.

The fear of the huge cost of a general treatment programme may well have been the underlying rationale for the health minister's resistance to the mother-to-child programme. But now the legal ground beneath her feet was shaken and the economic and moral claims for treatment were mounting.

CRY MURDER!

Now that the mother-to-child case was won, TAC members turned their attention to their next goal: access to antiretroviral therapy in the public health system. By now, TAC leader Zackie Achmat's health was failing, but he had taken a public stand, refusing to go onto antiretroviral drugs until they were available free to all who needed them. In July, Achmat was bedridden and his friends and supporters feared that he was dying. Nelson Mandela visited Achmat at his home to find out what would persuade him to change his mind, and emerged from the house to tell the press that he was going to take up Achmat's case with the president.[414] This event was reported across the world, giving publicity, and a human face, to the struggle for treatment.

By September 2002, the TAC had taken a decision to begin a civil disobedience campaign until the government provided antiretroviral therapy for all those in need. The campaign would entail volunteers actively breaking the laws of the land and offering themselves up for arrest in the style of the freedom volunteers of the 1950s. It was a huge step to take, and there were those who baulked at it. For example, trade union federation Cosatu, a partner in the TAC's campaign for treatment, drew the line at illegal acts against the democratically elected government.

In early October, on the occasion of the fourth anniversary of the Partnership Against AIDS, the government information service released a report on recent cabinet discussions about its AIDS strategy.[415] It spoke of a new engagement with the challenges of using antiretrovirals in the public health sector. Work had already begun, it said, on training health workers to deliver care, on guidelines and protocols, and on regulations 'to facilitate import and manufacture of cheap and generic drugs'. A technical task team drawn from members of the treasury and Department of Health had been appointed to address those challenges.[416]

A few days later, TAC leaders met[417] with the deputy president, Jacob Zuma, and agreed to suspend their plans for a civil disobedience campaign, to give the government more time to work on the framework of a treatment programme.

There was some confusion, however, about what they else they actually agreed. The joint statement issued after the meeting spoke of the importance of a process to negotiate a treatment framework. This would be done in Nedlac, the tripartite organisation representing business, labour and government. The TAC believed that this was the process that would shape the treatment programme, but evidently the government had other ideas. Although it participated in the Nedlac negotiations, it chose not to sign the final agreement, and went its own way.

Once again there was a contest over the issue of who should determine AIDS policy, with civil society groups petitioning the government for a foothold in the process.

While government officials maintained that they were working on the treatment plan, Tshabalala-Msimang's actions did not engender confidence on this matter. In early 2003 she invited denialist Roberto Giraldo to South Africa, to advise the government on nutrition and HIV. (This was the same Giraldo who had gone on record with his beliefs that nutritional supplements were superior treatment for AIDS than antiretroviral drugs.)[418]

After months of government inaction on the national treatment plan, the TAC revived the civil disobedience campaign, choosing March 21, Human Rights Day, for the launch.[419] It aimed to have 600 volunteers arrested in the first week, to symbolise the 600 South Africans who were dying each day of AIDS.

As on that fateful day in 1960, when protesters burnt their pass books and demanded to be arrested, TAC volunteers gathered at police stations around the country. There they laid charges of culpable homicide against the minister of health and the minister of trade and industry, and demanded to be arrested. This action passed without the tragic consequences of the Sharpeville protests of 1960, though in Durban police tear-gassed and beat peaceful demonstrators. It did, however, receive the media attention it was designed to create.

That weekend the government placed full-page advertisements in the newspapers detailing the extent of its HIV and AIDS programming. The TAC dismissed these as a 'wish list'.

The civil disobedience campaign marked the finality of the rift between the activists and the government. Relations had deteriorated to a point where parties swapped insults in public forums. The health minister's first public appearance after the launch of the civil disobedience campaign was disrupted by TAC activists blowing hooters and shouting 'Murder', 'Shut up' and 'Go to jail'. Achmat displaced the minister on the podium to read out his own statement, insulting her in derogatory terms. The minister refused to be deterred, and managed to complete her address flanked by police.

Next, the minister used the occasion of a cocktail party for important donors to attack the credibility of the protesters who were gathered outside. 'Our Africans say: Let us wait for a white man to deploy us... to say to us you must toyi-toyi here,' she said, apparently referring to Heywood, who was in the room.

When he shouted back 'You are lying, minister,' she thanked him for identifying himself.

Although the TAC suspended the civil disobedience campaign shortly after it began, it was questionable whether the rift could ever be repaired. The minister's credibility with the media was also at an all-time low. Like her predecessor, she could do no good. On occasions she was even attacked by journalists who were acting out of their own ignorance of the subject: like the time she asked them to speak of 'HIV and AIDS' rather than 'HIV/AIDS'. While they immediately imputed this to a belief that HIV did not lead to AIDS, in fact it was the international agency UNAIDS that had advised writers to stop using the 'slash' as it conflated HIV with illness and death.

Alongside the politics of the street, the TAC was also pursuing legal strategies to advance the cause of treatment. Since the success of the mother-to-child campaign, the government had good grounds to fear another court challenge. Geoff Budlender was penning frequent letters that had the indirect effect of pushing this message home. In parallel, it was pursuing Big Pharma directly in a legal case to reduce the price of antiretroviral drugs further — or to allow local generics manufacturers to make them.

We think it is too much

During the long legal and political battles over treatment access, the epidemic was continuing to unfold. Although by 1998 the exponential phase of the epidemic's growth had ended, HIV prevalence continued in a slow upward climb. The 2003 antenatal survey showed that 27,9 per cent of pregnant women had the virus in their blood. This national average masked large differences between the provinces and age groups.[420]

According to the brutal geometry of HIV, the epidemic curve was flattening out, but instead of this being good news, epidemiologists feared that it was merely proof of rising deaths. Mortality was kicking in, they warned, though it would not peak until 2010.

Research conducted by the South African Medical Research Council showed that mortality among young women was rising significantly. Their first report on the subject[421] showed that in the year 1999/2000, deaths of young women between the ages of

22 and 29 years were three and half times greater than in 1985. They estimated that AIDS was the single biggest cause of death in 2000, accounting for a quarter of all known deaths.[422]

HIV was fulfilling all the worst predictions made in the early years, wiping out young adults in their productive and reproductive years. A report by the United Nations Children's Fund estimated that by 2003 over a million South African children had already been orphaned by AIDS.[423]

On the ground, the tragedy was palpable. The hospitals were buckling under the strain, with some reporting that up to 90 per cent of their patient load was HIV related. Growing numbers of health professionals began to plead with the government to allow them to treat their dying patients with antiretroviral drugs. In July 2003, health professionals at Chris Hani-Baragwanath collected signatures from over 60 per cent of the hospital's medical staff asking for drugs and better training to prevent AIDS deaths. Nurses told the press, 'We are seeing people die, and we think it is too much.'[424]

The burgeoning death toll focused new attention on the economic impacts of HIV. The private sector was already feeling the burden of illness and death on productivity and healthcare costs. By 2002 Anglo American had estimated that the disease was costing its operations between $4 and $6 per ounce of gold.[425] Their economists believed this would rise to $9 if nothing was done to manage the impact. In response they announced their intention to implement an antiretroviral treatment programme for all employees. Dr Brian Brink, who headed the company's AIDS programme, had been pushing for such a programme for several years, but until now management had not been convinced. At first the drugs were too expensive, but as that challenge diminished and new regimens simplified the treatment, attitudes began to change. 'The weight of evidence in favour of treatment was beginning to build up and tip the balance,' says Brink. Soon came the day that Anglo CEO Tony Trahar called Brink into his office and said, 'You know, we have got to get on. We have got to do this.'

Before the announcement, Brink had made several failed attempts to get a meeting with the health minister and the director-general of health. He even faxed their plans to the president's office, but there was no response. But when the minister heard the news, she berated the company for entangling the government in its plans. She was most concerned that people who left Anglo's employ would be a burden on the public health system.[426]

The growing economic burden of illness and death began to focus more attention on the macro-economic impacts of the epidemic. Previous modelling exercises had come up with contradictory results, and it was widely believed that the economic impact of AIDS would be felt most keenly at the level of the community and family.

'It is a harsh economic reality that not all lives have equal value,' wrote economists Clem Sunter and Alan Whiteside in 2000.[427] 'If the majority of those who are infected are unemployed, subsistence workers or unskilled workers, then the impact on the national economy will not be as great as if they are skilled and highly productive members of society.' Some economists had even concluded that by removing unproductive members from the society, per capita income could actually rise. At worst, South African economists agreed, the epidemic would shave half a percentage point off annual growth for the next 14 years.

This type of economist thinking had long provided the underlying rationale for the government's refusal to provide treatment programmes. The argument went that many more 'life-years' could be saved by the prevention of new HIV infections than by spending money on expensive treatment. It was therefore the moral obligation of the government to spend the health budget wisely by investing more heavily in prevention programmes.

But as the scale of death to come became more manifest, these arguments lost their ring of truth. International economists began to revise their assumptions and came up with alternative scenarios that were discomforting to say the least. In July 2003, a new World Bank modelling exercise[428] predicted that if nothing was done, the epidemic would lead to the collapse of South Africa's economy in three generations. This study examined, for the first time, the economic consequences of the long-term loss of human capital, which would result in generations of orphans without parenting, education or social skills.

At the time, Finance Minister Trevor Manuel dismissed the report as an 'unfortunate scare story'. But this new take on the economy must have given pause for thought, because a few weeks later, in response to a question from businessmen on how they should deal with AIDS, Manuel advised them to step up

HIV and AIDS training and discussion about nutrition to extend the lives of affected people — and 'further down the line', the provision of antiretrovirals.

South African economists began discussing the economic cost-benefit of treatment in much wider terms. Professor Nicoli Natrass[429], at University of Cape Town's school of economics, criticised the government's approach which she characterised as a 'triage economy' that sought to ration scarce resource for AIDS. Natrass argued that the severity of the AIDS crisis called for a 'moral economy', and warranted the allocation of substantial new resources to deliver treatment programmes. These would not only save lives but enhance prevention efforts. 'AIDS is different,' she wrote, 'because it is a public health crisis which not only has deep social roots but challenges the very notion of what it means to be a society.'

Since the beginning of the new millennium, international thinking about HIV and AIDS had turned increasingly around the broader developmental impacts of the epidemic. It was now understood that security, governance and sustainable development would all be weakened by the impact of AIDS deaths. And with this knowledge came the understanding that expanding access to antiretroviral treatment was not just a moral obligation, but a necessity for the future of countries worst-affected by HIV.

International agencies like UNAIDS and the World Health Organisation began to argue more forcefully for expanding treatment programmes in low-income countries, and African politicians began considering the issue with the seriousness it deserved. Botswana, which at that time had the highest HIV prevalence in the world (at 32.9 per cent of antenatal attendees), kicked off with a pledge to offer universal access to antiretrovirals in the public health sector. Funds were to be provided by the government, in partnership with pharmaceutical companies and donors.

ONE MORE DEATH IS TOO MANY

Pressure on the government to deliver treatment was coming from all sides. In May, Cosatu began to consider mass action against the government. 'If they don't come to the party we'll even take our people to the streets,' said spokesperson Caroline

Scheepers. 'We can't afford the drugs, as the working class. Many people are dying.'

The first clear signal of change came in early July, when on the eve of President Bush's first South African visit, President Mbeki told CNN[430] that he didn't imagine that there would be any problem coming to an agreement on funding for antiretrovirals.

The combination of pressures and forces on the South Africa government to endorse the national treatment programme were finally hitting home. The moral, social and economic rationale for doing so was now clear. And with an election looming, there were fears that the ANC would lose support on this one emotive issue. Sources claimed that a group of senior ministers was working hard to effect a U-turn in government policy

On 8 August, a special meeting of the cabinet was convened to discuss the long-awaited report from the task-team investigating the treatment plan. They agreed to go ahead, and the Department of Health was instructed to come up with a detailed operational plan. 'Government shares the impatience of many South Africans on the need to strengthen the nation's armoury in the fight against AIDS,' the cabinet statement read.

Announcing the news to experts and activists at a conference in Durban, the KwaZulu-Natal health minister Dr Zwele Mkhize said, 'There is no question about this. It must be placed on record that this is not an ideological issue. With the rising mortality rate from AIDS, one more death is too many.'

By November 2003 the treatment plan was complete and the finance minister had allocated R5 billion for antiretrovirals over the coming three years. The long struggle for the right to treatment was over. The challenge of delivery was to begin.

Epilogue

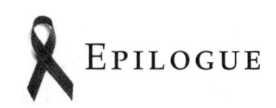

2005, and the band played on...

It's November 2005 and I am back in South Africa after several years' absence. The silence around AIDS has broken — everyone is talking about it, everyone knows someone who has died.

It is two years since the South African government pledged to provide antiretroviral therapy to all who need it. People I speak to have strongly divergent views on how well the programme is going. There are those in government health facilities who say they are working around the clock to save lives. So far nearly 100 000 people are receiving treatment at 183 sites[431]. This is the largest treatment programme on the continent and second only in the world to Brazil, which has had a decade's head start in providing drug therapy to people living with HIV.

Others are critical. There is resistance in the health department, they say, and the programme is rolling out far too slowly. After all, treatment is reaching only 21 per cent of the million who are in need. In percentage terms this puts South Africa way down the league table — between Lesotho and Cameroon (the average for the continent is 17 per cent).

It is clear that there are problems, not only on the supply side, but the demand side too. I hear so many tragic stories about individuals who choose to die a painful death rather than expose themselves to testing and treatment... young people with university degrees and professional careers included. So it seems that the climate of stigma and denial still prevails. Strong leadership is still needed from those who command authority and respect.

Towards the end of November, the Human Sciences Research Council releases the results of a major new household survey. Researchers have interviewed 23 000 men, women and children across the country and tested 16 000 for HIV. The national prevalence rate for all adults is just over 16 per cent, but it peaks alarmingly among women in the 25- to 29-year age group. One-third of young women in this age group have the virus in their blood. And it is people living in informal settlements around the cities and towns who have by far the highest levels of HIV. As with previous surveys of this nature, the majority of those interviewed (66 per cent) do not believe they are at risk of contracting HIV. And while the majority have heard of antiretroviral therapy, only about half of people interviewed say they would actively seek it out if they needed to — one-fifth being too afraid of side effects, or even death.[432]

December 2005... World AIDS Day. Health Minister Manto Tshabalala-Msimang is speaking on SABC radio. She is upbeat. We are winning the war against AIDS, she says. There is a gratifying increase in awareness and prevention is working among teenagers. But there are still many challenges ahead....

Listeners are invited to phone in with their questions. Some praise the minister for her good work. But not all of them agree. Caiaphas, for one, seems to think she owes the nation something of an apology.

'I have absolutely no apology to make to the nation,' the minister replies. 'I have always had a very open mind... on issues of nutrition, absolutely not. I have seen bedridden patients who have been given beetroot, garlic and olive oil and they have got better. I have seen patients improve on ARVs. You can't pin me to ARVs.'

Another caller asks about the vitamins that are being promoted by the Rath Foundation as a treatment for HIV. The previous day's papers carried a report that the Treatment Action Campaign has filed a court interdict to prevent Matthias Rath from promoting his medicines as an alternative to antiretroviral therapy, and from conducting unauthorised trials on people living with HIV.[433] The TAC is also asking the court to find that the health minister and her department have a duty to stop Rath doing this. The caller is puzzled and confused by these goings-on and asks the minister to explain.

Dr Tshabalala-Msimang assures him that vitamins and nutritional supplements are part of a comprehensive plan. They are not medicines and they don't have to be tested, she says, so there is really nothing wrong. She claims that Rath is not saying that 'vitamins alone' can cure.

This latter statement provokes a firestorm of attack. The opposition Democratic Alliance's spokesperson on health, Dianne

Kohler-Barnard, insists that Rath has categorically claimed that vitamins cure HIV. He is conducting illegal trials, she says, and people have died. Voices are raised. The programme starts to deteriorate into an angry shouting match. But the minister has the final word:

'I have said that ARVs do not kill. I will not be straight-jacketed to support ARVs only. It needs a multi-pronged approach — nutrition, food supplements and traditional medicines. People have three things to choose from.'

The new Medicines Act is at last in force. And as predicted in 1997, it has led to a weakening of the medicines regulatory body. The role and function of the Medicines Control Council[434] lies at the heart of this new controversy around the Rath vitamin cure. Allegations of misuse of pharmaceuticals have been made, but the Council is reluctant to act. Many are concerned about this turn of events: one legal expert describes the minister's actions in this regard as part of a calculated and coordinated 'war on science'.

Perhaps it is not so much a war on science as a postmodern attack on science, in which a critique of racialised views on sexuality and culture and an analysis of the vested interests of Big Pharma have shaped an alternative Africanist paradigm. History, and the people of this wounded land, will be the judge of it.

And as for the controversial section 15C of the Medicines Act, the much fought-for provisions have yet to be used. After a court challenge from the TAC, pharmaceutical companies eventually agreed that local generics manufacturers could make cheap copies of patented antiretrovirals for local use and for export to other African countries. Thanks to the TAC, and not the Medicines Act, the bulk of antiretrovirals dispensed in the State programme are being manufactured by a local pharmaceutical company.

The day I visit Busi Maqungo it is her son Lutando's third birthday. Falling pregnant by mistake in 2002, Busi thought about having a termination, but she feared that it would haunt her for the rest of her life. This pregnancy differed significantly from the last, as nevirapine was available, and Busi made sure she, and the newborn baby, took the drug. It was a long and anxious wait, but eventually Lutando was diagnosed HIV negative. 'Although I knew the drugs worked,' says Busi, 'I still couldn't believe it. It's just a miracle. One dose of nevirapine can save the life of a baby.'

While Busi is telling me about her life with HIV, Lutando is being entertained by his older brother in the adjacent room.

He soon tires of this (after all it is his birthday) and his assertive shouts blot out our voices on the tape. I learn that he has been nicknamed Luciano, for the fine tone of his voice.

Busi's courage to confront her HIV status has given her, and her boys, chances that they would not otherwise have had. They have recently moved from an informal settlement in the Cape Flats to a pristine housing estate on the edge of Cape Town. Busi has travelled far in life — from a childhood of abuse and abandonment in rural Transkei to the life of an international HIV advocate.

In a Johannesburg tea garden, Peter Busse is enjoying a banana milkshake. Since he left Napwa in 1999 he has rebuilt his career as an international consultant on HIV and AIDS. He uses participatory workshops to educate people about the personal and political implications of the epidemic. Members of the London Stock Exchange and university students in Canada are but two of his recent audiences.

Peter is reminiscing about the long, hard road of South Africa's AIDS response. For him the highs have been to do with the fantastic array of people he has worked with over the years. 'Also the positive people — despite all kinds of neglect they have been remarkable. When I first came out you could count on two hands the number of people who were open. And now there are vast amounts.'

The low of it all has been the incredible sense of expectation that came with the advent of democracy in 1994 — and then the scandals and the disappointments and the conflicts. 'Eleven years later you sit here and think, where did it all go wrong?'

Peter's personal journey with HIV has also had its highs and lows; he will never forget the graph drawn by the doctor on the day of his diagnosis. 'The main thing that sticks in my mind was... just draw a little picture, just draw a horizontal and a vertical, and from the top of the vertical, draw a line down 45 degrees, with an arrow. That is what Denis drew. So there was no possibility of it going up or reversing. That was the progression. Inevitably downwards... towards death.'

Earlier this year Peter celebrated his twentieth year of living with HIV with a huge party for all his friends. But recently his health has crashed. In the ten or so years I have known him, I have not seen him so gaunt. He needs to slow down, to take a rest. His friends are concerned; Peter has always managed his health in his own way, and nothing will prevent him from flying around the world to advocate for the people living with HIV.

A few weeks later Peter falls disastrously ill. Friends rally around, help is sought, but it is too late: his liver has failed. In the early hours of January 6, 2006 he dies in the Johannesburg General Hospital. *Hamba kahle* Peter, these pages are dedicated to you....

Leading South African AIDS denialist Prof Sam Mhlongo also dies, in a car crash, later in the year. Denialist bloggers[435] speculate how this may have occurred... 'I don't mean to sound paranoid, but I do believe that the AIDS mafia is capable of this,' one writes. 'Though, of course, their preferred method would have been to covertly do something to him to make him get sick, and then say it was "AIDS"... Something like what they "may" have done to Peter Mokaba.'

2007... STILL PLAYING

During a serious illness in late 2006 the health minister appears to lose her grip on the government's AIDS programme. While she is in hospital, the deputy president, the deputy health minister and the head of the AIDS directorate assume stewardship of the AIDS response.[436] They make peace with their critics in the trade unions and civil society organisations, with the activists and the experts and the TAC. A new and improved five-year national AIDS plan is released... a plan of promise, it is said.[437]

In March 2007, Tshabalala-Msimang undergoes a liver transplant, but it soon becomes clear that she is not planning to retire on the grounds of ill-health. Even before she returns to work she has engaged in a new conflict with the AIDS fraternity. She publicly withdraws from a major scientific conference on HIV and AIDS, on the grounds that she has not been accorded a proper place in the line-up of speakers.[438] Opening the conference, Deputy President Phumzile Mlambo-Ngcuka[439] chastises the organisers. 'This type of politics is very unhelpful,' she says, 'and doesn't contribute to the environment we are building to fight the battle together. Fight those battles elsewhere if you have to.'

A few weeks after the health minister has resumed office, reasons are found to fire her deputy, Nozizwe Madlala-Routledge, who has been credited with the new improved national AIDS plan.[440] This turn of events provokes the fury of the activists and widespread condemnation at home and abroad.

Calls are made for the minister to resign. The *Sunday Times* publishes articles alleging that the minister had been fired from a hospital job in her exile days, for stealing from patients.[441] They also claim to have medical records showing that the minister abused alcohol while in hospital for surgery during 2005. Court intervention is sought and won, and the *Sunday Times* is forced to return the minister's stolen medical records.

In his weekly article in the online journal *ANC Today*, President Mbeki comes to Tshabalala-Msimang's defence.[442] Recalling their shared journey into exile in 1962 and her subsequent commitment to the struggle, he eulogises her as a genuine heroine of the liberation struggle. In a second article, he tackles those who have criticised the minister's theories on HIV and nutrition. Mbeki writes that the media has been guilty of deliberately misrepresenting the minister's views in order 'to ridicule, discredit, defeat and completely exclude from all medical practice relating to HIV and AIDS, all arguments about the critical importance of good nutrition and other non-pharmaceutical interventions.'

'Consistently, and with no sense of shame,' he writes, 'some in our country and the rest of the world have waged a determined campaign to falsify and otherwise vulgarise what the ANC and our government have been saying... Among other things they have claimed that we were arguing that poverty and malnutrition cause HIV and AIDS, and that, medically, the AIDS syndrome could be addressed by tackling poverty and malnutrition, without resort to therapeutic interventions specific to the clinical indications manifested in each patient...

'Stripped of all pretence, the violent hostility to our movement, our government and our Minister of Health on the issue of HIV and AIDS derives and is centred on our deliberately careful approach to the use of antiretroviral drugs.'

Although this article is reported across the world, the mass media highlights the president's emotional defence of the minister they most love to hate. None seem to appreciate that this is the president's first major statement on HIV and AIDS since 2000. Nor that it is a clear acknowledgement of the science of AIDS.

Will the band play on until the last musician drowns?

Lesley Lawson,
London,
September 12, 2007

Endnotes and references

1. Garrett, L. 2000. *Betrayal of Trust*. New York: Hyperion.
2. Shilts, R. 1987. *And the Band Played On*. New York: St Martin's Press.

Prologue: 1996, MASHAYABHUQE – AIDS KILLS EVERYTHING

3. Sizakele and her mother were interviewed in the film, *Mashayabhuqe, AIDS hits everyone*, Directed by Lesley Lawson, produced by Robyn Hofmeyr, Jenny Hunter, Teaching Screens, broadcast on eTV on December 2, 1998.
4. The Nzama family were interviewed in the film *Mashayabhuqe*, 1998.

PETER
5. Yeoville — a down-at-heel inner-city suburb of Johannesburg where Peter had lived for several years.

Chapter One: FROM GAY PLAGUE TO AFRICAN AIDS

ISOLATED CASES
6. By the end of 1983 there had been 3 064 cases of AIDS reported in the USA. Of these, 1 292 people had died. The vast majority of these were gay men, although some cases in women, children and haemophiliacs had already been reported. At this time there was no test for HIV.
7. A good history of HIV and AIDS in this period is available online at:
   www.avert.org/his81_86.htm
8. Coen Slabber's statement on homosexuality was in 1983; this and other early statements of the NP government are quoted in:
   Grundlingh, L. 2001. 'A critical historical analysis of government responses to HIV/AIDS in South Africa' as reported in the media, 1983-1994. Paper presented at a seminar at Rand Afrikaans University, Friday May 25.
9. For an account of the legislation against homosexuality:
   Cameron, E. 1995. 'Unapprehended felons. Gays and lesbians and the law in South Africa' in *Defiant Desire*, eds M Gevisser and E Cameron. New York: Routledge.
10. Surveys on attitudes towards homosexuality and AIDS:
    - A 1987 survey of Cape Town residents found that 71 per cent believed homosexuality morally wrong. Quoted in Christiansen, E. 2000. 'Ending the

- apartheid of the closet: sexual orientation in the South African Constitution'. *J Int Law and Politics*, 32, 997.
- A survey of black university students found that 82 per cent believed gay men and women had AIDS: Quoted in Nicholas, L, Tredoux C & Daniels P. 1994. 'AIDS knowledge and attitudes towards homosexuals of black first-year university students: 1990-1992'. *Psychol Rep*, 75 (2) 819-23.
- Nkoli, S. 1995. 'Wardrobes: Coming out at a gay activist in South Africa' in *Defiant Desire*, eds M Gevisser and E Cameron. New York: Routledge.

11 Simon Nkoli was one of the accused in the Delmas treason trial, which ran from 1985 to 1989.

'AFRICAN AIDS'

12 In the early days of the epidemic it was common to refer to pattern I and pattern II countries. Pattern I countries were the American, European and Scandinavian countries, and Australia, where HIV was found primarily in men who had sex with men and injecting drug users. Pattern II countries were the countries of sub-Saharan Africa where HIV was found among heterosexuals, transmitted sexually, in unsafe blood and vertically from mother to child.

13 ABC *Nightline* story was broadcast in October 1986.

14 Primate origin of the virus:

Although there were several aspects of this hypothesis that were incorrect, later research shows that HIV skipped the species barrier for the first time in the 1930s. The virus HIV-1 is thought to have originated from a certain species of chimpanzee indigenous to central West Africa. A second virus, HIV-2 — which is currently prevalent in West Africa — is thought to have originated from a particular species of monkey. HIV-1 is thought to be more virulent than HIV-2.

15 An account of the current thinking and research about the origin of HIV is available at: www.avert.org/origins.htm

16 'Sex with monkeys' anecdote told by Dr Peter Piot interviewed in the film *6000 a day. The story of a catastrophe foretold*. Arte 2001.

17 'Injecting monkey blood/monkey toys' anecdote in Chirimuuta, R C, and Chirimuuta, R J. 1989. *AIDS, Africa and Racism*. London: Free Association Books.

18 'Nairobi hooker' story — 3/2/1987, *Guardian*, quoted in Chirimuuta and Chirimuuta, 1987, ibid.

19 Rosenberg, C. 1992. *Explaining Epidemics and other studies in the History of Medicine*. Cambridge: Cambridge University Press.

RACISM AND DENIAL

20 An account of the first symposium of AIDS in Africa is given in:

Misser, F. 1986. 'Trying to break the African connection'. *New African*. January, 13-14.

21 High HIV estimates made by Panos in 1986 are described in Chirimuuta & Chirimuuta, 1987, op cit.
22 African responses to the early epidemic in:
- Kibedi, W. 1987. 'AIDS: an African viewpoint'. *Dev Forum*. Mar, 15 (2): 1, 6.
- Misser, F & Brisset, C. 1987. 'Africa not interested in EEC help on AIDS'. *New African*. April, 16.
- Hitchcock, B. 1986. 'Clampdown on AIDS information in E Africa'. *New African*. January, 9-10.
23 Duesburg, P. 'Retroviruses as carcinogens. Expectations and reality'. *Cancer Research*, 1987 47, 1199-1220.
24 The spectrum of views of the denialists may be found on the website: www.virusmyth.net
25 Professor Kary Mullis won the Nobel Prize for Chemistry in 1993 for his invention of the polymerase chain reaction (PCR) method, which facilitated the process of making copies of DNA.
26 The first clinical trials of AZT for treating HIV were started in 1986. See Chapter Ten for more about AZT.
27 'Call of the Group for the Scientific Reappraisal of the HIV/AIDS hypothesis'. *Science*. Feb 17, 267, 1995.
28 National Institute of Allergy and Infectious Diseases. 2003. The evidence that HIV causes AIDS. Created November 1994, updated February 2003. Available at: www.niaid.nih.gov/factsheets/evidhiv.htm
29 *New African* articles suggesting alternative AIDS hypotheses:
- Misser, F. 1986. 'Malaria antibodies in their blood'. January.
- Misser, F. 1996. 'Africa has been the site of US experiments to test new viruses for biological warfare'. March.
- Also suggestions that HIV was invented by the Rhodesians and/or South African security forces in their struggle to maintain white supremacy in articles by Rake, 1998; Ankomah, B, March 2001.
30 An account of Mhlongo's experiences in London are given in:
Shenton, J. 2000. Interview with Professor Sam Mhlongo, *New African*. July-August.
31 False positives — it is widely acknowledged that early versions of the HIV test gave false positives. However the combination of tests currently used are said to be 99, 5 per cent accurate. www.avert.org/testing.htm

THE VIRUS CONTD...

32 HIV statistics available at www.unaids.org
33 No evidence of a hetereosexual epidemic in South Africa: Shoub, B. 1987. 'AIDS in South Africa — a time for action'. *SAMJ*. 71, 6 June 677.

Chapter Two: THE VIRUS UNDERGROUND

THE BREACH IN THE CORDON

34 Malawian miners could take up two-year contracts. They were the only ones allowed to do so.
35 Kark, S. 1949. 'The social pathology of syphilis'. *S Afr Med J.* 23:77-84. Reprinted in *Int J Epidemiology*. 2003; 32: 181-186.
36 The Chamber of Mines is the employer organisation for the mining industry.
37 The prevalence rate of HIV among mineworkers of different nationalities in 1986 was Malawi 3,76 per cent, Botswana 0,34 per cent, Lesotho 0,09 per cent, Mozambique 0,09 per cent, Swaziland 0,05 per cent, South Africa 0,02 per cent.
38 The results of the Chamber of Mines HIV surveillance are discussed in:
    - Jochelson, K, Mothibeli, M & Leger, J P. 1991. 'Human immunodeficiency and migrant labour in South Africa'. *Int J. Health Servs. 21 (1): 157-173.*
    - South African Institute for Race Relations. 1988. *Race Relations Survey 1987/88*, Johannesburg: SAIRR.
39 The formation of the WHO's GPA and the UN General Assembly from AIDS chronology, UN Chronicle. www.un.org
40 Regulations making AIDS notifiable and prohibiting 'aliens' with HIV reported in: South African Institute for Race Relations. 1989. *Race Relations survey 1988/89.* Johannesburg: SAIRR.

MEN ALONE

41 The Witwatersrand University project and interviews are described in Jochelson, Mothibeli & Leger. 1991. op cit.

THE MANY FACES OF DENIAL

42 Chamber comment quoted in Jochelson, Mothibeli & Leger, op cit.
43 Migrants more likely to have HIV:
    - Lurie, M, Harrison, A, Wilkinson, D, et al. 1997. 'Circular migration and sexual networking in rural KwaZulu-Natal'. *Health transition review.* Supp 3, (7) 17-27. Available at http://htc.anu.edu.au/pdfs/Lurie1.pdf
    - Lurie, M. 2002. 'Migration and AIDS in southern Africa: challenging common assumptions'. *A&M News*. October 4 2002: 11-12.
44 Campbell, C. 2003. *Letting them die. Why HIV/AIDS intervention programmes fail.* Oxford: James Currey.
45 Carletonville miners' HIV statistics:
    'A targeted intervention falls short'. 2005. *Horizon* December.
46 The results of the 2001 survey were never made public. However they are quoted in:
    Williams, B, Gouws, E & Frolich, J, et al. 'Lessons from the front'. UN-NGLS,

Voices from Africa. No date. Available at:
www.un-ngls.org/documents/publications.en/voices.africa/number10/8williams.htm

THE VIRUS EMERGES

[47] Martin, M, Schoub, B & Padyachee, G, et al. 1990. 'One year surveillance of HIV-1 infection in Johannesburg, South Africa'. *Trans R Soc Med Hyg*. Sept-Oct 84(5): 728-30.

[48] Testing of over 6 000 samples between 1988 and 1989:
Martin, D J, Schoub, B D, Padyachee, G N, Smith, A N, et al. 1990. 'One year surveillance of HIV-1 infection in Johannesburg, South Africa'. *Transactions of the Royal Society of Tropical Medicine and Hygiene*. Sep-Oct Vol 84 (5) 728-30.

[49] HIV prevalence was doubling rapidly in the late 1980s. Doubling times in male and female STI clinic attendees was 10,67 and 9,78 months respectively. Doubling time at family planning clinics was 6,55 months. Discussed in:
- Schoub, B D, Smith A N, Johnson, S, Martin, D J, Lyons, S F, Padayachee, G N, Hurwitz, H S. 1990. 'Considerations on the further expansion of the AIDS epidemic in South Africa — 1990'. *S Afr Med J*. Vol 77 (12), pp613-618.
- Friedland, I, Klugman, K, Karstaedt, A, et al. 1992. 'AIDS, The Baragwanath experience. Part 1 Epidemiology of HIV infection at Baragwanath Hospital, 1988 — 1990'. *SAMJ*. Aug 82 (2) 86-90'.

[50] Sher, R. 1989.' HIV in South Africa, 1982-88'. *SAMJ*. Oct 7 (7) 314-9.

[51] HIV and sexual networks:
The different subtypes of virus are not biologically connected to sexual orientation or race: there is no 'gay virus' or 'black virus.' The type of virus you might get — or indeed whether you get it at all — is dependent on the sexual networks to which you have been exposed. This also helps to explain the vexed question of why heterosexuals in the rich countries of the north (who are largely unconnected to gay or African sexual networks) have been disproportionately less affected by HIV and AIDS. They may have large amounts of unprotected sex, but there is little or no HIV in the sexual networks in which they play.

[52] A detailed discussion of the research into molecular epidemiology of HIV is available in:
Williamson, C & Martin, D. 2005. 'HIV-I Genetic Diversity' ed Abdool Karim, S S and Abdool Karim, Q. *HIV/AIDS in South Africa* Cambridge: Cambridge University Press.

THE SECOND EPIDEMIC

[53] 320 truck drivers were interviewed at five truck stops in KwaZulu-Natal: 56 per cent said they were HIV positive; 34 per cent said they always stopped for sex during a journey; 29 per cent had never used a condom with a sex worker;

70 per cent had wives or regular partner, and 65 per cent travelled regularly to high prevalence countries to the north. At the same truck stop, 56 per cent of the 194 sex workers were HIV positive. From:

> Ramjee, G & Gouws, E. 2001. 'Targetting HIV prevention efforts on truck drivers and sex workers'. *AIDS Bulletin*. April 2001, Vol 10 No 1.

54 HIV monitoring in Katimo Mulilo began in 1992: At 13,7 per cent, HIV prevalence among pregnant women there ranked with the worst hit countries to the north. (By comparison, the South African national average was 2,69 per cent.). Statistics from:
- UNAIDS.org
- *AIDS Analysis Africa*, 1997, Vol 17 (3).

55 High prevalence in Katimo Mulilo discussed in Webb, D. *HIV and AIDS in Africa*. Pluto Press, London, 1997.

56 Origins and genetic diversity of the virus is discussed in Williamson and Martin, 2005, op cit.

Toni

57 Toni Zimmerman was interviewed in the film, in the film *Mashayabhuqe*, 1998 op cit.

Chapter Three: Sex in the city

HIV in the city

58 Early HIV survey results in Hillbrow and other inner-city areas are described in:
- Schoub, B D, Smith, A N, Lyons, S F, Johnson, S, Martin, D J, Mc Gillvray, G, Padyachee, G N, Naidoo, S, Fisher, E L & Hurwitz, H S. 1988. Epidemiological considerations of the acquired immunodeficiency syndrome epidemic in South Africa.' *S Afr Med J*. Vol 74(4) 153-7.
- Schoub, B D. 1990. 'The AIDS epidemic in South Africa — perceptions and realities.' *S Afr Med*. J Vol 77 (12) pp607-608.
- Schoub, B D, Smith, A N, Johnson, S, Martin, D J, Lyons, S F, Padayachee, G N & Hurwitz, H S. 1990. 'Considerations on the further expansion of the AIDS epidemic in South Africa — 1990'. *S Afr Med* J. Vol 77 (12) pp613-618.

59 An account of the demographic changes in Hillbrow are given in:
> Morris, A. 1999. *Bleakness and light. Inner-city transition in Hillbrow*, Johannesburg. Johannesburg: Witwatersrand University Press.

Working lives

60 See Morris 1999, ibid, for an account of the growth of the sex industry in Hillbrow.

More on the sex industry in Hillbrow:

- Nairne, D. 1999. '"Please help me cleanse my womb". A hotel-based programme in a violent neighbourhood in Johannesburg'. *Research for Sex Work 2.*
- Wojcicki, J & Malala, J. 2001. 'Condom use, power and HIV/AIDS risk: sex-workers bargain for survival in Hillbrow/Joubert Park/Berea, Johannesburg'. *Social Science and Medicine* 53: 99-121.
- 11/4/2001, *Mail & Guardian*, 'One day I'll get a proper job'.
- Stadler, J & Delaney, S. 2004. 'The "healthy brothel": the context of clinical services for sex workers in Hillbrow.' History Workshop, African Studies Seminar, February 24.
- Dunkle, K, Beksinska, M, Rees, H, et al. 2005. 'Risk factors for HIV infection among sex workers in Johannesburg, South Africa'. *International Journal of STD and AIDS* V 16 (3): 256-261.
- Statistics for sex workers in Hillbrow from Stadler and Delaney op cit.

61 Askari/AIDS conspiracy:
- 12/11/1999, *Mail & Guardian*, 'Apartheid forces spread AIDS'.
- Also noted in: Truth and Reconciliation Commission Amnesty Hearings 6/9/1999.

62 De Kock's dismissal of askari/AIDS conspiracy is described in:
Shell, R. 1999. 'The silent revolution: the AIDS pandemic and the military in South Africa'. Conference paper 'Consolidating Democracy in South Africa', August 1999, Umtata.

63 Third force — During the dying years of apartheid during the period of political negotiations a covert third force was established to undermine the political settlement and destabilise the country with violent actions. The extent to which the leadership of the apartheid government was involved is still a matter of dispute.

64 For tales of Ferdi Barnard, the covert forces and sex work:
Pauw, J. 1997. *Into the heart of darkness. Confessions of apartheid's assassins.* Johannesburg: Jonathan Ball.

LOVE AND WAR

65 Discussion of masculinity and war:
- Herdt, G. 2003. 'Sexuality in times of war'. *American Sexuality Magazine* 1 (5) 2003.
- Hankins, C, Friedman, S, Zafar, T, et al. 2002. 'Transmission and prevention of HIV and sexually transmitted infections in war settings: implications for current and future armed conflicts'. *AIDS* v 16 (17): 2245-2252.

66 Amnesty Hearings of Truth and Reconciliation Commission:
- Daluxulo Luthuli hearing, 7/4/1998, available at:
  www.doj.gov.za/trc/amntrans/durban/dbn1.htm
- Israel Hlongwane hearing, 12/8/1998, available at:
  www.doj.gov.za/trc/amntrans/1998/98081114_hmm_hammar2.htm

- Discussion about rape and war, Caprivi trainee hearings, Pinetown magistrates' court. Available at:

    www.doj.gov.za/trc/amntrans/1999/990308_ptn_990308pn.htm
- Discussion of training of Caprivi cadres also in *Truth and Reconciliation Commission of South Africa Report*, Vol 6, Section 3, Chapter 3, 2003. Available at: www.info.gov.za/otherdocs/2003/trc

[67] Krog, A. 1999. *Country of my skull*, London: Vintage 277.

[68] Shell is an historian and demographer. At the time of his paper he was Associate Professor of Statistics at the University of the Western Cape. The paper can be read at:

   www.uwc.ac.za/portal/faculty_department/statistics/downloads/session4_Aids_and_the_Military.pdf

[69] 16/9/1999, *Mail & Guardian*, 'AIDS came to South Africa through migrant labour'.

Everyday love

[70] Mokwena, S. 1991. 'The era of the Jackrollers: contextualising the rise of youth gangs in Soweto.' Presented at Seminar 7, Centre for the Study of Violence and Reconciliation, University of the Witwatersrand.

[71] At the time of writing the paper Mokwena was a researcher at the Centre for the Study of Violence and Reconciliation.

[72] Rape and HIV in South Africa is discussed in:
- Walker, L, Reid, G& Cornell M. 2004. *Waiting to happen. HIV/AIDS in South Africa (the bigger picture)*. Cape Town: Double Storey Books.
- 24/10/2006, *Cape Times*, 'Shocking figures reveal rape trends in South Africa'.
- The Gender and Health Research Unit research showed that 19 per cent of South African men reported having raped a woman; the mean age of first rape was 17 years. Quoted in the South African Medical Research Institute. *Building a health nation through research*. Annual Report 2005/6.
- Wood, K & Jewkes, R. 1997. 'Violence, rape and sexual coercion: everyday love in a South African township'. *Gend Dev* 5 (2): 41-46.
- Kistner, U. 2003. Gender-based violence and HIV/AIDS in South Africa. A literature review for CADRE/Department of Health. January 2003. Available at: www.cadre.org.za

[73] Reports on Zuma rape trial:
- 16/2/2006, *BBC News online*, 'Crowds stand by Zuma in rape case'.
- 6/4/2006, *Mail & Guardian*, '100 per cent Zuluboy', Fikile-Ntsikeleo Moya.
- 8/4/2006, *Mail & Guardian*, 'Testimony pushes back AIDS battle'.
- 10/4/2006, *Mail & Guardian*, 'Taking a shower will not prevent HIV'.

AIDS in the city

[74] Journal articles describing how HIV came to Baragwanath:

- Friedland, I, Klugman, K, Karstaedt, A, et al. 1992. 'AIDS. The Baragwanath experience. Part I Epidemiology of HIV infection at Baragwanath Hospital, 1988 — 1990'. *SAMJ*. Aug, 82 (2): 86-90.
- Friedland & McIntyre. 1992. 'AIDS. The Baragwanath experience. Part II HIV infection in pregnancy and childhood'. *SAMJ* Aug, 82 (2): 90-4.
- Karstaedt, A. 1992. AIDS. The Baragwanath experience. Part III HIV infection in adults at Baragwanath hospital'. *SAMJ*, Aug 82 (2): 95-97.
- Allwood, C, Friedland, I, Karstaedt, A et al. 1992. 'AIDS the Baragwanath experience. Part IV Counselling and ethical issues'. *SAMJ* 1992, Aug 82 (2): 98-101.

Chapter Four: BAD BEHAVIOUR

DANGEROUS DISINFORMATION

75 Van Niekerk quote, 20/1/1988, *The Citizen*, Quoted in Grundlingh, 2001 ibid.
76 Parliamentary debate: Mopp, P & de la Cruz, D. April 1988, House of Representatives, Hansard 7296.
77 General discussion of the National Party response, media and condom distribution programmes:
- Grundlingh, L. 2001. 'A critical history of government responses to HIV/AIDS in South Africa as reported in the media, 1983-1994'. Paper presented at a Development Studies Seminar at Rand Afrikaans University, May 25, 2001.
- Grundlingh, L. 2002. 'Neither health nor education? An historical analysis of HIV/AIDS Education in South Africa'. Paper presented at a seminar at Rand Afrikaans University, April/May 2002.

78 Van Niekerk on the dangers of AIDS, *The Star, Business Day* 6/6/89, quoted in Grundlingh 2001, op cit.

COME BACK AFRICA

79 The Maputo conference was conceived and planned when the ANC was still a banned organisation in South Africa. However, by the time the conference took place the ANC had been unbanned.
80 Chris Hani was assassinated by a right-winger in 1993. Some believe his death deprived the country of a politician who could have broken the denial over AIDS and led the government's prevention programme.
81 Hani's speech has been quoted in:
- Marais, H. 2000. *To the edge. AIDS Review 2000*. Centre for the Study of AIDS. University of Pretoria.
- Abdool Karim, Q & Abdool Karim, S. 2002. 'The evolving HIV epidemic in South Africa'. *International Journal of Epidemiology* 31:37-40.

[82] Nzo document quoted in:
> 11/6/1999, *Mail & Guardian,* 'Aw c'mon you don't really believe those AIDS myths?'

[83] The first AIDS Advisory group that had been established in 1985 included only professionals such as research scientists and health workers.

[84] The Ugandan government's AIDS control programme is widely thought to have contributed to a decline in HIV prevalence in the early 1990s.

[85] The Holmshaw programme is described in Grundling 2001, op cit.

[86] Banning of safe sex videos, 5/3/93, *Mail & Guardian* cited in South African Institute of Race Relations. 1994. *A survey of race relations in South Africa,* 1993/4. SAIRR. Johannesburg.

[87] Yellow hand campaign discussed in Grundlingh 2002, op cit.

Making a plan

[88] Lightfoot, N. 1995. 'The aborted "yellow hand" campaign'. *AIDS Bulletin.* Jul; 4: 20.

[89] Nacosa launch described in:
> Whiteside, A. 1993. 'First step to a black-and-white policy on AIDS. South African Report 1'. *AIDS Analysis Africa.* Nov-Dec 3 (6) 2.

[90] Speech by Nelson Mandela to the National Conference on AIDS, October 23 1992. Available at: www.anc.org.za

Bad timing

[91] Right-wing campaigns and smear pamphlets discussed in:
- Jochelson, K. 2001. *The colour of disease... syphilis and race in South Africa. 1880-1950.* New York: Palgrave.
- Van der Vliet, V. 2004. 'AIDS: losing "the new struggle"?' *Daedalus* 130 (1): 151-84.
- Smear pamphlet fraudulently signed by Sisulu — *Mail & Guardian,* Oct 5, 1990.

[92] 27/12/1988, *Newsday,* 'S. Africa's new propaganda weapon', Laurie Garrett.

[93] The Conservative Party was the main right wing opposition to the National Party and had a large following among Afrikaans-speaking South Africans.

[94] CP demand for testing returning exiles: Hansard, Feb 26 1991, Cited in:
> South African Institute for Race Relations. 1992. *Race relations survey 1991/2.* Johannesburg: SAIRR.

[95] 27/9/1990, *New York Times,* 'AIDS rising fast among black South Africans'.

[96] Demotion of Holmshaw and Carswell, 7/30/1992, Advocate No 608. Available at www.aegis.com

[97] Carswell, W. 1993. HIV in South Africa. *The Lancet.* July 17; 342 (8864): 132.

[98] Viljoen, A T. 1989. 'Apartheid and AIDS'. *The Lancet.* 1989 Nov 25; 2 (8674): 1280.

[99] Annual antenatal survey statistics available from: www.doh.gov.za

100 Conclusions and reactions to the 1990 CIA report described in:
> 5/7/2000, *Washington Post*, Death Watch, the Global Response to AIDS in Africa, Barton Gellman.

THE VIRUS CONTINUED...

101 Today there is a consensus that an average of 1 per cent HIV prevalence in the general population represents a tipping point beyond which a general epidemic is difficult to contain.

102 For a description of growth of informal settlements, decline in marriage and female migration in the 1990s, see:
> Hunter, M. 2007. 'The changing political economy of sex in South Africa: the significance of unemployment and inequalities to the scale of the AIDS pandemic.' *Social Science and Medicine*, 64 (3): 689-700.

103 27/8/2003, *The view*, Apartheid's invisible women. Geographer's new book traces the lives of the women transforming transitory housing meant for men. Available at www.uvm.edu/theview

104 Elder, G. 2003. *Hostels, sexuality and the apartheid legacy. Malevolent geography.* Ohio University Press.

105 Human Sciences Research Council. 2005. *South African National HIV prevalence, HIV incidence, behaviour and communication survey, 2005*. Cape Town: HSRC Press.

106 Early research in KwaZulu-Natal:
- Abdool Karim, Q, Abdool Karim, S S & Mkomokazi, J. 1991. 'Sexual behaviour and knowledge of AIDS among urban black mothers. Implications for AIDS prevention programmes'. *S Afr Med J*. 80 (7): 340-3.
- Abdool Karim, Q, Abdool Karim, S S, Singh B, et al. 1992. 'Seroprevalence of HIV infection in rural South Africa'. *AIDS* Dec. 6 (12): 1535-9.
- Abdool Karim, Q. 2001. 'Barriers to preventing human immunodeficiency virus in women: experiences from KwaZulu-Natal, South Africa'. *Journal of the American Medical Women's Association*, December 2001. Available at: www.globalaging.org

Chapter Five: FREE AT LAST!

NEW BROOMS

107 Account of meeting with FW de Klerk:
> Cameron, E. 2005. *Witness to AIDS*. Cape Town: Tafelberg Publishers Limited, 124.

108 Kale, R. 1995. 'South Africa's Health: Restructuring South Africa's health care: dilemmas for planners'. *BMJ*; 310:1397-1399 (May 27).

109 19/6/1995, *Reuters*, 'S. Africa buys 97 million condoms to fight AIDS'.

Living positively

110 Peter Busse quote about disclosing his HIV status in the Nacosa meeting from: Beyond Awareness Campaign. 2000. *Living openly. HIV positive South Africans tell their stories.* HIV/AIDS and STD Directorate, Department of Health.

111 Between 1994 and 1997 the upper house of parliament was referred to as the Senate. It then became the National Council of Provinces.

112 21/6/1995, SAPA, quoted in ANC Daily News Briefing, www.anc.org.za

113 The GNP+ meeting in South Africa was held in March 1995.

Enemies in high places

114 Zuma 1994 health budget speech described in Kale 1995, op cit.

115 Zuma and tobacco industry:
Malan, M & Leaver, R. 2003. 'Political change in South Africa: tobacco control and public health policies'. World Bank.
www1.worldbank.org/tobacco/pdf/2850-Ch06.pdf

116 Zuma in the National Assembly, on drugs and drug prices, on 18/6/1996, SAPA, ANC Daily News Briefing

117 The practice of importing branded drugs from a cheaper source in another country is known as parallel importation. It later became the core of the dispute between the pharmaceutical industry and the South African government.

118 Underspending on the AIDS programme:
Marais, H. 2000. *To the edge. AIDS Review 2000.* Centre for the Study of AIDS. University of Pretoria, 26.

Florence

119 Florence Ngobeni's autobiographical accounts from:
- Experiences of an HIV/AIDS counsellor, South Africa. Available at: www.ippf.org
- How young people can make a difference, Talk to students at GWU, November 29, available at www.kaisernetwork.org

Chapter Six: A Song and Dance

Making a splash

120 Background to the *Sarafina* episode:
- 11/2/1996, *Sunday Argus,* 'New Shock over R14 million AIDS Play'.
- Phila Legislative Update, *The Sarafina II Controversy.* Number 3, June 1996. Accessed on 14/08/02 at www.hst.org.za/pphc/Phila/sarafina.htm
- Ngema tells a journalist, 'Everyone knows I love women and am not

shamed of it,' and is described by others as a womaniser in 27/6/1997, *Mail & Guardian*, 'Revisiting Ngema'.

GYM SLIPS AND PELVIC THRUSTS

121 Reports on the early controversy:
- SAPA daily reports, February 26 to March 14, 1996 available from ANC Daily News Briefings, www.anc.org.za
- 28/1/1996, *Sunday Times*, 'State Splurges R14 million on Pelvic Thrusts', Ivor Powell.
- 9/2/1996, *Mail & Guardian*, 'Health Minister Defends AIDS Musical'.
- 13/2/1996, *Cape Argus*, 'Department wants R15 a head for AIDS musical'.
- 8/3/1996 *Mail & Guardian*, '"I Should be Paid a Million Rands", Mbongeni Ngema Profile,' Mark Gevisser.
- 15/2/1996, *Cape Times*, 'Mandela intervenes in row over R14,7 m AIDS play'.
- 28/2/1996, *Cape Argus*,' IFP hit Zuma's decision on play'.
- 11/3/1996, *Cape Argus*, 'AIDS message not effective'.
- 22/3/1996, *Mail & Guardian*, 'Sarafina of the Health System', Mark Gevisser.

122 Freirian participatory theatre — Pauolo Freire was an influential Brazilian educationist and thinker in Marxist and post-colonial educational philosophy. He and others developed a form of participatory theatre that was aimed at engaging and empowering the audience.

123 Background on *Township Fever* from the film *The Fever, 1990*, directed by Francis Gerard, for BBC (Arena/Screenplay). I worked as a researcher on this film.

CRYING FOUL

124 1/3/1996, ANC Daily News Briefing, Mandela expresses confidence in Health Minister Zuma.

125 Department of Information and Publicity, African National Congress. February 28 1996. Parliamentary Hearing on *Sarafina 2*.

126 1/3/1996, *Cape Times*, EU 'did not know about *Sarafina 2*'.

127 1/3/1996, *Natal Witness*, compares funding of *Sarafina 2* with provincial AIDS budget.
- 11/3/1996, *Cape Times*, 'Zuma faces AIDS play showdown'.

128 Public protector's report on *Sarafina*:
Report in terms of section 8(2) of the public protector act 23 of 1994. Report no 1 (special report) *Investigation of the play Sarafina 2*. Public protector, Republic of South Africa. May 20 1996.

129 The report criticised Shisana for failing to formalise aspects of the oral agreement between Ngema and the Department of Health. Abdool Karim was criticised for failing to make a decision as to the source of the funding ie whether it was to come from the EU or from DoH funding.

130 ANC response to public protector's report:
> Department of Information and Publicity, African National Congress. June 5, 1996. Sarafina II Report.

131 The total unauthorised expenditure on *Sarafina* was R10 519 202. Of this R2 211 138 was recovered from Committed Artists and a further R51 000 was recovered by a special investigations unit. The 24th report of the standing committee on public accounts, August 2002 recommended that the remaining R10 468 202,30 be authorised by parliament to bring the matter to a close. By 2001, the legal costs incurred in attempting to recover state losses had amounted to R576 595. From 24th SCOPA report, August 2003.

The balance sheet

132 12/1/1997. ANC Daily News Briefing. Mandela, Address to the nation.

133 Crewe, M. 2000. 'South Africa: touched by the vengeance of AIDS'. *The South African Journal of International Affairs* Vol 742. Winter 2000: 23-35.

134 Bull terrier quote:
> 22/3/1996, *Mail & Guardian*, Sarafina of the Health System, Mark Gevisser.

Enter Big Pharma

135 Big Pharma is the name used by critics of the multinational research-based pharmaceutical industry.

136 On health restructuring:
> Kale, R. 1995. 'South Africa's Health: Restructuring South Africa's health care: dilemmas for planners'. *BMJ*. 310: 1297-1399.

137 Mandela blames Sarafina controversy on Big Pharma:
> 11/9/1996, 'Sarafina donation offer withdrawn', SAPA, from ANC Daily News Briefing, www.anc.org.za

138 Deeb replies:
> 14/9/1996, Don't blame us for Sarafina debacle: medicines body. SAPA, from ANC Daily News Briefing.

139 Zuma 'enemies of liberation' quote in Gevisser, *Mail & Guardian*, op cit.

140 UNAIDS was established in 1995 and replaced the now-defunct WHO Global Programme on AIDS.

141 UNAIDS, Global AIDS statistics, 1996. Available from www.unaids.org

142 Accounts of the Vancouver conference:
- Schouten, J. 1996. 'A Step summary of the XI International AIDS Conference', *Step Perspective* 8 (2).
- 8/7/1996, *Washington Post*, 'With fanfare global AIDS Conference gets underway'.
- 26/7/1996, *Mail & Guardian*, 'Zuma's revenge'.

Chapter Seven: HEARTS AND MINDS

A CURE FOR AFRICANS BY AFRICANS

143 Visser's description of the test results as described by SAPA, January 22 1997, ANC Daily News Briefing:

> Before he started the treatment John's PCR count (a measure of the virus in his blood) was just over 222 000. His CD4 count (an indicator of the strength of his immune system) was just 39. After three treatments his viral load was down to 30 000 and his CD4 had jumped to 138. Emma's PCR dropped from 1,2 million to about 236 000 in three treatments.

144 Gerwel quoted in:

> Power, S. 2003. 'The AIDS Rebel'. *The New Yorker*, May.

145 Mbeki's comments on the cabinet meeting:

> Mbeki, T M. 1998. 'ANC has no financial stake in Virodene'. *Mayibuye*, March 1998.

146 Key newspaper cuttings and other articles on Virodene breakthrough:
- SAPA news reports, January 22, 23, 24, 25, February 5, 6, March 11 1997, available from ANC Daily News Briefing.
- 22/1/1997, Associated Press, 'AIDS breakthrough questioned'.
- 23/1/1997, *Cape Argus*, '"Ceiling" on conventional treatment'.
- 23/1/1997, *The Star*, 'AIDS breakthrough'.
- 23/1/1997, *Cape Argus*, 'SA researchers stun fellows'.
- 23/1/1997, *Sowetan*, 'SA Scientists in HIV/AIDS breakthrough'.
- 23/1/1997, *Beeld*, 'Wonderkur vir vigs in SA ontdek'.
- 23/1/1997, *Business Day*, 'Pretoria university scientists present AIDS drug'.
- 24/1/1997, *Beeld*, 'Olga Visser'.

147 It emerged that Zigi and Olga Visser had already been involved in commercial transactions over her cryonics research and had set up a business together.

148 Interview with Zigi Visser: 26/1/1997, *Sunday Independent*.

THE OLGA AND ZIGI SHOW

149 Du Plessis interview in:

> 'Rebel with a cause'. 1997. *SAMJ*. March, Vol 87 (3) 263-264.

150 Visser's research had been supported by the Alcor Foundation and The Cryonics Institute in the US.

151 An account of Visser's correspondence and her performance at the Atlanta conference is given in:
- Charles Platt, Hearts, brains and minds. Available at:
  www.cryocare.org/index.cgi?subdir=ccrpt10&url=visser.html

152 17/06/2001, Mike Darwin, 'Olga Visser Fraud', email message. Available at: www.cryonet.org/cgi-bin/dsp.cgi?msg=16561

Side effects

153 Critical articles on Virodene:
- 24/1/1997, *Mail & Guardian,* 'AIDS "breakthrough" broke all the rules'.
- 26/1/1997, *Sunday Tribune*.
- 31/1/1997, *Mail & Guardian,* 'What's the active ingredient?'
- 31/1/1997, *Mail & Guardian,* 'Government aims to 'own' AIDS drug'.
- 27/2/1997, *Business Day,* '"AIDS drug" just an industrial solvent'.
- 28/2/1997, *Mail & Guardian,* Virodene 'cruel trick'.

154 6/2/1997, The halting of AIDS tests. ANC statement announces MCC's decision to halt Virodene tests, and encourages further work on the substance.

155 BC 1247 Peter Folb/Virodene Papers: B Correspondence with Dr N Zuma, Manuscripts and archives, University of Cape Town.

156 6/2/1997, *SAPA,* 'Zuma supports Virodene research'.
- 6/2/1997. Statement by Dr N C Zuma on Virodene controversy, Ministry of Health. Available at www.info.gov.za/speeches/1997

157 Sidley, P. 1997. 'SA research into AIDS "cure" severely criticised'. *BMJ.* 314:769.

158 3/7/1997, *Mail & Guardian,* 'Virodene researchers guilty of misconduct'.

159 5/5/1997, Independent Newspapers, 'Fund for Virodene research'.

Compassionate release

160 14/2/1997 *Mail & Guardian,* 'AIDS agony over drug'.

161 BC 1247 Peter Folb/Virodene papers. Correspondence between Prof Peter Folb and Dr N Zuma B1.1, 1997 - 18/7/1997; 21/8/1997; Archives and manuscripts, University of Cape Town.

Themba

162 Themba is not his real name. He was interviewed in *HIV/AIDS and Development,* Lesley Lawson. SAIH/INTERFUND. 1997.

Chapter Eight: Drug Wars

Zuma vs Big Pharma

163 One of the influential books making the case against Big Pharma was:
Muller, M. 1982. *The health of nations — a north-south investigation.* London: Faber and Faber Ltd.

164 Brand-name drugs, generic drugs and intellectual property rights:
In very simple terms: brand-name drugs are marketed by the pharmaceutical companies that develop them. The originator of a drug takes out a patent that gives the company exclusive rights to make and sell the drug for a certain length of time. Once the patent expires, the manufacture of cheaper

ENDNOTES AND REFERENCES 299

copies by other pharmaceutical companies is allowed. These copies are called generic drugs.

Thus the pharmaceutical industry is divided into the research-based pharmaceutical industry and the generics industry. The generics industry is able to make drugs for a lower price because they do not have to bear the costs of research.

In 1994, the World Trade Organisation was established, to regulate world trade. It required all members to strengthen their patent laws. A new agreement, the TRIPS agreement (Trade related aspects of intellectual property rights) gave patent holders 20 years of exclusive rights to market their drugs. In this time generic alternatives can not be made or distributed. Before the WTO and TRIPS many poor countries had weak patent laws and were thus able to make generic drugs more freely.

165 The process of drug policy reform is discussed in detail in the following:

Gray, A, Matsebula, T & Blaauw D, et al. 2002. *Policy change in a context of transition. Drug Policy in South Africa, 1989-1999.* Centre for Health Policy. School of Public Health, University of the Witwatersrand, Johannesburg.

166 Regulations withdrawn:

4/5/1997, *Business Day*.

167 The conflict between the Minister and the PMA in early 1997 is described in the following document:

Public Protector (1997) *Report on the propriety of the conduct of members of the ministry and Department of Health relating to statements in connection with the prices of medicines and the utilisation of generic medicines in South Africa.* Report No 6 of the Public Protector, November 21, 1997.

168 The first Medicines Bill was called the Medicines and Related Substances Amendment Bill 30, of 1997.

169 The dispute over South Africa's drugs reform policy is chronicled in:

2/6/1997, *Business Day*, US pharmaceutical companies to tackle Zuma on proposed bill.

170 Discussion about the bill:

Phila Legislative Update, Medicines and Related Substances Control Amendment Bill, 1997. May 1997. Available at:

www.hst.org.za/pphc/Phila/medbill.htm

171 Meetings between Big Pharma and the SA government are chronicled in:

Love, J. *Time-line of Disputes over Compulsory Licensing and Parallel Importation in South Africa, August 1999, Consumer Project on Technology.* Available at:

www.cptech.org/ip/health/sa/sa-timeline.txt

172 29/7/1997. Letter from Ralph Nader, James Love and Robert Weisman to Vice President Gore regard U.S. policy toward South Africa pharmaceutical policies: Available at www.cptech.org/pharm/goreonsa.html

BAD MEDICINE

173 4/5/1997, *Business Times (Sunday Times* supplement*)*, Vested interests resist reform in medicines.

174 The second bill was called the Medicines and Related Substances Control Amendment Bill No 90, of 1997.

175 17/5/1997, Folb letter to Zuma on Medicines Bill. BC1247 Peter Folb/Virodene papers, E. Court cases, EI The Pharmaceutical Manufacturer's Association of South Africa and 41 others vs the President of South Africa and 9 others. Manuscripts and archives, University of Cape Town.

176 Folb statement at Medicines Bill hearings; September 17. In Fob/Virodene papers, E1, op cit.

IT'S THE WORDING!

177 Joseph letter, quoted in Love *Timeline 1999*, op cit.

178 Comments of the Consumer Project on Technology to the Portfolio Committee on Health, Cape Town. James Love, October 6, 1997.

179 SA, a test case: Letter to Ms Sybil Harrison, USTR, from Shannon SS Herzfeld. February 16, 1999. Available at:

www.cptech.org/ip/health/phrma/301-99/301-letter.html

180 Letter from Director Bada Pharasi to DG of Health March 13, 1997, quoted in Arbitration Award, Commission for Conciliation, Mediation and Arbitration, CCMA hearings July to November 1988, In 'Dismantling of the Medicines Control Council', Folb/Virodene papers, op cit.

MORE SIDE EFFECTS

181 A good account of the early debate about the use of antiretrovirals in low-income countries is given in:

27/12/2000, *Washington Post*, 'An unequal calculus of life and death', Barton Gellman.

182 23/11/1997, *Sunday Independent Online*, 'Police called in as banned drug poisons AIDS patients'.

183 AIDS Law Project research on unlawful use of Virodene described in:

17/11/1997, Letter from Fatima Hassan (Attorney) and Mark Heywood (Head: AIDS Law Project) to Medicines Control Council. In B1 correspondence with Dr N C Zuma Folb/Virodene papers op cit.

184 Visser statements on Virodene being a cure, and research being hampered by medical authorities with vested interests are quoted in an AIDS Law Project letter to the Medicines Control Council, Folb/Virodene papers op cit.

185 21/11/1997, *Independent Online (IOL)* 'Virodene doctor suspected of still treating AIDS patients'.

186 Sidley, P. 1997. 'Researchers' offices raided over banned AIDS drug'. *BMJ*.

(December 6) 315: 1485-1488.
187 Folb's view on Virodene and the continued illegal testing: Confidential fax from Folb to Zuma., 5/12/1997, B1 correspondence with Dr N C Zuma, Peter Folb/Virodene papers op cit.
188 12/3/1998, *Business Day*, 'Human trials with Virodene carried out in Portugal'.
189 4/3/1998, *Business Day*, 'Virodene's sour taste'.
190 Zuma to Youth League:
- 2/12/1997, *Pretoria News*, 'Give them Virodene'.
- 2/12/1997, *Sowetan*.

NONHLANHLA
191 Nonhlanhla Mbokazi was interviewed in the film *Mashayabhuqe*, 1998, op cit.

Chapter Nine: POISONED BARBS

BEHIND CLOSED DOORS
192 Bannenberg comment:
>10/10/1997, *Mail & Guardian*, 'Drugs regulator takes on Zuma'.
193 Peter Folb background:
>Peter Folb's full-time job was professor of Pharmacology at the University of Cape Town, and he had presided over the Council during the period of political transformation. Like many left-leaning academics of this era, he had been personally involved with the internal opposition to apartheid in the 1980s, contributing his medical and professional skills. A known ANC supporter, he had also been appointed by the minister to serve on the committee that designed the new National Drugs Policy.
194 Restructuring the Medicines Control Council:
- Kariem, S. 1988. 'Medicines Control Council Statement'. *SAMJ*. 88 (8): 923.
- Folb, P. 1988. 'Medicines Control Council, Setting the record straight'. *SAMJ*. 88 (10).
195 Also Folb's account, including conversations with Dukes:
>Peter Folb. Virodene papers. BC 1247, Manuscripts and archives, University of Cape Town. D1 CCMA arbitration between Schlebusch, Bruckner and Department of Health: D1.1 Correspondence and copies of reports, D1.2 Applicants bundle of documents.

ZUMA UNDER ATTACK
196 Milestones in the dispute over the Medicines Bill are detailed in Love timeline, 1999, op cit.
197 19/2/1998, *Business Day*, 'Coalition contests drugs law in court'.

198 The 6 per cent allegation:
- 2/3/1998, *Mail & Guardian*, 'Protector called in to probe ANC-Virodene link'.
- 4/4/1998, *Cape Argus*, 'Virodene shares for ANC were a 'black empowerment' move'.
- 6/3/1998, *BBC News*, 'ANC probed over banned AIDS drug'.
- 6/6/1998, *Mail & Guardian*, 'Virodene "general" denies ANC link'.

199 Zuma statement on DP:
3/3/1998, SAPA, quoted in ANC Daily News Briefing.

200 Folb fax to Zuma, December 5 1997. B.1 Correspondence with Dr N C Zuma. In Folb/Virodene papers op cit.

201 The faxes sent by Zigi Visser to George Chaane of the ANC's legal desk on December 11 and 12 1997 are discussed in:
13/3/1998, *Mail & Guardian*, 'Virodene's unanswered questions'.

202 ANC on Mike Ellis:
3/3/1998, Further statement on Virodene allegations. African National Congress statement. Available at www.anc.org.za/ancdocs/pr/1998/pr0303b.html

'UNBOUNDED CONTUMELY'

203 Mbeki, T. 1998. 'The war against Virodene'. *Mayibuye*, March. Available at: www.anc.org.za/ancdocs/pubs/mayibuye/mayi9801.html

204 Firing of Schlebusch and Bruckner described in Folb/Virodene, CCMA papers, op cit.

205 Many years later, it emerged that there was no evidence of misconduct on the part of the registrar and his deputy and the CCMA heard in their favour.

206
- 24/4/1998, *Mail & Guardian*, 'Zuma replaces Medicines Control Council head'.
- 27/3/1998, *Mail & Guardian*, 'Zuma shuts down pesky medicines council'.
- 30/3/1998, *Mail & Guardian*, 'Dissolving MCC not related to Virodene'.

SANCTIONS LOOM...

207 Clinton in parliament:
26/3/1998, *CNN*.

208 Hlongwane quote:
26/3/1998, *Associated Press*, Controversial laws discussed by US commerce secretary available at:
http://lists.essential.org/1998/pharm-policy/msg00017.html

209 Tom Bombelles: 27/3/1998, *SABC*, quoted in Love timeline 1999, op cit.

210 Submission of PhRMA for the National Trade Estimate Report on Foreign Trade Barriers, NTE, 1998.

211
- 6/2/1998, *Business Day*, 'Congressmen call for action against SA's Medicines Act'.
- 25/2/1998, *Business Day*, 'US drug industry wants to put South Africa on priority watch list'.

- 29/3/1998, *New York Times*, 'South Africa's Bitter Pill for World Drug Makers', Donald G Mc Neil.
212 The Special 301 Process, USINFO, available at http://164.109.48.86/products/pubs/intelprps/301.htm
213 15/7/1998, *Business Day*, 'US withholds benefits over Zuma's bill', Simon Barber.

One week in Geneva
214 The World Health Assembly represents all the health ministers of member states and is the governing body of the World Health Organisation.
215 WHA: EB101.R24, Revised Drug Strategy, available at:
   http://lists.essential.org/1998/pharm-policy/msg00018.html
216 Meeting and PhRMA statement outlined in Love timeline 1999, op cit.
217 US Memo on meeting:
   May 27 1998. Cable from US Mission in Geneva to the US Department of State. Revised Drug Strategy at WHO: Atmospherics of the Debate, and Recommended Plan of Action. DOC_NUMBER: 1998GENEVA03470. Available at: www.cptech.org/ip/health/who/confidential.rtf
218 - 11/5/1998, *The Star*, 'Zuma poised to sack Shisana'.
   - 12/5/1998, *Dispatch Online*, 'Report says Zuma wants Shisana out'.

Something new out of Africa
219 - 7/5/1998, *Dispatch Online*, 'Zuma ditched subordinates over Sarafina'.
   - 19/6/1998, *Mail & Guardian,* 'Virodene's new black owners'.
   - 20/6/1998, *Dispatch Online*, 'Black group buys rights to Virodene'.
220 10/7/1998, *Mail & Guardian*, 'Virodene man's link to drugs, car'.
221 Rees statement:
   - 26/6/1998, *Mail & Guardian*, 'Tax rands help fast-track Virodene'.
   - 20/6/1998, *Mail & Guardian*, 'Virodene, still no permission for human trials'.
222 17/12/1998, ANC Daily News Briefing, MCC rejects application for Virodene clinical trials.
223 Mbeki, T. 1998. *The African Renaissance South Africa and the World*, April 9. Available at www.enu.edu

Chapter Ten: 'Pills cost pennies'

Suffer the children
224 Zwi, K J, Pettifor, J M & Soderlund, N. 1999. 'Paediatric hospital admissions at a South African urban regional hospital. The impact of HIV, 1992–1997'. *Ann Trp Paediatr* 1999 Jun; 19 (2): 135-42.
225 Stein, A, Krebs, G & Richter L, et al. 2005. 'Babies of a pandemic'. *Archives of*

Diseases in Childhood. 90 (2) 116. Available at:
http://adc.bmjjournals.com/cgi/content/full/90/2/116

226 Cadman, J. 1998. 'Vertical transmission. Research at the retrovirus conference'. March 1998. *The Body.* Available at www.thebody.com

227 TAC, MTCT Timeline details SA NGO and activist action on mother-to-child prevention. Available at www.tac.org.za

AZT – BACK STORY

228 The background to the issue of drug pricing and intellectual property rights is well described in the following:

27/12/2000, *Washington Post*, 'An unequal calculus of life and death'. Barton Gellman.

229 ACT UP — AIDS Coalition to Unleash Power. A US activist group formed by HIV-positive people in 1987 to demand greater coherence in national AIDS strategies to fight for access to drugs. The 1989 NY stock exchange protest brought the drug price down from $10 000 to $6 400 per person per year.

230 17/1/1990, *New York Times*, 'US halves dosage for AIDS drug'.

231 The first encouraging results from AZT trials were published in August 1989. The next day the value of manufacturer Burroughs Welcome rose 32 per cent. The drug cost $7,000 per person per year in the USA. More detail on the back story of AZT available at: www.avert.org

232 PMTCT trials:

The first trials that showed that AZT was effective in reducing perinatal transmission were called the ACTG 076 trials. The first ACTG trial, which reported in 1994, involved starting the mother on AZT when she was 14 weeks pregnant, as well as for the first six weeks of the baby's life. Several subsequent trials shortened the duration of AZT. The Thai regimen, which was reported in 1998, cut the treatment down considerably — starting at 36 weeks of pregnancy. Other milestones in successful PMTCT trials were:

Petra trial (reported 1999) which tested a combination of AZT and 3TC; HIVNET 012 (1999) which tested nevirapine; Saint trial (2000) compared nevirapine with the AZT/3TC combination.

233 The history of drug trials for therapies to prevent mother-to-child transmission of HIV is well described in the following:

McIntyre, J & Gray, G. 2002. 'What can we do to reduce mother to child transmission of HIV?' *BMJ* 324:218-221.

234 The manufacturer of AZT at the time of the first ACT UP protests was Burroughs Wellcome. Through a merger this became Glaxo Wellcome in 1995. Another merger in 2000 resulted in Glaxo Smith Kline.

235 22/8/1997, *Mail & Guardian*, Cheap HIV drugs for pregnant women. A major

drug company negotiates with the health department to lower the price of the drug AZT for pregnant women to prevent them passing the disease to their children.

236 Peter Young discount quote:
> 5/3/1998, Company to offer AZT at steep discount to Third World, CNN, 0033 GMT.

BRIDGING THE GAP

237 US AIDS deaths toll decline described on p 472 in Garret, L, *Betrayal of trust*. New York: Hyperion.

238 The attitudes in this period towards treatment vs prevention on the part of international health actors are described in Gellmann 2000, op cit.

239 Geneva conference:
- 25/6/1998, UPI, 'AIDS conference tries to close gaps'.
- 28/6/1998, Reuters, 'Geneva conference targets wealth gap'.
- Lancet letter quoted on: www.actupny.org/reports/Geneva.html

THEY BROKE OUR HEARTS

240 11/10/1998, *Sunday Times*, 'Save our babies Dr Zuma'.

241 15/10/1998, *Africa News Service*, 'Zuma defends AZT policy'.

242 Partnership against AIDS:
- 1/10/1998 ANC Daily News Briefing, www.anc.org.za/anc/newsbrief/
- 7/10/1998 — 9/10/1988, ANC Daily News Briefing, ibid.

243 18/11/1998, *Sunday Times*, 'Awareness is the only cure for the spread of AIDS', Nkosazana Zuma.

244 Florence Ngobeni quoted in:
> 6/7/2000, *Washington Post*, 'Free of apartheid, divided by disease', Jeter, J.

NKOSI

245 Nkosi and Gail Johnson and teachers were interviewed in the film,
> *Talking about sex, HIV and AIDS*, Teaching Screens for National Departments of Health and Education, 1997. Director Lesley Lawson.

246 The full text of Nkosi's speech to the International AIDS Conference available at: www.nkosishaven.co.za

Chapter Eleven. A state of denial

THE CUTTING EDGE

247 The staff and patients at Murchison hospital were interviewed in the film,
> *Mashayabhuqe, AIDS hits everyone*, Teaching Screens, 1998.

AIDS, THE NEW STRUGGLE

248 Nelson Mandela's speech at the World Economic Forum, Davos, 3 February 1997. Available at: www.anc.org.za/ancdocs/history/mandela/1997/sp970203.html

249 Rose Smart took over leadership of the AIDS Directorate in 1996.

250 National programme faltering:
> This was due to a lack of managerial capacity rather than insufficient funds. Between 1994 and 1997, the AIDS programme consistently under-spent its budget allocation. The challenges were complicated by the quasi-federal system that gave immense powers to provincial governments, and meant that the directorate had little say over how programmes were executed.

251 For more on budgets and under-spending in this period see:
> Marais, H. 2000. *To the edge. AIDS review 2000*. Centre for the Study of AIDS, University of Pretoria.

252 A good review of these events and the government structures for HIV is given in: Strode, A & Grant, K. 2004. *Understanding the institutional dynamics of South Africa's response to HIV/AIDS*. IDASA.

LIFE SKILLS

253 Interview with Aloma Foster from 'Talking about sex, HIV and AIDS' op cit.
> Evaluation of Teacher training programme, Northern Province, CASE, July 1998. Khulisa Management Services. 2000. *Evaluation of HIV/AIDS programme in secondary schools*. November 2000.

THE MATERIALITY OF EVERYDAY SEX

254 Zwane's study is described in a submission to the Truth and Reconciliation Commission, available at:
> www.doj.gov.za/trc/submit/gender.htm

255 Hunter. 2002. The materiality of everyday sex: thinking beyond prostitution. *African Studies* 61 (1) 100-119.

256 Luke, M & Kurz, K. 2002. Cross-generational and transactional sexual relations in sub-Saharan Africa. Available at www.icrw.org

257 Dunke, K, Jewkes, R & Brown, H *et al*. 2004.Transactional sex among women in Soweto, South Africa: prevalence, risk factors and association with HIV infection.

258 Research on AIDS and poverty and sexual networking and poverty were discussed at a conference in Durban in 2006. A good summary of these discussions can be found at www.aidsmap.com

259 Smart, T. 2006. PEPFAR: Greater wealth, not poverty, associated with higher HIV prevalence in Africa, according to survey, August 2, 2006.

260 Smart, T. 2006. PEPFAR: Epidemiologist presents a scientific rationale for focusing on Abstinence and Being Faithful in sub-Saharan Africa.

Endnotes and References

An epidemic of AIDS hysteria

261 The role of the media and civil society organisations and the general climate of denial in 1998 discussed in:
Lawson, L. 1998. Millennium Megabomb, *Leadership* 17 (4).
262 *New African* denialist articles are described in the endnotes for Chapter One.
263 16/9/1998, *The Citizen*, Charles Geshekter. Available at:
www.virusmyth.net/aids/data/cghysteria.htm
264 Ankhoma, B. 2001. AIDS: rhetoric and reality, *New African* March 2001.
265 Dr Piot World AIDS Day speech available at:
www.hri.org/news/world/undh/1998/98-12-01.undh.html

Chapter Twelve: Positive lives

Death by stoning

266 Articles dealing with the death of Gugu Dlamini and subsequent court case:
- 28/12/1998, Associated Press, 'HIV-positive South African woman murdered'.
- 24/1/1999, *Sunday Times*, 'Residents flee as AIDS sparks war'.
- 14/8/1999, *Sunday Independent*, 'Dlamini case dropped for lack of proof'.
- 16/8/1999, Associated Press, 'Charged dropped'.
- 31/8/1999, *The Mercury*, 'AIDS worker killing fiasco under review'.
- 29/9/1999, *Mail & Guardian*, 'AIDS martyr's killers may face justice'.
- 10/1/1999, *Sunday Times*, 'Callers threatens victim of killer virus'.
- 10/12/2000, *Sunday Times*, 'AIDS martyr honoured by council'.
- 11/1/2001, *The Star*, 'Activists bemoan Dlamini inquest postponement'.
- 12/1/2001, *Dispatch*, 'Dlamini family afraid to testify in court'.
- 18/7/2001, *The Star*, 'Murdered AIDS activist, family seeks justice'.
- 22/7/2001, *City Press*, report on inquest.
- 19/8/2001, *Sunday Times*, 'Statue to honour AIDS martyr'.
- Minutes of AIDS Consortium meeting 31/2/1999.
267 4/3/1999, *Mail & Guardian*, 'Mbeki launches AIDS train'.

Treatment action

268 Quotes from Achmat and various TAC activists from 'TAC. Treatment Action Campaign. An Overview'. Available at www.tac.org.za
269 11/12/1998, *Cape Argus* reported former human rights commissioner Dr Rhoda Kadalie's presence at the fast. Her comments related to the recent $4.6 billion arms procurement programme, the largest public procurement deal in post-apartheid South Africa.
270 24/3/1999, *Cape Times*, article on Zuma at branch meeting.
271 29/4/1999, *Mail & Guardian*, 'AIDS organisations demonstrate at Glaxo Wellcome'.

272 29/4/1999, *The Star*, 'Mbeki wants lower price for anti-AIDS drug'.
273 2/5/1999, *Sunday Independent*, 'Zuma pledge on cost of anti-HIV drug'.
274 2/5/1999, *Sunday Times*, 'Zuma rejects cheap AZT'.
275 7/5/1999, *Mail & Guardian*, 'Ministry refuses anti-HIV drug discount'.

Broedertwis

276 Later conflict between TAC and Napwa:
  TAC Newsletter 30 March 2004, Condemn the threats by NAPWA against AIDS Activists. Mark Heywood, TAC treasurer. Available at www.tac.org.za
277 Heywood quote on 1999 Napwa/TAC conflict in:
  Heywood, M. 2005. The price of denial. Available at www.tac.org.za
278 Minutes of the Napwa Board meeting held at Johannesburg International Airport Conference Centre, May 20, 1999.

Chapter Thirteen: Securing the future

Watching out

279 USTR statement on SA at WHA:
  5/2/1999, *US Government efforts to negotiate the repeal, termination or withdrawal of article 15 (C) of the South African Medicines and Related Substances Act of 1965.* US Department of State report.
280 In 1995 Ralph Nader founded an organisation called Consumer Project on Technology, which focused on intellectual property rights, and had a particular interest in compulsory licencing. James Love was the director of the organisation.
281 Discussion of the March meeting in Geneva and other key calendar events:
  Love timeline, 1999, op cit.
282 Eric Sawyer was a founder member of ACT UP/New York and had been active in US treatment access issues since the late 1980s.
283 16/4/1999, Interview with Eric Sawyer, HIV/AIDS Human Rights Project. John James, available at www.aids.org
284 11/4/1999, *Reuters*, Groups say US hurts world access to AIDS drugs.

The Charm offensive

285 The story of Secure the Future is based on the account in the article:
  - 29/12/2000, *Washington Post*, 'The limits of $100 million', Bill Brubaker; and
  - 6/5/1999, Wall Street Journal, 'Bristol-Myers Squib heeds call to bolster the war against HIV in Africa'.
286 The other countries participating in Secure the Future were Botswana, Namibia, Lesotho and Swaziland.

ENDNOTES AND REFERENCES 309

287 Nono Simelela took over from Rose Smart as AIDS directorate chief at the beginning of 1999.

288 30/4/1999, PhRMA supports USTR on South Africa. Available at:
http://lists.essential.org/pharm-policy/msg00104.html

289 WHA resolution and Roberts' statement in:
24/5/1999, *Third world network*, Health Assembly adopts new revised strategy. Available at www.twnside.org.sg/title/assembly-cn.htm

GORE'S GREED AND THE FED-UP QUEERS

290 Sawyer interviewed in:
24/4/1999, *San Francisco Chronicle*, 'New crusade to lower AIDS drug costs'.

291 Love, J. 1999. Clinton/Gore top staffs: pharmaceutical background. *AIDS Treatment News* #317, April 16, 1999.

292 Sawyer on Gore:
23/6/1999, *Baltimore Sun*, 'AIDS protesters track Gore on campaign trail'.

293 Gore and genocide statement: *ZMagazine*, Scott McLarty, available at:
www.zmag.org

294 Gore Zaps — Described on ACT UP website, www.actupny.org

295 10/7/1999, *Observer*, 'Gore accused of working against cheap AIDS drugs', Julian Borger.

296 23/8/1999, *New York Times* editorial, 'Drugs for AIDS in Africa'.

297 21/2/2001, *Cameraone*, 'Act up groups "Zap" 2000 campaigns'.

298 12/8/1999, *Business Day*, 'Drugs patent wrangle nears end', Simon Barber.

299 7/7/1999, *Cape Argus*, 'Gore accused of AIDS drug profit policy', Rich Mkhondo.

DRAMA WITH SAMMDRA

300 Gray, A, Matsebula, T, Blaauw, D, Schneider, H & Gilson, L. 2002. *Policy change in a context of transition: Drug policy in South Africa 1989-1999.* Johannesburg, South Africa: Centre of Health Policy, University of Witwatersrand.

301 21/7/1999, *Cape Times*, 'Loophole freeing dozens of drug dealers'.

302 23/7/1999, *Independent Online*, 'Court sets aside invalid new drug law'.

AID FOR AFRICA

303 19/7/1999, White House press release, Vice President Gore announces administration will seek $100 million initiative — a record increase — in funds to fight global AIDS. Available at www.fedglobe.org

304 Removal from Watch List and other events described in: Love timeline, 1999, op cit.
- 17/9/1999, Joint understanding between the governments of South Africa and the United States of America, Issued by Department of Trade and Industry. Available at www.polity.org.za.
- 23/9/1999, Five common mistakes by reporters covering the US/South

Africa disputes over compulsory licensing and parallel imports, James Love, Consumer Project on Technology, available at www.cptech.org

305 1/12/1999, White House Press release, President Clinton announces new cooperative effort to help poor countries gain access to affordable medicines.

Chapter Fourteen: WHERE THE TRUTH LIES

WE CAN DO THIS!

306 Profiles:
- Mantombazana Tshabalala-Msimang. www.polity.org.za
- 01/09/2003, Profile, Dr Who? Available at www.iafrica.com

307 PhRMA statement on discussions with new MoH:
Submission of the Pharmaceutical Research and Manufacturers of Amercia (PhRMA) for the National Trade Estimate Report on Foreign Trade Barriers (NTE), 2001. November 27, 2000.

308 The PMA temporarily suspended the lawsuit on September 9 1999.

309 In July 1999 the results of HIVNET 012 study were announced. This showed that a single 200mg tablet of the antiretroviral drug nevirapine, given to mothers in labour, followed by a single 2mg dose to the newborns within 72 hours of delivery demonstrated similar results to the short course AZT in reducing the transmission of HIV from mother to child.
- 23/7/1999, *Mail & Guardian*, 'Ban on AZT under review'.

310 - 6/8/1999, *Dispatch*, 'Health dept to fight AIDS using Ugandan model'.
- 8/8/1999, *Sunday Times*, A nation coming to terms with AIDS. Once the HIV capital of Africa, Uganda had become the continent's inspiration for combating the spread of the disease.

311 Nevirapine pricing:
18/7/1999, *Sunday Independent*.

A NEW KIND OF POISON

312 President Mbeki's address to the National Council of Provinces, 28/10/1999. Available at www.info.gov.za/speeches/1999/991028409p1004.htm

313 Controversy about AZT:
- 28/10/1999, *IOL*, 'Mbeki justifies caution on "toxic" AZT'.
- 28/10/1999, *IOL*, 'Mbeki is wrong, AZT is safe, says Glaxo'.
- 30/10/1999, *Sunday Independent*, 'Mbeki sparks row over AIDS drug'.
- 7/11/1999, *IOL*, 'AIDS drug sparks human rights debate'.
- 1/12/1999, *The Mercury*, 'Mbeki attacked again for AZT decision'.

314 Dr Tshabalala-Msimang's initial comments on AZT in:
28/10/1999, *SAPA*, Mbeki warns about AZT, available at ANC Daily News

Briefing, www.anc.org.za

315 Brink's article *AZT: A medicine from hell*, October 1998 is available at www.tig.co.za. It was published in *The Citizen* on March 17, 1999. Dr Desmond Martin's reply was published on March 31, 1999.

316 Researcher James Myburg alleges that the Vissers alerted Mbeki to the Brink AZT debate in *The Citizen*. However Brink maintains that he passed the work directly onto Roberts who gave it to the president.

(Myburg's allegation was made by at an interdisciplinary AIDS seminar series in Oxford University on 23/11/05. Quoted in Nattrass, J. 2006. *AIDS, Science and governance: the battle over antiretroviral therapy in post-apartheid South Africa*. Available at: www.aidstruth.org/nattrass.pdf)

317 Brink's account of why the case was dismissed at:
www.indymedia.ie/article/70676?print_page=true

318 Statement to the National Assembly by Dr M E Tshabalala-Msimang MP, Minister of Health, on HIV/AIDS and related issues. November 16 1999.
Available at www.info.gov.za/speeches

319 The study to which the minister referred was being conducted at Chris Hani-Baragwanath hospital by researchers Drs James McIntyre and Glenda Gray. Dubbed the Saint trial, the study aimed to compare the efficacy of nevirapine to that of a two-drug combination of AZT and 3TC.

Gore's greed revisited

320 Love quote:
24/11/1999, *San Francisco Chronicle*, World Trade showdown/activists, industry split over AIDS drugs.

321 The legal consequences of the ambiguity in the wording of 15 C of the Medicines Act are clearly outlined in the following essay:
Chung T (2002) *Shocking the conscience of the world. International norms and the access to AIDS treatment in South Africa*. Essay presented in partial fulfilment of a Juris Doctor Degree. Harvard Law School. Available at:
leda.law.harvard.edu/leda/data/450/Chung.rtf

Talking to the denialists

322 The eight questions Mbeki was asking were allegedly:
1. What means and methods are used in the Public Health System to test the 'HIV status' of individuals?
2. What definition is used, again in the public health system, to classify a person as being afflicted with AIDS?
3. Of the people determined to have died of AIDS, what 'opportunistic disease' was identified as having been the immediate cause of death?
4. Would there be any record of the treatment that such people would have

received for these diseases, including the health profiles of such people at the point they started experiencing continuous bouts of diarrhoea, coughing, weight loss, etc?

5. Has any research been done on the health profiles of the populations where allegedly it has been found that there are large numbers of 'HIV positive people' (eg in KZN)?

6. Has any research been done on 'HIV-positive' infants, children and orphans with regard to their health profiles, those of their mothers and families, as well as the lifestyles and socio-economic circumstances of the mothers and families?

7. On what do we base the statistics we publish occasionally on the incidence of HIV and AIDS, and how do we arrive at the projections?

8. Are there any anti-HIV/AIDS drugs that are dispensed by the public health system on a regular basis, including to medical workers who might be exposed to needle pricks?

Source: 2/3/2000, Talked with the President, David Rasnick. Available at : www.virusmyth.net

323 Brink, A. 2004. *'Just say Yes Mr President': Mbeki and AIDS*, 2004. Available at: www.dr-rath-foundation.org.za/pdf-files/justsayyes.pdf

324 The Minister and Geshekter's meeting is described in Rasnick 2000, op cit.

325 4/2/2000, Mbeki State of the Nation address to parliament. Available at: www.info.gov.za/speeches/2000/000204451p1001.htm

326 28/2/2000, *SAPA*, 'Expert panel will look at AIDS with fresh eyes'.
- 2/3/2000, Statement on the proposed establishment of an Expert Advisory Panel on HIV/AIDS. Issued by the Minister of Health.

327 The President's March 15 letter to his critics described in:
25/3/2000, *Sunday Independent*, 'Mbeki digs in heels over HIV/AIDS'.
This article was in turn reported internationally by Agence France Press on March 26, 2000.

328 Mbeki's letter to Clinton available at:
www.pbs.org/wgbh/pages/frontline/aids/docs/mbeki.html

329 Impact of Mbeki's letter to Clinton:
19/3/2000, *Washington Post*, South African President escalates AIDS feud, Barton Gellman.

330 May 2000, *New African*, 'Around Africa', column by Huw Christie.
- 14/4/2000, *Cape Argus*, 'Don't snub AIDS talks because of Mbeki', available at int.iol.co.za

More poison

331 8/2/2000, *The Star*, 'Health minister rejects AZT probes'.

332 Proceedings of the National Assembly, Wednesday April 5, 2000. Available at: www.parliament.gov.za

ENDNOTES AND REFERENCES 🎗 313

333 9/4/2000, *Sunday Times*, 'Doctors slam minister for blaming deaths on drug'.
334 6/4/2000, *SAPA*, 'Manufacturer puzzled by Nevirapine death claims'.

Chapter Fifteen: BEHOLD A PALE HORSE

WISE MEN AND FOOLS

335 Composition of the President's Advisory Panel. Source: *Presidential AIDS Advisory Panel Report*, March 2001, available at
www.info.gov.za/otherdocs/2001/aidspanelpdf.pdf

Invited by the president and present at both panels:
Professor Salim S Abdool-Karim; Dr Stefano M Bertozzi; Dr Harvey Bialy; Dr Awa Marie Coll-Seck; Dr Etienne de Harven; Dr Ann Duerr; Professor Peter Duesberg; Dr Christian Fiala; Dr Helene Gayle; Dr Roberto A Giraldo; Dr ET Katabira; Dr Claus Koehnlein; Dr Manu VL Kothari; Dr Clifford Lane; Dr Marsha Lillie-Blanton; Dr Malegapuru W Makgoba; Professor Sam Mhlongo; Professor Ephraim Mokgokong; Professor Stephen Owen; Dr Jorge Perez; Dr David Rasnick; Mr David Scondras; Dr Joseph Sonnabend; Dr Zena Stein; Dr Gordon Stewart.

Invited by the president and only present at the first panel:
Dr W Chalamira-Nkhoma; Dr Andrew Herxheimer; Professor Luc Montagnier; Dr Walter Prozesky; Dr Mark D Smith; Dr Stefano Vella; Dr Jose M Zuniga.

Invited by the president and present only at the second panel:
Dr Stephen Chandiwana; Professor Roy Mugwera; Professor Eleni Papadopoulos-Eleopoulos; Prof Heinz Spranger; Dr Valender Turner.

Invited by the president but could not attend:
Professor Françoise Barre-Sinoussi; Dr Robert Gallo; Dr Kaptue; Dr Souleymane M'Boup; Professor Fred Mhalu; Professor Valerie Mizrahi; Professor Pierre Mpele; Dr Paranjape; Dr Praphan Phanuphak; Professor Robert Root-Bernstein; Dr Kary Mullis.

Invited by the secretariat and present only at the second meeting:
Professor Jerry Coovadia; Professor Charles Geshekter; Dr Glenda Gray; Dr Anthony Mbewu; Professor James McIntyre; Dr Lynn Morris; Dr Dan Ncayiyana; Dr Philip Onyebujoh; Dr Priscilla Reddy; Professor Barry Schoub; Professor Allan Smith; Dr Jimmy Volmink; Professor Alan Whiteside; Dr Carolyn Williamson; Mr Winston Zulu.

336 *The fool* — poem by Patrick Henry Pearse (1879–1916).
337 Accounts of the panels:
- The President's speech: Remarks at the first meeting of the Presidential AIDS Advisory Panel. May 6, 2000. Pretoria. Available at:
www.anc.org.za/ancdocs/history/mbeki

- 25/5/2000, *New York Press*, 'A contrary conference in South Africa', Celia Farber, available at www.virusmyth.net
- Sidley, P. 2000. 'Mbeki appoints a team to look at cause of AIDS', *BMJ*. 320:1291, May 13.
- 5/7/2000, *Village Voice*, 'Debating the obvious: inside the South Africa government's controversial AIDS panel', Mark Schoofs, July 5, 2000.
- *Presidential AIDS Advisory Panel Report*, March 2001, available at www.info.gov.za/otherdocs/2001/aidspanelpdf.pdf

Acting out

338 5/7/2000, *Village Voice*, 'Debating the obvious: inside the South Africa government's controversial AIDS panel', Mark Schoofs, July 5, 2000.

339 1/7/2000, *SAPA/AFP*, '5 000 scientists sign statement over cause of AIDS row'.

340 3/7/2000, *SAPA*, 'Mbeki's office consigns Durban declaration to dustbin'.
- 8/9/2000, *Mail & Guardian*, 'All the President's Scientists, Diary of a round-earther', Anonymous.

341 *Presidential AIDS Advisory Panel Report*, March 2001, available at: www.info.gov.za/otherdocs/2001/aidspanelpdf.pdf

342 Christie, H. 2000. 'Suspend all HIV testing, Mbeki panel recommends'. *New African*, September.

343 On December 1 2005, Dr Manto Tshabalala-Msimang told a caller during an SABC radio phone-in that the research recommended by the president's panel was continuing.

344 26/2/2007. Harvey Bialy: GIGO — or why HIV antibody tests in South Africa are worthless. http://barnesworld.blogs.com/barnes_world/2007/02/index.html

Breaking the silence

345 Mbeki-bashing quote:
3/7/2000, *SAPA*, 'Mbeki's office consigns Durban Declaration to dustbin'.

346 Description of the march:
- ACT UP New York, www.actupny.org
- TAC overview, www.tac.org.za

347 9/7/2000, Speech of President Mbeki at the opening session of the Thirteenth International AIDS Conference, Issued by: Office of the Presidency. Available at www.anc.org.za/anc/newsbrief

348 Reports on the conference:
- 10/7/2000, *CNN*, 'Hundreds walk out on Mbeki at AIDS conference'.
- 10/7/2000, *Washington Post*, 'Hundreds walk out on Mbeki'.
- 10/7/2000, *Newsday*, 'Focus on poverty, not HIV/AIDS'.
- 30/11/2001, *BBC News*, 'Nkosi's story'.
- 21/7/2002, *The Citizen*, 'Durban Report: Shovelling out the AIDS controversy'.

Endnotes and References 315

- Cohen, M. 2000. 'Commentary: the meaning of the opening ceremony'. *Medscape Today,* available at www.medscape.com/viewarticle/418898
- Nkosi's speech, available at www.nkosishaven.co.za

The ja-nee president

349 11/9/2000, *Time,* 'You cannot attribute immune deficiency exclusively to a virus'. Available at www.time.com/time/europe/magazine/2000/0911/mbeki.html

- Mbeki's response to questions about HIV/AIDS in an interview with *Time* magazine, Government Communication and Information System. Available at www.gcis.gov.za
- 10/9/1999, *Reuters,* 'South Africa's Mbeki clings to controversial AIDS stance'.
- 10/9/2000, *Associated Press,* 'Mbeki: HIV not the only cause of AIDS'.
- 7/9/2000, ABC, 'AIDS issue leads to on-air spat' transcript available at: www.abc.net.au
- 5/9/2000, *Mail & Guardian,* 'AIDS: It's an Illuminati Plot'.
- 8/9/2000, *Mail & Guardian,* 'Govt AIDS nut linked to Ku Klux Klan'.

350 Nujoma told and ILO conference in June 2000 that AIDS 'is an artificial disease… it is the result of certain countries producing chemical means to kill other humans, other nations.' Nujoma called on ILO members to join forces to make 'those who have invested in chemical war spend that money instead on the fight against this disease'.

- 15/6/2000, *Inter press service,* 'ILO conference approves maternity rights treaty'.
- 8/9/2000, *Mail & Guardian,* 'Cosatu: End scientific speculation on HIV/AIDS'.
- 13/9/2000, *Cape Times,* 'Say HIV causes AIDS, leaked paper tells Mbeki'.
- 14/9/2000, *BBC,* 'SA government steps into AIDS row'.
- 14/9/2000, *The Star,* 'HIV might very well cause AIDS, Mbeki'.
- 15/9/2000, *UPI,* 'South African government takes out AIDS ads'.
- 22/9/2000, *Mail & Guardian,* 'ANC concern over Mbeki fiasco'.
- 22/9/2000, *Cape Times,* 'AIDS debate losing its steam'.

Losing their grip

351 PEP for rape survivors: In the late 1990s, along with the demand for AZT to prevent HIV transmission from mother to child, there had been a strong demand for the drug to be available to rape survivors. It was already common practice in Europe and the US to offer a short course of antiretrovirals in this context.

352 Debate on the president's budget vote, National Assembly, 13/6/2000, Leon challenges Mbeki over AZT for rape survivors:

- 9/6/2000, *Sunday Times,* 'Mbeki vs Leon'.
- 6/10/2000, *Mail & Guardian,* 'What Leon and Mbeki has to say'.

353 Grip provided a cocktail of AZT and 3TC to rape survivors.

254 Grip saga:
- 22/10/2000, *Sunday Times*, 'MEC boots anti-rape project out of hospital'.
- 2/11/2000, *The Star*, 'Health MEC probes AIDS NGO'.
- 19/2/2001, *Africa Eye News Service*, 'Mpumalanga prosecutes anti-rape doctors'.
- 3/2/2003, *Sunday Times*, 'Now rest your case Miss Manana'.

355
- 6/10/2000, *Mail & Guardian*, 'Mbeki fingers the CIA in AIDS conspiracy'.
- 1/10/2000, *Cape Times*, 'No drug conspiracy, AIDS group tells Mbeki'.
- 6/10/2000, *Mail & Guardian*, 'What the president said'.
- 6/10/2000, *Guardian*, 'CIA and drug firms out to get me, Mbeki says'.

356 Gumede, W M (2005) *Thabo Mbeki and the soul of the ANC*. Zebra Press. Cape Town.

357
- 15/10/2000, *Sunday Times*, AIDS: Mbeki backs off.
- 17/10/2000, *Associated Press*, 'Mbeki to scale down AIDS debate'.

Chapter Sixteen: IN THE COURT OF PUBLIC OPINION

DEFIANCE!

358 1/10/2000, *Cape Times*, 'No drug conspiracy, AIDS group tells Mbeki'.

359 The defiance campaign is described in:
- Treatment Action Campaign, An overview. Available at www.tac.org.za
- Defying the Drug Cartel, The South African Campaign for access to essential medicines, An interview with Zackie Achmat, *Multinational Monitor*, Jan/Feb 2001, Vol 22 — Number 1&2.
- 17/10/2000, TAC Press release, 'TAC announces the Christopher Moraka Defiance Campaign against patent abuse'.

360 Fluconazole is the generic name of the drug; Pfizer's branded version is named Diflucan.

360 17/10/2000, *Cape Times*, 'Rebels show smuggled drugs cost R100 less'.

362 20/6/2000, TAC Press release, 'Pfizer donation protects profits while people with HIV/AIDS die!'

363 20/10/2000, *Cape Times*, 'AIDS activist hands himself over to the police'.

364 9/10/2000, *Reuters*, 'Mbeki's scepticism sparks anger, denial'. Sue Thomas.

BIG PHARMA VS MANDELA

365 The five-company treatment access initiative was announced on May 11, 2000. The events that led up to it, and the entry of the generics industry, are described in the article:

> 28/12/2000, *Washington Post*, 'A turning point that left millions behind', Barton Gellman.

Endnotes and References 317

366 Cipla offers, 23/2/2001, MSF press release.
367 Tumbling drug prices:
- 21/2/2001, *BBC News*, 'Glaxo offers cheaper AIDS drugs'.
- 6/3/2001, *Wall Street Journal*, 'Price war breaks out over AIDS drugs in Africa as generics present challenge'.
- 7/3/2001, *BBC News*, 'US firm offers cheap AIDS drugs'.

368 SA refusal to settle court case in:
27/11/2000, Submission of the Pharmaceutical Research and Manufacturers' of America (PhRMA) for the National Trade Estimate Report on Foreign Trade Barriers (NTE).

369 14/1/2001, *Independent Online*, 'Drug firms to fight AIDS battle in court'.
370 Anti-Pharma articles in the UK press:
- 14/1/2001, *Guardian*, 'Drug giants sue to cut HIV lifeline'.
- 12/2/2001, *Guardian*, 'Evil triumphs in a sick society'.
- 12/2/2001, *Guardian*, 'A lot of very greedy people', John le Carré.
- 12/2/2001, *Guardian*, 'The profits that kill'.
- 12/2/2001, *Guardian*, 'At the mercy of drug giants'.

371 Le Carré, J. 2000. *The Constant Gardener*, Hodder & Stoughton.
372 1/4/2001, *CNN*, 'Drug companies: South Africa spurned AIDS drug offers'.
373 23/04/2001, *Business Day*, 'The court of public opinion', Pat Sidley.

The case that wasn't

374 Coverage of the court case:
- 7/3/2001, *Guardian*, 'Pretoria puts pressure on drug giants'.
- 16/4/2001, Reuters, 'S Africa set to lock horns with drug industry'.
- 5/3/2001, *Independent Online*, 'Medicines Act is illegal.'
- 22/4/2001, *Observer*, 'Drugs: Round one to Africa'.
- SAPA news reports April 18 — April 19, 2001

375 Affidavit of James Packard Love in the matter between the Pharmaceutical Manufacturers' Association of South Africa and others and the President of the Republic of South Africa and others. Case No 4183/98 April 2001. Available at: www.cpt.org
376 20/4/2001, *Business Day*, 'Silent trump card gives state winning hand'.
377 19/4/2001, *Independent online*, 'Good news, bad news for AIDS patients'.
378 Heywood, M. 'Debunking conglomo-talk: a case study of amicus curiae as an instrument for advocacy, investigation and mobilisation'. *Law Development and Democracy*. Available at www.tac.org.za

'Dr No'

379 Accounts of the meeting: TAC statement, June 12 2001, available at:
www.tac.org.za

- 15/6/2001, *Mail & Guardian*, 'AIDS battle to return to court'.
- Heywood, M. 2003. 'Current developments, Preventing mother to child HIV transmission', *South African Journal of Human Rights*. 19(2): 278-315. Available at: www.tac.org.za

380 The cost of R1,99 per child was given in a report by an MoH consultant: 18/7/2000, *Mail & Guardian*, 'It costs R1,99 to save a child'.

381 TAC affidavits and court case available at www.tac.org.za

Toxic shock

382 The 2001 Virodene story:
- 19/7/2001, *Wall Street Journal*, 'Tanzanian military helped company skirt drug regulations to test Virodene', Mark Schoofs.
- 2/9/2001, *Business Day*, 'AIDS drug has SA pair thrown out of Tanzania'.
- 9/9/2001, *Mail & Guardian*, 'SA AIDS quacks given the boot'.
- 14/9/2001, *Mail & Guardian*, 'Virodene quacks amass huge debt'.

383 Oxihumate:
- 2/10/2001, SAPA, 'Oxihumate not illegal: Health Dept'.
- 3/10/2001, *Mail & Guardian*, 'AIDS treatments: from dry-cleaning fluid to fertiliser'.
- 5/10/2001, *Mail & Guardian*, 'The AIDS fertiliser hits the fan'.

384
- 5/6/2002, *Mail & Guardian*, 'The ANC's Virodene backers'.
- 28/6/2002, *Mail & Guardian*, 'Results of trials to be released'.
- 22/6/2002, *City Press*, 'Project Virodene dying despite aid'.
- 5/7/2002, *Mail & Guardian*, 'Who's bankrolling Virodene?'

385 Address by President Thabo Mbeki at the inaugural ZK Matthews memorial lecture, University of Fort Hare, October 12 2001.
www.info.gov.za/speeches/2001/011016442p1001.htm

Chapter Seventeen: Little white crosses

The mother-to-child story so far...

386 Nevirapine price quoted in the National Assembly April 5, 2005. Available at: www.parliament.gov.za

387 In the South African Nevirapine Trial (SAINT), 1 306 mother and infant pairs were randomised to either nevirapine during labour and post-delivery, or multiple doses of AZT/3TC during labour and for one week after delivery to mother and baby. In both treatment arms, about 40 per cent of infants were breast-fed. Eight weeks after birth, there was no significant difference observed between the rate of HIV infection or death across the two treatment arms, with a rate of 14,3 per cent in the simpler nevirapine arm and 12,5 per cent in the more involved and expensive dual therapy arm.

388 7/7/2000, *IOL online*, 'SA sceptical about free HIV drug offer'. Available at: www.iol.co.za

389 Moodly, D. 2000. 'The Saint trial: nevirapine (NVP) versus zidovudine (ZDV)+lamivudine (3TC) in prevention of peripartum HIV transmission'. Int Conf AIDS 2000, Jul 9-14; 13:16 (abstract no. LbOr2).
- 11/7/2000, *The Star*, '"Saint" lightens gloom of AIDS conference'.

390 Heywood, M. 'Current developments', op cit. Available at: www.tac.org.za/Documents/MTCTCourtCase/Heywood.pdf

Making a plan

391 9/5/1999, *Sunday Times*, 'Zuma in dramatic AZT about-turn. Hospital's go-ahead to distribute drug'.
- 20/1/2002, *Sunday Times*, 'Doctors defy drug ban'.

392 21/9/2000, Statement by the Gauteng Premier's committee on AIDS, available at www.info.gov.za/speeches/2000
- 22/5/2001, *Business Day*, 'Gauteng goes ahead with AIDS project'.

Back to court

393 Affidavits of Busi Maqungo (August 2001), Prof P A Cooper (November 2001) and other court papers available at www.tac.co.za

394 14/12/2001, *The Independent on Saturday*, 'Nevirapine not enough, says TAC'.

Dr No strikes back

395 6/3/2002, Minister of Health's statement to parliament on the National PMTCT research sites. Available at:
www.info.gov.za/speeches/2002/0203081046a1001.htm

396 28/1/2002, AFP, 'AIDS drugs may be in S African provincial hospitals by July'. Involvement of Mandela:
- 7/2/2002, *BBC*, 'Mandela urges "war" on AIDS'.
- 8/2/2002, *Sunday Times,* 'Mandela rebukes government on AIDS'.
- Sidley, P. 2002. 'Mandela presents his concern about AIDS policy to ANC committee'. *BMJ*. February 23, 324-446.

397
- 19/2/2002, *The Star*, 'Health Minister slams Shilowa's AIDS plan'.
- 19/2/2002, *The Star*, 'Tshabalala-Msimang stands alone'.

398 24/3/2002, *The Star,* Nevirapine hitch is academic not medical.

399 ANC Youth League statement in Heywood, Current developments, op cit.
- 27/3/2002, *The Star*, What did Manto and Maduna really say?

Of sheep and geese...

400 Giraldo, R (2001) Scientific data against the use of nevirapine in pregnant

women, infants, children, and anybody else. October 2001. Available at: www.virusmyth.net
401 10/3/2003, *IOL online*, Manto not interested in dissident's HIV views.
402 28/9/2001, *Mail & Guardian*, 'Coal-fired AIDS muti tested on soldiers'.
- 2/10/2001, *Associated Press*, 'South African firm begins marketing nutritional supplement'.
- 5/10/2001, *Mail & Guardian*, 'HIV/AIDS fertiliser hits the fan'.
- Botes, M, Dekker J & Van Rensberg, C. 2002. 'Phase 1 trial with oral oxihumate in HIV-infected patients'. *Drug development research* 57 (1): 34-39.

403 8/3/2002, *Mail & Guardian*, 'AIDS dissident Allen linked to Mokaba'.
404 22/3/2002, *Mail & Guardian*, 'AIDS drugs killed Parks, say ANC'.
405 *Castro Hlongwane, Caravans, Cats, Geese, Foot & Mouth And Statistics: HIV/AIDS and the Struggle for the Humanisation of the African*, March 2002. Available at: www.virusmyth.net/aids/data/ancdoc.htm.
406 30/3/2002, *New York Times*, 'An AIDS sceptic in South Africa feeds simmering doubts'.
- 4/4/2002, *The Star*, 'Revolution is his trade be it war or medicine'.

407 20/3/2002, *SAPA*, 'ANC reaffirms support of government HIV/AIDS policy'.

Chapter Eighteen: THE MORAL ECONOMY

THE TURNABOUT
408 7/4/2002, *Sunday Times*, 'HIV/AIDS: Judgement Day!'
409 Mbeki article:
Mbeki, T, Health Month, *ANC Today* 2 (14) 5-11 April 2002.
- 6/4/2002, *Cape Argus*, 'Mbeki's latest rant'.
- 19/4/2002, *Mail & Guardian*, 'What bent Mbeki'.

410 17/4/2002, Statement of Cabinet on HIV/AIDS, available at www.doh.gov.za

BORN FREE
411 Sachs, A. 2005. The judicial enforcement of socio-economic rights. Available at: www.lawsociety.ie
412 Tshabalala-Msimang's poison quote:
8/7/2002, *Newsday*, 'Rage over 'Poison' as AIDS treatment. South Africa's fears disputed by others'.
The minister later denied that she said this.
413 The first case that placed social and economic rights before the Constitutional Court was the Grootboom case. In October 2000, the judgement established that the government had an obligation to realise the 'right to housing' for those desperately in need.

Cries of murder!

414 27/7/2002, *IOL online*, 'Madiba to take up Achmat's case with Mbeki'.

415 9/10/2002, ANC Daily News Briefing, Partnership against AIDS marks fourth anniversary. Government Communication and Information Systems. Available on www.anc.org.za

416 16/10/2002, *The Star*, 'Government vows to lead national AIDS battle'.

417 16/10/2002, Statement on meeting between deputy president and the Treatment Action Campaign, available at www.tac.org.za

418
- 20/1/2003, *The Mercury*, 'Manto hosts AIDS dissident despite criticism'.
- 21/1/2003, *The Mercury*, 'Rave reviews for Manto's dissident'.

419 TAC Civil Disobedience Campaign Update, March 26, 2003. Available at: www.tac.org.za
- 16/3/2003, *Independent Online*, 'We are going to put the government on trial,' available at www.iol.org.za
- 21/3/2003, *The Star*, 'AIDS activists turn up the heat on ministers'.
- 21/3/2003, *Guardian*, 'AIDS protesters accuse Pretoria ministers of manslaughter'.
- 24/4/2003, *Mail & Guardian*, 'AIDS activists demonstrate countrywide'.
- 25/3/2003, *Mail & Guardian*, 'TAC disrupts Manto's speech'.
- 26/3/2002, *Business Day*, 'Health Minister unfazed by irate activists'.
- 26/3/2003, *The Mercury*, 'Time for hugs is over, TAC tells Manto'.
- 5/4/2003, *Mail & Guardian*, 'The long walk to civil disobedience' (Letter by Achmat).
- 11/4/2003, *Mail & Guardian*, 'The madness of Queen Manto'.

We think it is too much

420 The HIV prevalence rate peaked at 37,5 per cent of women in KwaZulu-Natal, and nationally among young women (25-29 year age group) at nearly 30 per cent. From:
> Department of Health. 2006. National HIV and syphilis antenatal seroprevalence survey in South Africa, 2005.

421 South African Medical Research Institute. 2001. The impact of HIV/AIDS on adult mortality in South Africa. September 2001.

422 At the time of writing, new research showed that deaths of young women (ages 20-39 years) had more than tripled during the period 1997 to 2004. This emerged from a report by Statistics South Africa, reported in *Mail & Guardian* on 8/6/2006.

423 UNICEF, UNAIDS, USAID. 2004. *Children on the Brink*. UNICEF, New York, July 2004.
- 4/8/2003, *Reuters*, 'SA pandemic enters the valley of death'.

424 31/7/2003, *Cape Times*, 'Baragwanath staff beg Manto: Give us drugs'.

[425] 6/8/2002, *Mail & Guardian*, Anglo to give staff anti-AIDS drugs.
[426] 15/8/2002, *The Star*, 'Dr No takes swipe at Anglo for its AIDS plan'.
[427] Whiteside, A & Sunter, C. 2000. *AIDS. The challenge for South Africa*. Human & Rousseau Tafelberg.
[428] Bell, C, Gersbach, H & Devarajan, S. 2003. *The long-run economic costs of AIDS: theory and an application to South Africa*. World Bank Policy Research Working Paper No 3152. October.
- 28/7/2003, *Reuters*, 'World Bank AIDS report on SA sparks furore'.
- 29/7/2003, *Business Day*, 'World Bank Study on AIDS a scare story'.
- 30/7/2003, *Kaiser Daily HIV/AIDS report*. World Bank report on AIDS, South African economy prompts debate over foreign investment, antiretroviral therapy.

[429] Prof Nicoli Natrass is director of the AIDS and Society Research Unit in the School of Economics at the University of Cape Town.
- Natrass, N. 2004. *The Moral Economy of AIDS in South Africa*. Cambridge University Press, United Kingdom.

ONE MORE DEATH IS TOO MANY

[430] Mbeki to CNN quote in:
- 6/5/2003, *Mail & Guardian*, 'Cosatu threatens street action over AIDS'.
- 9/7/2003, *Cape Argus*, 'Mbeki hints at roll out of anti-AIDS drugs'.
- 15/8/2003, *Mail & Guardian*, 'AIDS: ministers revolt'.
- 6/8/2003, *Independent Online*, 'AIDS summit ends with new call for treatment'.
- 7/8/2003, *The Star*, 'Government makes dramatic AIDS pledge'.
- 10/8/2003, *Sunday Argus*, 'Activists applaud dramatic AIDS drug pledge'.
- 1/10/2003, *Daily News*, 'AIDS treatment plan on its way to cabinet'.
- 10/10/2003, *Business Day*, 'Cabinet unveils antiretrovirals plan'.
- 13/11/2003, *The Star*, 'Is state dithering about AIDS over?'

Epilogue: AND THE BAND PLAYED ON...

[431] ART figures for October 2005 in:
- *Progress on global access to HIV antiretroviral therapy. A report on "3 by 5" and beyond*. World Health Organisation, March 2006.
- HSRC. 2005. *South African National HIV prevalence, HIV incidence, behaviour and communication survey*. Human Sciences Research Council, HSRC Press.

[432] Arguments against seeking out ART were: bad side effects, (12,4 per cent); expense (9,8 per cent); fear of discrimination (9,3 per cent); fear of death (8,5 per cent); lack of confidentiality (6,9 per cent); not HIV positive (6,6 per cent); do not want to have an HIV test (3,3 per cent); do not believe in HIV (1,9 per cent).

433 29/11/2005, *IOL*, 'TAC takes Rath and health minister to court'.
434 Events in 2006 suggest that the Council is taking orders from the director-general of Health, a man with no medical background. See:
- 7/7/2006, *Mail & Guardian*, 'Health department DG frees seized Rath drugs'.
- 21/7/2006, *Mail & Guardian*, 'Hands off' Rath query, MCC ordered.
- Berger, J. 2006. 'HIV/AIDS and South Africa's war on science'. Paper delivered at the XIV International AIDS Conference, Toronto, Canada, August 13-18.

435 Bloggers discussing Mhlongo's death on: newaidsreview.org
436 24/12/2006, *Sunday Independent*, 'Hail to Nozizwe, the beetroot slayer'.
437
- 17/4/2007, *Mail & Guardian*, 'A plan of promise'.
- 6/6/2007, *Mail & Guardian*, 'UN praises South Africa's AIDS plan'.
- 13/6/1007, South African AIDS Conference signals new unity, a chance for progress, Keith Alcorn, NAM, available at www.aidsmap.com
- 18/6/2007, *Health-e*, 'Is AIDS denialism defeated?' Kerry Cullinan.

438 6/6/2007, *Business Day*, 'Offended Minister snubs AIDS gathering'.
439 Speech delivered by the Deputy President P Mlambo-Ngcuka at the opening of the third South African AIDS conference, Durban, June 5 2007. Available at: www.gov.za
440 Sidley, P. 2007. 'SA health minister sacked after attending AIDS conference'. *BMJ*. 335 (7615): 321.
441
- 12/8/2007, *Sunday Times*, 'Manto hospital booze binge'.
- 19/8/2007, *Sunday Times*, 'Manto: a drunk and a thief'.
- 31/8/2007, *Sunday Times*, 'Judge backs media freedom'.
- 8/9/2007, *New York Times*, 'Taking on apartheid, then a nation's stance on AIDS'.

442 Mbeki, T. 2007. *ANC Today*, Volume 7, No. 34. 31 August – 6 September 2007 'Letter from the President: True heroines & heroes – our health workers'. 'What the media says: Nutrition, AIDS, health, politics and profit'.

TIMELINE

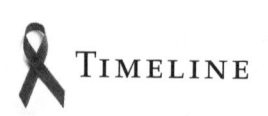

DATE	VIRUS, SCIENCE, GLOBAL RESPONSE	SA EPIDEMIC AND RESPONSE
Before 1980s	HIV transfers to humans in Africa around 1930. HIV enters the US around 1970	
1981	AIDS, or 'GRID', is first identified in the US. First cases are found among gay men, and then injecting drug users	
1982	The syndrome is first described by CDC and the name AIDS is created; cases are identified in Europe among gay men. Heterosexual cases are found among Africans in France, Belgium and some central African countries	July — First SA gay men identified as having AIDS
1983	AIDS is first reported among women who are not drug users, as well as children, in the US. AIDS is formally identified in Central and East Africa. The cause of AIDS is still unknown, but scientists are more confident that there is an infectious agent	January — Two gay men die of AIDS-related illness
1984	HIV, the virus that causes AIDS, is isolated. Western scientists become aware that AIDS is widespread across Africa	National Party government appoints AIDS advisory group
1985	January — First blood test for HIV is licensed. October — Rock Hudson becomes the first public figure known to have died of AIDS. Western scientists become more aware of AIDS or 'slim' disease in Uganda and other African countries. AIDS has been reported in every country of the world	
1986	First public information campaigns on AIDS launched in the UK. International news media report on 'African AIDS'. First clinical trials of AZT to treat AIDS	Influx control legislation repealed
1987	WHO launches Global Programme on AIDS. Major public education campaigns on AIDS across the world, using scare tactics like images of the 'grim reaper'. March — Duesberg publishes first denialist article. October — UN General Assembly special session on AIDS. November — UK's Channel 4 broadcasts first denialist film	May — 1986 Chamber of Mines research shows large number Malawian mineworkers test HIV positive. June — Heterosexual cases noted outside the mines. October — Legislation introduces compulsory testing for all foreign workers; those with HIV become prohibited immigrants

TIMELINE 325

Date	Virus, science, global response	SA epidemic and response
1988	International AIDS Summit — 118 health ministers attend, $37 million is promised December 1 — First World AIDS Day	Racist Conservative Party smear pamphlets use AIDS Malawian miners repatriated First government-sponsored AIDS education poster promoting monogamy and condoms
1989	New WHO director puts brakes on AIDS programme	
1990	March — Dr Jonathan Mann leaves WHO and GPA goes into decline	April — ANC health conference in Maputo discusses HIV and AIDS National Party's 'yellow hand' campaign Exaggerated prophesies about SA epidemic surface in the media May 1990 — two HIV positive askaris alleged to have been deployed in Hillbrow brothels August 1990 — The Pretoria Minute agrees on suspension of armed struggle and return of exiles October — First antenatal HIV survey; 0,76 per cent of pregnant South African women are HIV positive (published 1991) Number of AIDS cases among heterosexuals equals homosexual cases for the first time
1991	A CIA report on the impending global AIDS disaster is ignored	AIDS testing and counselling centres established in SA
1992		July — National Party government AIDS programme stalled October — Nacosa forms a united front against AIDS
1994	AIDS in now the leading cause of death of young Americans Concorde study shows that AZT does not have lasting impact on HIV	April — First democratic election July — New ANC government accepts Nacosa's national AIDS plan and doubles budget AIDS becomes a presidential lead programme Napwa formed as a volunteer organisation Health Minister Zuma strengthens new anti-smoking laws; work begins on the design of a national drugs policy
1995	January 1 — World Trade Organisation established; TRIPS agreement governs pharmaceutical patents UNAIDS established to coordinate the UN response to AIDS	AIDS directorate established in Department of Health December 1 — Premiere of *Sarafina II*
1996	July — International AIDS conference in Montreal — Triple drug antiretroviral therapy described Successful results of PMTCT trial described; Zuma heckled	January — *Sarafina* debacle hits the press February — Irregularities in *Sarafina* tender and funding exposed June — Public Protector's report on *Sarafina* Mid 1996 — Zuma meets Virodene scientists October — Row over tobacco advertising November — First new pharmaceutical regulations rejected

Date	Virus, science, global response	SA epidemic and response
1997	April — Pharmaceutical industry begins campaign against South Africa's plans to reform pharmaceutical sector July — US PhRMA meet with Zuma team in Washington Mid-year — Glaxo offers AZT deal to SA October 4 — US ambassador writes to SA government about his government's opposition to Medicines Bill	January — Virodene unveiled at cabinet meeting February — Mandela tells Davos conference that AIDS is one of the biggest challenges to the new SA May — Medicines Bill in parliament June — Parliamentary hearings on Medicines Bill July — Virodene doctors found guilty of misconduct August — Nacosa review; new Medicines Bill tabled in parliament; Mbeki meets Folb and Virodene researchers; Medicines Control Council (MCC) decide against compassionate release of Virodene September — Zuma tells parliament she intends to make AIDS notifiable; parliamentary hearings on new Medicines Bill; Medicines Bill passed November — MCC raids on Vissers' house December — Allegations of illegal use of Virodene continues; MCC allows further research on Virodene; Mbeki intervenes in dispute among Virodene shareholders; Mandela signs Medicines Act into law but it is not promulgated
1998	January — World Health Assembly (WHA) recommends the adoption of the Revised Drug Strategy February — International conference hears scientific evidence for how HIV-1 jumped the species barrier from chimpanzee to humans February — Short course AZT found to reduce transmission of HIV from mother to child (Thai regimen) March — Glaxo announces global discount on AZT; US ramps up the pressure on SA Medicines Act; Clinton addresses SA parliament May — USTR puts SA on Special 301 Watch List; Shisana leads WHA in drugs debate as lead negotiator for African countries June — US holds four trade items hostage for special tariffs July — Twelfth International AIDS conference in Geneva profiles success of triple therapy and treatment inequities November — UNAIDS chief Piot says southern Africa is facing an unprecedented AIDS emergency	January — MCC review begins February — Pharmaceutical companies file interdict against promulgation of Medicines Act March — Democratic Party (DP) accuses ANC of having financial interests in Virodene; Mbeki slams MCC and other critics of Virodene in press article MCC review team reports; top officials fired and Folb demoted April — Mbeki speaks about African Renaissance June — Shisana leaves government, new MCC director says that a special committee has been created to work on Virodene June — Virodene sold to new owners September 16 — *The Citizen* carries an article by dissident 'The epidemic of AIDS hysteria' October — Government launches 'Partnership against AIDS'; Zuma says no to national PMTCT December — Gugu Dlamini killed; TAC formed; new MCC rejects application for clinical trials of Virodene

TIMELINE 327

Date	Virus, science, global response	SA epidemic and response
1999	April — SA on US Watch list again May — Secure the Future launched June — US activists disrupt Gore campaign July — Inexpensive drug nevirapine found to be effective in preventing MTCT; Gore announced new AIDS spending; USTR says it no longer has objections to SA strategy as long as it is Trips compliant September — US takes SA off Watch List November — AIDS outstrips all other causes of death in Africa for the first time; International journalists write about now-suspended SA medicines litigation for the first time December — Clinton commits US to affordable medicine strategy	March — Debate on AZT in the Citizen; TAC launch treatment action campaign for PMTCT March 10 — Virodene researchers found to have conducted illegal trials. March 19 — Conflict between Virodene shareholders April — Judge Edwin Cameron announces that he is HIV positive; Joint statement by Zuma and TAC; New Medicines Act passed without contentious clauses (SAMMDRA) June — Thabo Mbeki becomes president, Dr Manto Tshabalala-Msimang becomes Health Minister July — Tshabalala-Msimang says she is reviewing AZT decision August — Tshabalala-Msimang visits Uganda, signs pact on drugs lobby and investigates nevirapine September — SA pharmaceutical companies suspend litigation against Medicines Act October — Mbeki tells National Council of Provinces that AZT is a dangerous drug; Tshabalala-Msimang tells journalists that it weakens the immune system and causes birth defects, orders MCC to review AZT December — Denialist historian Geshekter at Medunsa 'Rethinking Core Concepts about HIV and AIDS'; Tshabalala-Msimang meets with Geshekter
2000	January — CIA report warns that AIDS represents a security threat; Gore addresses UN Security Council special session on AIDS March — Pfizer zapped by US activists over fluconazole/diflucan prices May — Five-company initiative accelerating access to antiretroviral drugs announced July — Thirteenth International AIDS Conference held in Durban; International activists protest SA governments AIDS policy; Boehringer makes free nevirapine offer – free for five years in developing countries September — Mbeki gives ambiguous interview to Time magazine; Indian Generic company CIPLA announces low prices for generic drugs	January — New National AIDS Council appointed which excludes AIDS experts and AIDS NGOs. (SANAC); Mbeki consults staff and advisers about dissident views, talks to US denialists on telephone February — Tshabalala-Msimang rejects MCC reports on AZT March — International panel to review SA's AIDS policy is announced April — Pfizer fluconazole donation agreed; Mbeki writes to Clinton; Tshabalala-Msimang tells parliament that SA women died in nevirapine trial May — First meeting of president's advisory panel, one third of participants are denialists who question whether HIV leads to AIDS July — Second meeting of president's advisory panel; 5000 AIDS experts sign Durban declaration that HIV leads to AIDS; TAC launches major treatment protests; Tony Leon and Mbeki have public disagreement about rape and ART prophylaxis September — Denialist treatise circulated in DoH; Government takes out newspaper advertisements saying that HIV leads to AIDS; Cosatu calls on government to stop speculation about the cause of AIDS; Mbeki tells ANC MP caucus that there is a conspiracy around antiretroviral drugs and that TAC is funded by the drug companies October — TAC's Zackie Achmat smuggles Fluconazole into SA from Thailand; NGO (GRIP) under attack for delivering ART rape prophylaxis

Date	Virus, science, global response	SA epidemic and response
2001	May — Global Fund to fight AIDS, TB and Malaria launched June — UN General Assembly devoted to HIV/AIDS (UNGASS) November — Doha Declaration interprets WTO rules in favour of affordable medicines	March 5/6 — Medicines Act court case begins April — Pharmaceutical companies withdraw their interdict against Medicines Act June — TAC write to minister of health asking to make nevirapine/PMTCT available in the public sector; she says no August — TAC begins legal case for PMTCT; Tshabalala-Msimang visits Tanzanian clinic where Virodene is being tested September — Virodene researchers deported from Tanzania and arrive back in SA saying they have excellent results October — Mbeki's speech to Fort Hare students November — TAC PMTCT case begins; interim ruling in their favour; Tshabalala-Msimang challenges ruling in constitutional court
2002	March — US experts question Uganda nevirapine PMTCT trials July 7-12 — Fourteenth International AIDS Conference in Barcelona. Mandela speaks on importance of leadership	January — Department of Health study recommends expanding PMTCT beyond trial sites; Minister of Health rejects February — Mandela engages with PMTCT issue March — 'Castro Hlongwane' document outlining an SA denialist position is debated in ANC circles April — Judge makes further ruling in favour of TAC's PMTCT case; Mbeki writes angry article in ANC Today; ANC NEC recommits to orthodoxy that HIV leads to AIDS; Cabinet confirms that they will abide by court ruling on PMTCT July — Final judgement in favour of PMTCT August — Anglo American mining company announces ART programme for employees; September — TAC decides on civil disobedience campaign to push for universal access to antiretroviral therapy in the public health system October — Government commits to new engagement on treatment; civil disobedience campaign suspended
2003		March — TAC revives civil disobedience campaign September — TAC, Cosatu and 9 others lodge complaint with Competition Committee over drug prices, requesting non-exclusive voluntary licence. November — Government announces plan to roll out ARVs nationally
2004	June – US government programme, Pepfar, begins first round of funding, pledge to provide $15 billion for HIV/AIDS over 5 years	March – Napwa members disrupt AIDS Consortium meeting April – Tshabalala-Msimang retained as health minister in new cabinet; Madladla-Routledge becomes new deputy health minister September – government is criticised for slow ARV rollout. Fewer than 12,000 are on ARVs, compared with the March target of 53,000 October – TAC begins campaigning for access to government ARV rollout plan

Date	Virus, science, global response	SA epidemic and response
2005	January – WHO says 700,000 people in low-income and transitional countries are receiving antiretroviral therapy July – G8 calls for universal access to HIV services	January – Mandela announces his son has died of an AIDS-related disease March – 44,600 are on ARVs in public sector and 60,000 in private sector July – 40 injured at peaceful protest about ARV rollout November – HSRC survey shows adult HIV prevalence at 16%; TAC interdict against Rath
2006	March – WHO says 1.3 million receiving antiretroviral therapy, thus missing the global '3 by 5' target June – High level UN meeting signs new Declaration of Commitment on HIV/AIDS August – SA stand at international conference on AIDS in Toronto criticised for displaying garlic, lemons and beetroot; 80 international scientists write to Mbeki asking him to fire Tshabalala-Msimang over her management of the AIDS crisis December – study shows that male circumcision reduces HIV infection risk by 50%	February – Mbeki disputes that large numbers of civil servants are dying from AIDS-related illnesses; Jacob Zuma rape trial begins May – Zuma acquitted of raping young HIV-positive woman October – Tshabalala-Msimang hospitalised with pneumonia
2007	January – microbicide found to be ineffective in clinical trial September – major vaccine trial halted as ineffective December – UNAIDS revises global figures for people living with HIV to 33.2 million, 2.1 million estimated to have died from HIV/AIDS in 2007	February – Tshablala-Msimang hospitalised again; Radebe appointed acting health minister March – new national AIDS plan is announced; Tshabalala-Msimang has liver transplant June – Tshabalala-Msimang snubs Durban conference, returns to work August – Deputy minister of health, Nozizwe Madlala-Routledge fired; Sunday Times articles allege that Tshabalala-Msimang is a drunk and a thief

Annual antenatal survey results

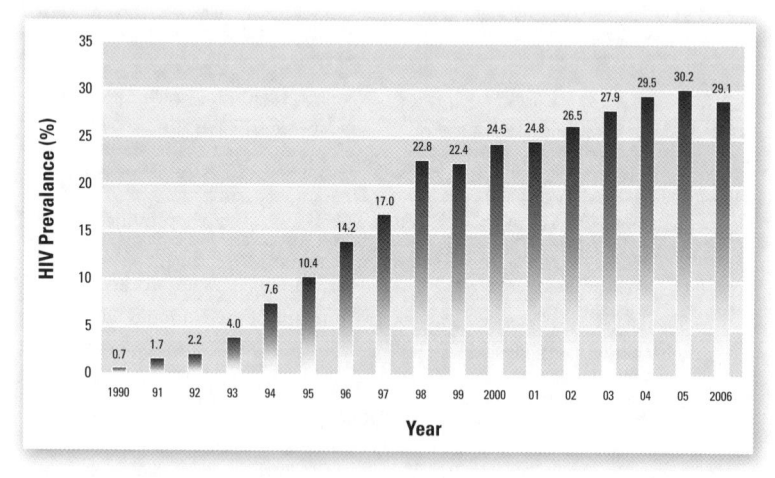

FIGURE 1: HIV Prevalence estimates, 1990–2006
SOURCE: National Department of Health (2007) National HIV and syphilis prevalence survey, South Africa 2006. NDoH. Pretoria

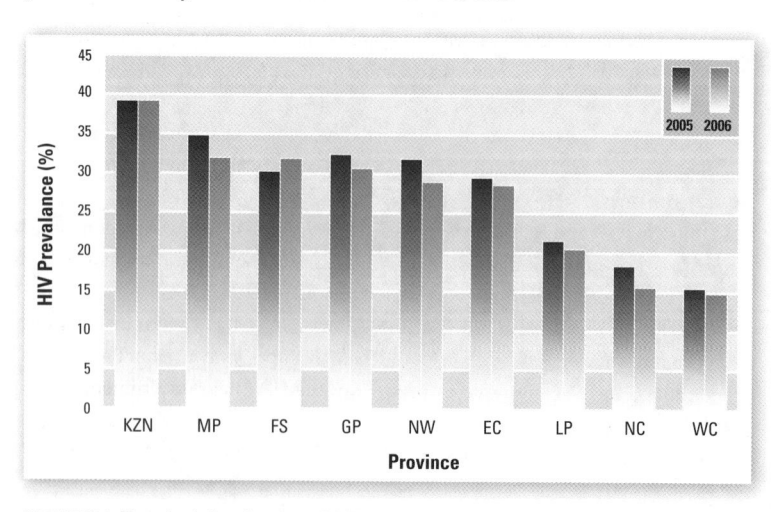

FIGURE 2: Provincial estimates, 2005–6
SOURCE: National Department of Health (2007) National HIV and syphilis prevalence survey, South Africa 2006. NDoH. Pretoria

Dramatis Personae

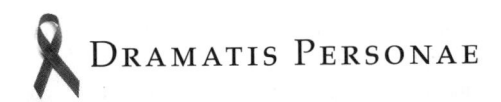

Characters appearing throughout the text

ABDULLAH, DR FAREED – Director of Western Cape province health department's AIDS programme until 2006

ABDOOL KARIM, DR QUARRAISHA – Epidemiologist who worked for the Medical Research Council and was first director of the National Directorate for HIV/AIDS and STDs (1995–1996); currently associate professor of Clinical Epidemiology at the Mailman School of Public Health, Columbia University, New York

ABDOOL KARIM, PROF SALIM – Epidemiologist, engaged in vaccine and microbicide research, currently professor of Clinical Epidemiology at the Mailman School of Public Health, Columbia University, New York and director of CAPRISA, South Africa

BRINK, ANTHONY – South African AIDS denialist, lawyer, writer and researcher

BRINK, DR BRIAN – Medical senior vice president of the Anglo American group

BUDLENDER GEOFF – Prominent human rights lawyer, involved in several TAC cases

BUSSE, PETER – Gay HIV-positive activist and counsellor, founder member and first director of Napwa (National Association of People Living with AIDS) (died 2006)

CAMERON, JUSTICE EDWIN – Gay lawyer with long-standing engagement in HIV issues, now a judge in the Supreme Court. The only prominent public figure in South Africa to have revealed that he is HIV positive

CREWE, MARY – Second director of the Community AIDS Centre in Hillbrow, currently director of the Centre for the Study of AIDS, University of Pretoria

DE KLERK, FW – Reforming last president of the apartheid government (1989-1994)

DEEB, MIRRYENA – Chief executive officer of the Pharmaceutical Manufacturers' Association

DLAMINI-ZUMA, DR NKOSAZANA – First minister of health in the ANC-led government (1994–1999), now foreign minister

DUESBERG, PROF PETER – Californian retrovirologist, one of the founders of AIDS denialism

ELLIS, MIKE – A long-standing leader in the Democratic Party/Democratic Alliance, former spokesperson for health

EVIAN, DR CLIVE – Medical doctor with long-standing involvement in HIV and AIDS care, first director of the Community AIDS Centre in Hillbrow

FLOYD, DR LIZ – Medical doctor with long standing engagement with HIV, currently director of the Multisectoral AIDS Unit for the province of Gauteng

FOLB, PROF PETER – Pharmacologist, former head of University of Cape Town Pharmacology Department, former chair of the Medicines Control Council, now director of the Traditional Medicines Research Unit at the SA Medical Research Council

HEYWOOD, MARK – Director of the AIDS Law Project and founder member and treasurer of the Treatment Action Campaign (TAC)

GRAY, DR ANDY – Pharmacist and senior lecturer at the University of KwaZulu-Natal

GRAY, DR GLENDA – Co-director of Perinatal HIV Research Unit, Chris Hani-Baragwanath Hospital, Soweto

JOHNSON, NKOSI – Born Xolani Nkosi, spokesperson for children living with HIV who came to international fame when he addressed the 13th International AIDS Conference in Durban, 2000 (died June 2001)

LEON, TONY – Leader of the official opposition party, the Democratic Alliance (formerly Democratic Party), from 1994 to 2007

LOVE, DR JAMES – Economist, expert in intellectual property rights, director of Consumer Project on Technology, Washington-based NGO started by Ralph Nader

MAKHALEMELE, MERCY – HIV-positive activist and organiser

MANDELA, NELSON – Liberation hero and first president of South Africa's ANC-led democratic government (1994–1999)

MAQUNGO, BUSI – HIV-positive activist and TAC member

MAZIBUKO, LUCKY – HIV-positive activist and journalist

MBEKI, THABO – Second president in South Africa's democratic government (1999–)

MCINTYRE, DR JAMES – Co-director of Perinatal HIV Research Unit, Chris Hani-Baragwanath hospital, Soweto

MELLORS, SHAUN – Long-standing HIV-positive activist and first South African to go public with his HIV status, in 1987

MHLONGO, PROF SAM – Head of Family Medicine and Primary Care, Medunsa University, medical doctor and denialist (died October 2006)

MOKABA, PETER – Charismatic ANC leader and parliamentarian, AIDS denialist (died 2002)

NKOLI, SIMON – Gay HIV-positive activist engaged in anti-apartheid, gay and AIDS politics (died November 1998)

Dramatis Personae 333

NGOBENI, FLORENCE – HIV-positive activist and counsellor at Perinatal HIV Research unit, Chris Hani-Baragwanath Hospital, Soweto (1996–2000)

NTSALUBA, DR AYANDA – Second director-general in the Department of Health (1998–2003)

PARKER, DR WARREN – One of the architects of the Department of Health's multi-media campaign, Beyond Awareness

PIOT, DR PETER – Director of UNAIDS, the agency that coordinates the UN response to HIV and AIDS

RASNICK, DR DAVID – Chemist and US AIDS denialist

ROBERTS, DR IAN – Special advisor to minsters Zuma and Tshabalala-Msimang (1996–2000)

SERWADDA, PROF DAVID – Ugandan doctor who first identified the virus in that country

SAWYER, ERIC – HIV-positive activist, ACT UP, New York

SCHOUB, PROF BARRY – Virologist, director of the National Institute for Communicable Diseases, Johannesburg

SHER, DR REUBEN – Immunologist, involved with HIV issues from the early 1980s (died 2007)

SHISANA, DR OLIVE – First director-general in the Department of Health, under Dr Zuma (1995–1998), now president and chief executive officer of the South African Human Sciences Research Council (HSRC)

SIFRIS, DR DENIS – A gay doctor active in the first epidemic as an activist and medical practitioner

SIMELELA, DR NONO – Third director of HIV/AIDS and STDs in the Department of Health

SMART, ROSE – Former director of the Pietermaritzburg ATICC and second director of HIV/AIDS and STDs in the Department of Health

TOMS, DR IVAN – Gay activist engaged in political and HIV issues from the 1980s. Now Executive Director of City Health, Cape Town

TSHABALALA-MSIMANG, DR MANTO – Second minister of health in the ANC-led government

VENTER, DR RINA – Minister of Health in FW De Klerk's cabinet

VISSER, OLGA – Inventor of the controversial AIDS medicine, Virodene, established Virodene Pharmaceutical Holdings with her husband, Zigi Visser

WHITESIDE, PROF ALAN – Economist and director of Health Economics and HIV-AIDS Research Division (HEARD), University of KwaZulu-Natal, Durban

ZIMMERMAN, TONI – HIV-positive activist and educator

ZUMA, JACOB – Former deputy president of South Africa and head of the SA National AIDS Council (1999–2003)

Glossary and abbreviations

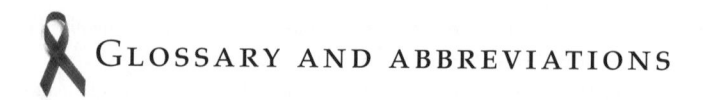

AFRICANIST – a specialist in African history, culture and politics.

ANC – African National Congress

ART – antiretroviral therapy

ARVS – antiretroviral drugs

ASKARI – former, 'turned' ANC guerillas used by the right-wing in the political struggle

ATICC – AIDS Testing, Information and Counselling Centre

BARRIER NURSING – isolation procedures that are used when nursing patients with contagious diseases, including physical separation of patients and the wearing of protective clothing by health workers

CDC – Centers for Disease Control

DA – Democratic Alliance (South Africa)

DP – Democratic Party (South Africa)

CRYONICS – speculative life support technology, seeks to preserve human life at low temperatures

CRYOBIOLOGY – the study of living tissue at low temperatures

CRYO-PRESERVATION – the preservation of living tissue at low temps

GPA – WHO's Global Programme on AIDS

IFP – Inkatha Freedom Party

IN VITRO – an experiment conducted outside the body (eg in a test tube)

IN VIVO – an experiment conducted on living tissue

MASHAYABHUQE – Zulu phrase meaning 'it hits everything'

MSF, OR DOCTORS WITHOUT BORDERS – is a non-profit medical humanitarian organisation

MOFFIE – a derogatory term for homosexuals

NAPWA – National Association of People living with AIDS

NGO – non-governmental organisation

PARALLEL IMPORTATION – the practice of importing branded drugs from countries where they are cheaper

PHRMA – the organisation representing the pharmaceutical industry in the United States

PMA – Pharmaceutical Manufacturers' Association (South Africa)

PMTCT – preventing mother-to-child transmission of HIV, also referred to as MTC or vertical transmission

SAIMR – South African Institute for Medical Research

SANAC – South African National AIDS Council

SANGOMA – traditional healer

SHEBEEN – unlicensed bar
STI – sexually transmitted infection
TAC – Treatment Action Campaign
TRIPS – Trade-Related aspects of Intellectual Property Rights (World Trade Organisation)
UNAIDS – United Nations Programme on HIV/AIDS
VCT – voluntary counselling and testing
WHA – The World Health Assembly represents all the health ministers of member states and is the governing body of the World Health Organisation
WHO – World Health Organisation
WTO – World Trade Organisation

Sources

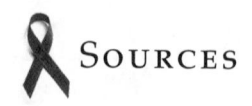

Print

I have drawn shamelessly on a wide variety of published primary and secondary sources, ranging from academic journal articles to newspaper articles and the grey literature of NGOs and AIDS agencies. These I have identified when referring to specific events or information.

However, my thinking has also been enriched and influenced in a more general way by the work of many writers, researchers and journalists who have gone before me, and are not always credited throughout the text. In particular I would like to name Mary Crewe, Hein Marais, Helen Schneider, Jamie Love (the CPT website), Barton Gellman and John Jeter (*Washington Post* series), Mark Schoofs and Helen Epstein (*New York Review of Books*).

I also refer throughout to previous publications of my own. These are:

HIV/AIDS and Development. 1997. Teaching Screens. Johannesburg: SAIH, Interfund.

'Millennial Megabomb'. *1998. Leadership*. 17.

Film

I have worked on several documentaries that have provided real-world contact and insights into the meanings of HIV and AIDS. In some chapters I refer to experiences and interviews from the research and shooting of these films.

They are:

Mashayabhuqe, AIDS hits everyone. 1996, 1998. Director Lesley Lawson, Producers Robyn Hofmeyr and Jenny Hunter. Teaching Screens (Broadcast ETV December 1998).

Talking about Sex, HIV and AIDS. 1997. Director Lesley Lawson, Producers Robyn Hofmeyr and Jenny Hunter. Teaching Screens. (Educational film series for Departments of Education and Health)

6 000 a day – An account of a catastrophe foretold. 2001. Director/Producer Phillip Brooks, Consultant Lesley Lawson. Dominant 7. Broadcast Arte December 2001

INTERVIEWS

Abdool Karim, Quarraisha (December 2005)
Abdool Karim, Salim (December 2005)
Brink, Brian (January 2006)
Abdullah, Fareed (December 2005)
Brouard, Pierre (November 2005)
Budlender, Geoff (January 2006)
Busse, Peter (October 1996, April 1997, June 1998, November 1998, November 2005)
Cooper, Peter (January 2006)
Crewe, Mary (October 1996, April 1997, November 2005, March 2007 – telephone interview)
Ellis, Mike (December 2005)
Evian, Clive (November 2005)
Folb, Peter (December 2005)
Floyd, Liz (January 2006)
Foster, Aloma (March 1997)
Geffen, Nathan (December 2005)
Gray, Andy (December 2005
Hardy, Bill (November 1998)
Heywood, Mark (November 2005)
Hermanus, May (November 2005)
Jochelson, Karen (February 2006)
Johnson, Gail (March 2007)
Lambert, Julian (July 2006)
Leclerk-Madlala, Suzanne (December 2005)
Mbokazi, Nonhlanhla (November 1996)
Makhalemele, Mercy/Cowper, Masi (October 1996, April 1997, March 2006)
Macqungo, Busi (January 2006)
McKerrow, Neil (November 1996)
McIntyre, James (January 2006)
Mazibuko, Lucky (January 2006)
Mellors, Shaun (December 2005)
Ngobeni, Florence (April 1997, November 1998, March 2007)
Nzama, Gertrude (November 1996)
Nzama, Pendulike (November 1996)
Nzama, Ntombizakona (November 1996)
Nxumalo, Sam (November 1996)
Parker, Warren (November 2005)
Randera, Fazel (December 2005)
Sawyer, Eric (March 2001)
Schneider, Helen (November 2005)
Schoub, Barry (January 2006)
Serwadda, David (April 2001)
Sher, Reuben (November 2005)
Sifris, Dennis (November 2005)
Smart, Rose (November 2005)
Swart, Kenau (January 2006)
Toms, Ivan (January 2006)
van der Watt, Herman (January 2006)
Webster, Eddie (November 2005)
Whiteside, Alan (December 2006)
Young, Peter (March 2001, April 2007 – telephone interview)
Zimmermann, Toni (November 1996)

Several people talked to me on condition that they would not be named or quoted.

Acknowledgements

Thanks to Judge Albie Sachs and Dr Mark Hunter for permission to quote at length from their work, and to Robyn Hofmeyr and Jenny Hunter of Teaching Screens for access to the material from the films.

I would also like to thank all those whose support and encouragement allowed me to write this book. Particular thanks to those who enabled my 2005–6 field trip with their generous and various forms of support. They are: Adrienne Bird and Tony Vis; Gille de Vlieg; Korki Bird and Rob Dyer; Mary Ann Cullinan; Aninka Claassens and Geoff Budlender; Richard and Penny Dowden; David and Lily Goldblatt; Jenny Gordon; Peter and Jenny Lawson; Caroline and Rick Menell; and Debbie Stewart and Steve Harding.

Finally, thanks and appreciation to the team at Juta/Double Storey, particularly Colleen Hendriksz and Glenda Younge, and my editor Gail Jennings.

INDEX

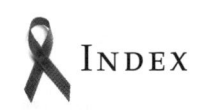

A
abandonment, 14, 79
ABC Nightline, 27
Abdool Karim, Dr Quarraisha
   Director of Directorate of HIV/AIDS and Sexually Transmitted Diseases, 85, 88, 92, 94–5, 96
   involvement in community-based malaria survey, 78–9
   on National AIDS Convention of South Africa (1992), 73
   on translating National AIDS Plan into implementation strategy, 86
   response to *Sarafina II* debacle, 97, 99, 100, 102, 162
Abdool Karim, Prof Salim, 214–15, 295
Abdullah, Dr Fareed, 150, 255–6, 267, 331
abortion on demand, 90, 105
abstinence, 66, 69, 99
academic debate, 39, 42, 44, 59, 60–1, 68–9, 211, 213
Achmat, Zackie, 87, 181–5, 187, 238–9, 247, 268–9
ACT UP (AIDS Coalition to Unleash Power) protests, 30, 151, 193, 196, 197, 199, 227, 229, 303
African AIDS, 147, 163–4, 172, 287
African National Congress (ANC)
   and Department of Health, 102, 266
   attendance at Maputo health conference (1990), 68–9, 291
   chairing of parliamentary health portfolio committee, 101
   civil strife with Inkatha Freedom Party, 14, 67
   collusion with researchers, 137
   denialism, 243
   entrapment in brothels, 55
   gains from sale of Virodene, 138
   guerrilla forces, 46, 53, 59, 74, 75
   health desk, 71
   involvement in sanctions campaign, 142
   links to black empowerment consortium, 250–1
   mass media coverage of, 83
   military wing, 145
   National Executive Committee, 262, 263
   National Health Committee, 263
   political alliance, 233
   relations with Democratic Party, 214–15, 255
   view of Mike Ellis, 105
   Youth League, 133, 260–1, 262
African Renaissance, 146, 147
Afrikaans speakers, 22, 74, 106, 135, 292
AIDS activists
   awareness of deep political resistance to HIV in South Africa, 246
   creation of adverse publicity for Pharma action, 242
   preoccupation of Northern activists, 154–5
   rejection of Virodene, 131–2
   relationship with Dr Nkosasana Dlamini-Zuma, 156, 188–9, 191
   report-back on National AIDS Plan, 163
   response to delays in roll-out of antiretroviral therapy, 208, 209
   response to *Sarafina II*, 99, 103, 107
   silent protest at international AIDS conference (Durban, 2000), 218
   wearing of specially designed T-shirts as advocacy statement, 182 (*see also names of specific activists*, eg Busse, Peter)
AIDS advisory board, 37
AIDS advisory group, 70, 75–6, 291
AIDS, Africa and Racism (Richard and Rosalind Chirimuuta), 28
AIDS awareness campaign, 64, 65–6, 68, 86, 95, 157
AIDS Charter, 72
AIDS community, 103
AIDS Consortium, 68, 178, 185
AIDS directorate, 254, 305, 308
AIDS education
   AIDS Testing and Information Centre, SAIMR, 24
   involvement of Dr Ivan Toms in, 25
   materials, 51, 66, 70, 75, 162
   of miners, 42
   of women, 93
   Sarafina II debacle, 95–7, 105
   shock tactics, 40–1
   workshops, 159, 171–2
AIDS Law Project, 131, 178–9, 181
AIDS prevention programmes
   in KwaZulu-Natal, 56
   involvement of Simon Nkoli and Peter Busse in, 32–3
   of South African government 21, 22, 68, 72, 101, 157, 158, 170, 189, 203, 233–4
   of Ugandan government, 291
   of World Health Organisation, 29
AIDS strategy group, 72
AIDS testing, information and counselling centres (ATICCs), 24, 32, 48, 66, 70, 334

AIDS train, 179, 183
AIDS Unit, 70–1
Alcor Foundation, 297
Allen, Anita, 229, 262
amicus curiae, 242, 243, 244
ANC Today, 265, 282
Anglo American Group, 36, 41, 272–3
Ankomah, Baffour, 173
Annan, General Kofi, 213, 244–5
annual antenatal surveys, 11, 55, 76, 77, 83, 330
antenatal clinics, 61, 63, 158, 169, 257
antiretroviral therapy (ART)
   access to treatment, 181
   arguments against seeking out, 322
   complexity of regimen, 107, 154
   cost of, 130, 243, 247
   denialists' doubt of efficacy of, 254
   efficacy of, 210
   European and US practice, 315
   government's approach to, 251, 252, 264, 266
   health professionals' plea to government for, 272
   President Thabo Mbeki's approach to, 230
   Prof. Peter Folb's explanation of to Dr Jacob Zuma, 118
   prolongation of life by, 222
   promotional campaign, 263
   public health sector provision of, 188, 245–6, 248, 268–9, 279
   toxicity of, 216
askari role in HIV transmission, 54, 55, 59, 334
Australian Broadcasting Corporation 243
AZT (zidovudine)
   clinical trials, 285, 303–4, 309–10
   controversial nature of, 151
   cost of, 157, 184, 253
   demand for for rape survivors, 315
   discount on, 156
   Glaxo agreement, 213, 215
   Mbeki–Rasnick conversation about, 212
   provision of, 182, 203–7, 211, 255, 256
   reduction of incidence of HIV transmission from mother to child, 107, 150, 228–9, 237
   toxicity of, 210, 226, 234–5
   treatment of babies with, 225

B

Bannenberg, Dr Wilbert, 128, 135
Baqwa, Selby, 102
Barber, Simon, 198
Barnard, Dianne Kohler, 278–9
Barnard, Ferdi, 55
barrier nursing, 25, 334
basic AIDS literacy, 104, 173

behaviour change, 97, 104, 150, 166, 170
Behold a Pale Horse (William Cooper), 232
Beyond Awareness, 162
Bialy, Harvey, 225, 227
Big Pharma (*see* pharmaceutical industry)
biological warfare, 31, 232, 315
black HIV-positive people, 25–8, 33, 75
blood, 24, 29, 70, 78, 110
Boehringer Ingelheim, 216, 254, 255
Bombelles, Tom, 141
brand-name drugs, 106, 123, 241, 298
breast-milk substitutes, 63, 207
Brink, Anthony, 205, 210, 229, 310, 331
Brink, Dr Brian, 36, 37, 40, 272, 331
Bristol-Myers-Squibb (BMS), 130, 194, 195, 241
British Medical Journal, 116
Brouard, Peter, 53–4, 97, 117
Brown, Gordon, 244
Bruckner, Christel, 140, 301
budget
   cost of Virodene roll-out, 110, 117
   Department of Health, 66, 70, 75, 87, 88, 156, 162, 182, 266
   for AIDS testing, 67–8
   for Murchison Hospital, 160
   for prevention programmes, 21
   for *Sarafina II*, 95, 96, 98–100, 102, 104
   HIV prevention, 86
   Mpumalanga Health Department, 235
   of rural homesteads, 10
   of single-woman headed households, 77
   presidential priority programme, 83
   underspending, 92, 305
   US AIDS funding, 199
Budlender, Geoffrey, 248, 259, 267–8, 271, 331
Burroughs Wellcome, 303
Business Day, 198, 242
Business Times, 124
Busse, Peter
   about responses to *Sarafina II*, 99
   and Napwa, 88, 180, 185, 187, 188
   attendance of meeting with parliamentary health portfolio committee, 89
   contribution to the Directorate of HIV/AIDS and Sexually Transmitted Diseases, 85
   coordination of counselling services at Community AIDS Centre in Hillbrow, 50, 51
   co-writing of counselling section of National AIDS Plan, 73, 83–4
   criticism of irresponsibility of mass media, 171
   disclosure of own HIV status, 87
   establishment of first AIDS prevention organisation in black townships, 32–3

overview of, 331
participation in first meeting of South African National AIDS Convention (1992), 72
personal experience of AIDS, 20, 186, 280–1
response to death of Simon Nkoli, 181
support gained from AIDS Testing and Information Centre, SAIMR, 24
suspicions regarding Virodene breakthrough, 111
workshop involvement, 11

C

Cabinet, 236, 266, 269, 275
Cameron, Justice Edwin, 72, 84, 87, 181, 331
Campbell, Prof. Catherine, 42
cancer, 13–14, 130, 151, 152
Carswell, Dr Wilson, 70, 75
case studies
    Dlamini, Gugu, 177–80, 181, 182
    Emma, 109–10, 297
    John, 20, 109, 296–7
    Mbokazi, Nonhlanhla, 134
    Mellors, Shaun, 64, 87
    Micky, 229
    Ngobeni, Florence, 93, 216–17, 240, 264
    Njokwe, Musa, 178
    Sizakele, 9, 16
    Themba, 120
    Xolani, Nkosi, 159
CD4 count, 296–7
Centers for Disease Control (CDC), 26, 225, 334
Chamber of Mines, 36–7, 40, 286
Channel 4 television station, 31
Chaskalson, Arthur, 267
child care, 9, 14–15, 90, 150, 211
Chris (of *Friends for Life*) 12
Chris Hani-Baragwanath Hospital
    as site of beginnings of heterosexual epidemic, 43, 62
    Perinatal HIV Research Unit, 63, 93, 103, 108, 149–50, 158, 239–40
    petition for drugs and better training to prevent AIDS deaths, 272
    provision of AZT, 256
    research conducted at, 225, 253, 310
CIA, 76, 232, 235
Cipla, 241
The Citizen, 172–4, 206–7, 210, 229, 310
civil disobedience campaign, 269, 270
clients (*see* sex industry)
clinical trials, 115, 116, 145, 146, 216, 247, 249, 254, 261, 285
clinics, 23, 43, 52, 67, 249, 287
Clinton administration, 141, 174, 196, 200, 208–9, 213
CNN, 243, 275

Collier, Dr Bill, 184
collusion, 137, 211
commercial sex workers (*see* sex industry)
Community AIDS Centre (Hillbrow), 44, 49, 50–4, 66–7, 73, 85, 97, 111, 117
compassionate access to unregistered drugs, 117–18, 119
compulsory licensing, 126, 128–9, 192–3, 209, 243, 246, 308
Concorde study, 151
concurrent relationships, 169–70
condoms
    ANC Health Desk promotion of use of, 69
    as prevention measure in *Sarafina II*, 99
    budget for, 211
    demand for, 51
    distribution of, 170
    homosexual use of, 22
    in Declaration of Partnership against AIDS, 157
    in government AIDS awareness campaigns, 65–9
    in life skills programme, 166
    lack of power of women to insist on use of, 79
    poor quality of free government supply of, 85–6
    preference for unprotected sex, 15, 169
    promotion of use of, 39, 41, 53, 134
    suspected reduction of fertility and power by, 68
conference (Durban, 2006), 306
confidentiality of status, 13, 25, 41, 50, 73, 87, 163
Conservative Party, 36–7, 75, 292
conspiracies, 30, 54, 68, 121, 139, 216, 232, 235–6, 238
Constitutional Court, 199, 259, 260, 265, 266, 320
consultation, 73, 86
Consumer Project on Technology, 143, 192, 193, 196, 205, 243, 308
Cook, Dr Albert, 26
Cooper, Dr Peter, 158, 256–7
Cooper, William, 232, 258
Coovadia, Dr Jerry, 214–15, 224
cordon sanitaire, 32, 35
Cornell, Morna, 185
Cosatu (Congress of South African Trade Unions), 100, 172, 233, 239, 269
costs
    Big Pharma interests, 121
    discounts, 234
    estimated by Anglo American, 272
    health
    budget coverage, 188
    of AIDS as occupational hazard in mining, 40

of antiretroviral therapy, 154, 245, 254
of AZT, 150–2, 157, 184, 303
of fluconazole, 181–2
of generic drugs, 122, 130, 192, 238–9, 241
of medicines, 106
of nevirapine, 257
of patented drugs 242, 298
of prevention of mother–to–child transmission programme, 207–8
of primary health care package, 89
of public health crisis 274–5
of Virodene, 110, 117
counselling, 11–12, 24, 32, 49, 51, 54–5, 93, 120, 149, 153, 258
courage, 42, 93, 134, 138, 141, 181, 280
Crewe, Mary, 11, 50, 67, 72, 73, 76–7, 85, 104, 111, 166, 233, 331
cryobiology, 112–13, 334
Cryonics Institute, 297
cryonics research, 112–14, 115, 297, 334
cryopreservation, 112, 116, 334
Cryopreservation Technologies, 116
culture, 39–40, 201

D

Daley, William, 141
death and dying, 14, 15, 16, 19, 43, 56, 66, 69, 75, 93, 97, 117, 134, 149, 157
death rates, 149, 225
Declaration of Partnership Against AIDS, 157
Deeb, Mirryena, 106, 122, 242, 331
defiance campaign against drug company profiteering, 238
De Klerk, F.W., 84, 89, 331
De Kock, Eugene, 54, 55
Dellums, Ronald, 194
Democratic Alliance (DA), 234, 255, 278–9, 334
Democratic Party (South Africa) (DP), 72, 91, 101–2, 105, 116, 123, 137, 138, 214, 215, 334
Democratic Party (USA), 196–7
democratisation of health care, 68–9, 88, 105
demystification, 87, 201
denial
  approach of Chris Hani to, 291
  approach of Dr Manto Tshabalala-Msimang to, 231, 232, 253–4, 281
  in ANC literature, 262–3
  in gay clubs, 22
  hostility from gay community due to, 64
  in Constitutional Court case, 261
  influence of, 209–15
  in mass media, 172–4
  presence at international AIDS Conference (Durban, 2000), 229
  presentation of views at conference (Pretoria, 2000), 219–27
  President Thabo Mbeki's views, 230
  racism and, 28–31
  rejection of fundamentals of AIDS science, 206
Department of Health
  AIDS prevention programmes, 21–2
  and WHO, 118, 129
  awareness of President Thabo Mbeki's denialism, 243
  budget, 75
  commitment to government's AIDS programme, 164
  connection to Medicines Control Council, 136
  cooperation with department of education on life skills programme, 165
  criticism of Western Cape health department for dispensing ART to HIV-positive pregnant women in Khayelitsha, 256
  cross-party think-tank on HIV and AIDS, 71
  directorate for HIV and AIDS, 162–3
  Dr Abdool Karim's directorship, 85
  findings of first national HIV survey, 77
  mass AIDS awareness campaigns, 65–6
  oral agreement with Mbongeni Ngema, 295
  portfolio of, 89
  progress report on pilot sites for PMTCT programme, 259
  provision of free health care for children under six years of age and pregnant women, 90
  resistance to roll-out of antiretroviral therapy, 277
  responsibility for AIDS programme, 84
  specialised AIDS unit, 70
  technical task team on use of antiretrovirals in public health sector, 269, 275
  unauthorised expenditure on *Sarafina II*, 102
  underspending of AIDS budget, 92
depression, 48, 150
diagnosis of HIV and AIDS, 9, 20, 29, 34, 64, 87
Diflucan, 160, 316 (*see also* Fluconazole)
dimethylformamide (DMF), 115, 132
Directorate for HIV and AIDS, 111
Directorate of HIV / AIDS and Sexually Transmitted Diseases, 85
disclosure, 44, 48, 64, 87, 89, 176–8, 181, 185, 187
discrimination, 12, 69, 87
Dispatches, 31
Dlamini-Zuma, Dr Nkosasana
  agreement on medical cooperation with Cuba, 89–90, 99–101

alliance with Pharmaceutical Manufacturers' Association, 199
and alleged antagonism to private health sector, 138
and antiretroviral therapy, 181, 185, 189
and AZT, 204, 253, 255
and Directorate of HIV/AIDS and Sexually Transmitted Diseases, 85, 94–5
and Medical Research Council, 71
and Medicines Act, 141
and Medicines and Related Substances Amendment Bill (No. 30 of 1997), 123–6
and Medicines and Related Substances Control Amendment Bill (No. 70 of 1997), 127, 129–30, 136
and Medicines Control Council, 135
and National Drug Policy, 106–7, 122
and reduction of price of AIDS drugs, 191
and *Sarafina II*, 97, 103, 105, 156
and Virodene trials, 110–11, 115–17, 118, 121, 132, 133, 137, 139–40, 156
and World Health Organisation, 196
as health minister in ANC government, 83
attendance of annual meeting of World Health Assembly, 142, 143, 144
attendance of Seventh International Global Network of People Living with AIDS (GNPA), 88
budget vote, 87
call on rural women to lobby their male-dominated communities for better sexual health and rights, 179
chair of the AIDS strategy group, 72
decision to make AIDS a notifiable disease, 163
exchange of views with Zackie Achmat, 184
opposition of pharmaceutical industry to reforms of, 153
promotion to post of Foreign Minister, 202
rejection of Secure the Future, 194–5
retrenchment of inherited bureaucracy, 92
struggle for the right to affordable medicine, 200
support of parallel and importation and compulsory licensing, 128
Doctors Without Borders (*see* Médecins sans Frontières (MSF))
Doha Declaration, 246
domestic workers, 37, 74
donor funding, 76, 88, 94, 102, 240, 250–1
The Dorchester (hotel), 52
drug discounts, 152–3, 155, 156, 184, 185, 194, 240, 241
drug policy, 106, 142
drug pricing, 121, 122, 124, 128, 130, 131, 155, 158, 185, 191, 200, 244, 247

drug schedules, 198–9
drug smuggling, 238–9
drug trials, 150, 215, 250
Duesberg, Prof. Peter, 30, 212, 222, 225, 331
Dukes, Prof. Graham, 135, 140
Du Plessis, Prof. Dirk, 109, 112, 115
Durban Declaration, 214, 223–4

E

economy, 29, 273
Edendale Hospital (Pietermaritzburg), 55
Edenvale Hospital, 108
Elder, Prof. Glen, 78
Ellis, Mike, 72–3, 91, 101, 105–6, 123, 128, 137, 138–9, 332
Enerkom, 250, 262
epidemic status, 26–7, 28, 32, 44, 160, 161, 211, 271, 287, 292, 321
essential drugs list, 91
ethics, 248, 254, 258
European Union, 97, 100, 102, 124, 128, 295
Evian, Dr Clive, 23–4, 44, 49–50, 67, 77, 85, 332
executive committee, 124–5
expert opinion, 10, 132
expert panel of inquiry, 212
exponential growth curve, 11, 76

F

false positives, 285
family planning, 50, 67–8, 287
Farber, Celia, 223
fear, 22, 37, 40–1, 44, 58, 62, 64, 65, 86, 88, 108, 119, 149–50, 159, 165
federal system, 92, 305
Fed-Up Queers, 197
Fiala, Dr Christian, 222
films about HIV and AIDS, 9–11, 12–13, 15, 31
financial support, 9, 10, 16, 79
Floyd, Dr Liz, 69, 72, 170, 332
fluconazole, 181–2, 238, 239, 240, 316 (*see also* Diflucan)
Folb, Prof. Peter
  chairmanship of Medicines Control Council, 112, 115–16, 118–19, 125–6, 136, 140, 300–1
  overview of, 332
  rejection of Virodene and Medicines and Related Substances Amendment Bill (No. 30 of 1997), 127, 132, 135
Food and Drug Administration, 128, 151, 267
'Forty Rand' scheme, 63
Foster, Aloma, 165
Fouéré, Erwan, 97
Freireian participatory theatre, 99, 294
Friends for Life, 12
full barrier nursing, 25, 334

funding, 19, 116, 140, 153, 199, 250, 252, 256, 295, 297

G

Garrett, Laurie, 74
Gauteng AIDS directorate, 170
Gauteng Health Committee, 116
Gauteng premier's committee on AIDS, 257
Gauteng regional health department, 151
Gay and Lesbian Organisation (GLOW), 32
gay community, 21, 22, 25, 28, 43, 44, 64, 163
Gayle, Dr Helene, 225
gay political activism, 23, 30, 32, 68
Geffen, Nathan, 245–6
gender-based violence, 61, 167
gender politics, 41, 59, 60, 164
generic drugs, 106, 122, 123, 126, 130, 192, 193, 238–9, 298
Gerwel, Jakes, 110
Geshekter, Prof. Charles, 172–4, 210, 211
Giraldo, Dr Roberto, 261–2, 270
Glaxo Smith Kline (*see* Glaxo Wellcome)
Glaxo Wellcome, 151, 153, 155, 184, 205–6, 213, 215, 241, 244, 256, 303
global advocacy agenda, 88, 230
Global March for Treatment, 227–8
global pledge to universal access to AIDS treatment, 246–7
Global Programme on AIDS (GPA), 36, 76, 286, 296, 334
global registration, 250
Golden Key, 52
Gore, Al, 124, 196–7, 198, 199
governance, 106, 146
government
    and AIDS community, 81, 175
    and AZT, 215, 235, 256, 266
    and fluconazole, 239
    and National AIDS Plan, 73, 83, 94, 163
    and *Sarafina II*, 103
    and US government, 124, 144
    close political relationship with tobacco industry, 90
    expert panel of inquiry, 214
    human resources, 92, 96
    lack of prioritisation of AIDS, 13, 43, 100
    ousting of Shaun Mellors, 64
    politicisation of AIDS, 101
    public education campaigns, 65–6, 70–1
    relationship with Democratic Party, 105
    relations with US, 241
    reluctance to fund prevention programmes, 13
    restructuring of public health sector, 84–5
    secrecy regarding AIDS statistics, 44
    social contract with civil society, 156, 189
    support of Virodene research, 110, 132, 137, 138
    suspicion of Nationalist Party preventative measures, 68, 72, 75
    technical advisory group on HIV and AIDS, 24
    and antiretroviral treatment, 242–3, 245, 246, 247, 268, 294
graphs, 13, 20, 225, 280
Gray, Dr Andy, 127–8, 198, 332
Gray, Dr Glenda, 108, 150, 216, 256, 260, 310, 332
Greater Nelspruit Rape Counselling Programme (Grip), 234–5, 315
Grey's Hospital, 149
Grip (Greater Nelspruit Rape Counselling Programme), 234–5, 315
Group for the Scientific Reappraisal of the HIV/AIDS Hypothesis, 30
Guardian, 27–8, 242
guilt, 190, 196
Gumede, William, 236

H

Hani, Chris, 69, 291
Hardy, Dr Bill, 160
health conference (Maputo, 1990), 68–70, 291
Health Gap, 227
The health of nations – a north–south investigation (M. Muller), 297
health policy, 106, 135
health system, 84, 89, 90
Hermanus, May, 41
heterosexuals, 32, 44, 173, 220–1, 284, 287
Heywood, Mark
    and Napwa, 182, 183, 185, 186, 188
    and Treatment Action Campaign, 243, 244, 246, 247, 248, 257, 258, 259, 270–1, 332
    as AIDS Law Project director, 181, 202–3, 209
    participation in 13th International AIDS Conference, 228,
HIV
    effect on bone marrow, 206
    effect on brain, 110
    lack of prioritisation of, 15
    monitoring, 32, 35, 43, 46
    mother-to-child transmission (MTCT), 48, 63, 98, 107, 149–52, 156, 157–8, 181, 182, 183, 184, 188–9, 190, 203, 205, 207, 208, 215–16, 228–9, 237, 239–40, 247, 248, 249, 253, 254, 255, 257, 258, 259, 260, 261, 263, 268, 279–80, 284, 309–10, 315
    positive people, 11, 17, 25–8, 88, 93
    surveillance, 286
    surveys, 22–3, 45, 49, 55, 78, 283, 286, 288
    target, 15
    terminology, 8, 21
    testing 11, 20, 23, 25, 26, 29, 31, 34, 36, 48,

49, 50, 51, 70, 71, 75, 120, 149, 163, 211, 224, 225, 226–7, 258, 270, 292
transmission, 12, 21, 26, 28, 34, 54, 55, 58–9, 173, 284, 287
Hlongwane, Israel, 57–8
Hlongwane, Pat, 178
Hlongwane, Vincent, 141, 153
Hodgkinson, Neville, 31
Holmshaw, Dr Manda, 70, 75
home-based care, 10, 15, 82, 161, 201
homophobia, 21–3, 24, 25, 26, 283, 287
homosexuality and AIDS, 21, 22, 29, 220–1, 283, 284
hope, 111, 116
Hospital Pharmacists Association, 127
hospitals, 9–10, 14, 25–6, 43, 87, 111, 149, 216, 235, 239, 256, 272 (*see also names of specific hospitals*, eg Chris Hani-Baragwanath Hospital)
Huismans, Prof. Henk, 116
human resources, 85, 86, 89–90, 92, 94–5
human rights, 14, 39, 41, 68, 73, 75, 163, 182
Human Sciences Research Council, 78, 277–8
human trials, 145
humiliation, 58
Hunter, Dr Mark, 168, 169
hypotheses, 13, 27, 29–30, 46

I

indigenous cure, 121, 163–4
infant mortality, 155–6
infrastructure, 84, 153, 154–5
injecting drug users, 21, 26, 28, 30, 284
Inkatha Freedom Party (IFP), 14, 55–7, 67, 99, 334
intellectual property rights
 and Big Pharma, 195, 208, 241, 242, 298
 and TRIPS, 121–2
 approach of US government to, 200, 213
 as protected by 301 Watch List, 142
 conflict with public health, 246
 Consumer Project on Technology, 243, 308
 debate regarding in World Health Assembly, 144
 in Medicines Act dispute, 141, 193–4
 in Medicines and Related Substances Amendment Bill (30 of 1997), 127, 128, 129
 in 'TRIPS-plus' agreement, 192
inter-ministerial committee on AIDS, 164
International AIDS Conference (Atlanta, 1985), 27
International AIDS Conference (11th, Vancouver, 1996), 107
International AIDS Conference (12th, Geneva, 1998), 155
International AIDS Conference (13th, Durban, 2000), 159, 214, 218, 224, 227–9, 254
International AIDS Conference (Barcelona), 267
International Classification of Diseases, 228
International Labour Organisation, 232, 315
international symbols, 70–1
Internet, 172, 204, 210, 212, 220, 223, 227
intervention strategy, 72
intimate partner violence, 61
in vitro tests, 109, 334
'inzile' politics, 70, 164
isibhaya sika bab'wakhe, 61

J

Jochelson, Karen, 38–9
Johannesburg City Health Department, 49
Johannesburg General Hospital, 23, 24–5, 49, 108, 158, 256–7
Johnson, Gail, 159, 228–9
Johnson, Nkosi, 159, 228–9, 332
joint advocacy strategy, 193
Joint United Nations Programme on HIV/AIDS (UNAIDS), 107
Joni, Jennifer, 179
Joseph, James, 128

K

Kadalie, Dr Rhoda, 182, 307
Kalafong Hospital, 215, 262
Kark, Sydney, 36, 41–2
Karrim, Dr Saadiq, 263
Katimo Mulilo, HIV prevalence in, 46, 287–8
Kaunda, President Kenneth, 32, 74, 88
Khamphepe, Judge, 58
Kitua, Dr Andrew, 250
Klaaste, Dr Aggrey, 176
Krog, Antjie, 58
KwaZulu-Natal as epicentre of HIV and AIDS epidemic, 10, 55, 78, 83, 168

L

Lambert, Dr Julian, 84
Lambert, Patricia, 232
The Lancet, 75–6, 155
Landauer, Dr Kallie, 109, 112
laws
 exclusive rights on Taxol, 130
 making AIDS a notifiable disease, 163
 patent, 298
 pro-abortion and anti-smoking, 105
 authorising removal of promiscuous people from community, 65
 requiring compulsory HIV testing for all foreign workers, 37
 right to pre-test counselling under, 11–12
Lazarus effect, 107, 154
Le Carré, John, 242

Leclerc-Madlala, Prof. Suzanne, 60
Leon, Tony, 215, 234, 332
Letting them die (Catherine Campbell), 42
life expectancy, 107, 174
life insurance cover denial, 34
life skills, 164–6, 203
lobbying, 23, 127
love, 58, 61
Love, Dr James, 124, 128, 143, 192, 196, 197, 208, 243, 244, 308, 332
Luthuli, Daluxolo, 57

M

Madlala-Routledge, Nozizwe, 281
Mail & Guardian, 62, 100, 105, 106, 135, 145, 185, 221–2, 251, 262
Maisela, Max, 250–1
Makgoba, Prof. William, 211
Makhalemele, Mercy, 63, 82, 88, 89, 108, 148, 185, 187, 218, 332
malaria, 10, 31, 78
malnutrition, 13, 211, 261
Manana, Sibongile, 234–5
mandatory testing for African immigrants, 29, 41
Mandela, Nelson
 approach to AIDS epidemic, 83
 criticism of pharmaceutical companies, 244
 criticism of *Sarafina II*, 103, 105, 296
 donning of 'HIV-positive' T-shirt, 182
 leadership of, 89, 92
 opening of national AIDS Convention of South Africa, 72
 overview of, 332
 presidential address of World Economic Forum (Davos, 1997), 161–2
 awarding of McIntyre and Gray for pioneering work on preventing vertical transmission, 260
 public support of Dr Manto Tshabalala-Msimang, 101, 106
 response to activism, 218
 retirement from active politics, 202
 signing of Medicines Act into law, 133, 136–7, 199, 208
 support for President Thabo Mbeki, 229–30
 support for Zackie Achmat, 269
 use of deputy, 84, 88, 146, 156–7
Mankahlana, Parks, 224
Mann, Dr Jonathan, 36
Manuel, Trevor, 183, 273–4
Maqungo, Busi, 190, 237, 238, 258, 267, 279–80, 332
marches, 243, 257
Mark (of *Friends for Life*), 12
martial rape, 56–8, 167
masculinity, 42, 56, 60–1, 167, 169

mashayabhuqe, 16, 57, 334
mass media
 AIDS-related headlines and lead stories, 21, 26–8, 35, 176, 185, 242
 attack on *Sarafina II*, 98, 103, 104–5, 106
 clarification of government position in, 233
 coverage of AZT, 254
 coverage of Dr Nkosasana Dlamini-Zuma's battle against high drug prices, 122, 124
 coverage of Dr Olive Shisana, 144, 145
 coverage of global day of action against drug company profiteering, 243
 coverage of intellectual property rights, 194
 coverage of Karim's and Covaadia's siding with Democratic Party, 214–15
 coverage of Medicines Act, 208–10
 coverage of President Thabo Mbeki's denunciation of opposition to Virodene as conspiracy, 139
 coverage of President Thabo Mbeki's denunciation of vested interests of AIDS establishment, 213
 coverage of South African trade dispute by international, 197
 coverage of Virodene issues, 110, 111, 115, 249, 250–1
 denunciation of toxicity of AZT, 204–5
 inaccuracies in reporting, 29–30
 lack of sound health reporting, 192, 252
 neglect of AIDS issues, 171
 Olga Visser's writing up of research for, 113
 outing of Shaun Mellors in, 64
 overlooking of Medicines Bill/Act key issues, 127, 136–8
 portrayal of denialism in, 31, 220, 227
 US coverage of Glaxo's global discount offer on AZT, 153
 visualisation of 'African AIDS' by Western, 147
mass sterilisation campaign, 68
Matsoso, Dr Precious, 210
Mazibuko, Lucky, 34, 176, 186, 188, 201, 232–3, 252
Mbeki, President Thabo
 and AZT, 184, 203–4, 310
 correspondence with Tony Leon, 234
 delivery of Declaration of Partnership against AIDS, 157
 lecture (University of Fort Hare, 2001), 251
 overview of, 332
 relations with US, 196, 275
 stance on HIV and AIDS, 31, 40, 74, 88, 151, 179, 202, 209–10, 211–12, 213–14, 220, 228, 229–30, 232, 233, 235–6, 239–40,

243, 245, 265, 311
  support of Dr Manto Tshabalala-Msimang, 282
  support of Virodene research, 109, 118, 132, 139, 146–7
McIntyre, Dr James, 44, 62, 63, 103–4, 150, 216, 226, 256, 260, 310, 332
McKerrow, Dr Neil, 14, 149
Medical Research Council, 71, 78, 85, 133
medical neglect, 62, 64
Medicines Act
  Big Pharma lawsuit, 153, 189, 200, 203, 208, 209, 240–1, 243, 253, 254–5, 279, 311
  Dr Olive Shisana's involvement with, 145
  legislation to replace, 191
  listing of South Africa on Special 301 Watch List due to, 195
  significance of, 146, 247
  threat of sanctions due to, 142
  US criticism of, 141, 143–4
Medicines and Related Substances Amendment Bill (No. 30 of 1997), 122, 299
Medicines and Related Substances Control Amendment Bill (No. 90 of 1997), 124, 125, 126–8, 129–30, 131–2, 133, 135, 136, 299
Medicines Control Council (MCC)
  and AZT, 205, 215
  and nevirapine, 216, 247, 253, 260, 261
  and Oxihumate, 262
  and Rath vitamin cure, 279
  and Virodene, 111, 112, 115, 116, 118, 119, 130–1, 132, 139–40, 145, 146, 249
  control of Minister of Health over, 124, 133
  criticism of Medicines and Related Substances Amendment Bill (No. 30 of 1997), 126, 127
  review of role of, 135–6
medicines regulatory authority, 140
Médecins sans Frontières (MSF), 193, 334
Medunsa University, 210, 227
Mellors, Shaun, 24–5, 88, 186, 187, 332
Merck, 128, 229, 241, 244
Mhlongo, Dr Sam, 31, 210, 225, 261, 281, 332
migrant labour, 35–6, 38–42, 45, 46–7, 55, 59, 72, 166, 286
military clinics, 249, 251, 262
military forces, 53, 56, 59
mineworkers' vulnerability to AIDS, 19, 35, 38–9, 43, 45, 286
minimum standards for protection, 193
ministerial veto, 126, 127
Mkhize, Dr Zwele, 275
Mkhondo, Rich, 198
Mlambo-Ngcuka, Deputy President Phumzile, 281

modelling exercises, 273
Mokaba, Peter, 262–3, 266, 281, 332
Mokwena, Steve, 60, 289–90
monogamous relationships, 66
Moore, Peter, 153
Moose, Ambassador George, 143–4
Mothibele, Monyaola, 38–9
Mpumalanga Health Department, 235
Msimang, Mendi, 251
MTC (*see* preventing mother–to–child transmission of HIV)
Muller, M., 298
Mullis, Prof. Kary, 30, 285
multinationals, 106, 107, 121, 122, 136, 260–1
multiple partners, 79, 169
municipal authorities, 77–8
Murchison Hospital, 160, 161
Myburg, James, 310

N

Nader, Ralph, 94, 192, 308
National AIDS Commission, 62
National AIDS Convention of South Africa (Nacosa), 71–3, 75, 84, 86
National AIDS Plan, 72, 73, 76, 83, 84, 86, 87, 92, 104, 156, 163, 164–5, 202, 281
National AIDS Programme, 94
National Association of People Living with AIDS (Napwa), 87, 88, 89, 108, 178, 180, 182, 184, 185, 186, 187, 188, 334
National Drugs Policy, 90–1, 122, 125, 300–1
national HIV survey, 77
National Institute of Virology, 224
National Party, 21, 64, 65, 67–8, 73, 90, 116
National Progressive Primary Health Care (NPPHC) network, 69, 71, 94
national treatment plan, 71, 259, 275, 305
National Union of Mineworkers (NUM), 37, 38, 39, 41
Natrass, Prof. Nicoli, 274, 322
Ndwedwe, 16
Nedlac, 269
negotiations, 41, 71, 72–3, 144
nevirapine (NVP)
  availability of, 248, 258, 279
  Big Pharma's offer of, 240
  clinical trials, 203, 247, 254, 304, 309–10
  cost of, 207, 253
  government roll-out of, 266
  government's drug of choice for prevention of mother-to-child transmission, 215–16, provision by hospital doctors, 257
  provision by Western Cape Health Department, 255
  TAC resistance to, 261
  US withdrawal of registration of, 260
New African, 31, 172, 173, 214

Newsweek, 26
New York Press, 223
New York Stock Exchange protest (1989), 151, 303
New York Times, 197, 263
Ngema, Mbongeni, 95, 97–8, 99, 100, 102, 295
Ngobeni, Florence, 149–50, 158, 183, 333
Ngubane, Prof. Sihawu, 62
Nkoli, Simon, 23, 32, 33, 180–1, 182, 284, 332
non-governmental organisations (NGOs)
    awareness of HIV and AIDS, 56, 70
    collaboration with government, 83–4
    failure to relate constructively to epidemic 13, 171–2
    film to forewarn, 9–10, 15
    funding crisis, 94
    national AIDS response, 71
    relationship between Department of Health and, 162–3
    resistance to white-headed, 40
    response to *Sarafina II*, 98, 99–100, 104
    specialising in HIV and AIDS, 68, 181
    (*see also specific NGOs*, eg National Progressive Primary Health Care (NPPHC)
notifiable disease, 37, 163, 286
Ntsaluba, Dr Ayanda, 202–3, 245, 258, 333
Nujoma, President Sam, 232, 315
nutrition, 261, 262, 282
nutritional supplements, 250, 261, 270, 278
Nxumalo, Joshua, 145, 250
Nxumalo, Sam, 56
Nzama family, 16–17
Nzama, Gertrude, 17
Nzama, Ntombizakhona, 17
Nzama, Pendulike, 17
Nzo, Alfred, 69

O

Observer, 208, 244
Office of Health Promotion, 75
origin of HIV and AIDS, 28–9
orphans, 10, 14, 15, 272, 273
outreach programmes, 52, 67
ownership, 69–70, 99
Oxihumate, 250, 262

P

parallel importation, 123, 124, 125, 126, 128–9, 192–3, 209, 243, 246, 293–4, 334
Parker, Dr Warren, 95, 96, 97, 162, 333
parliamentary debate, 65, 123, 127, 138, 139, 141, 203–4, 207, 212, 216, 259–60
Parliamentary Health Portfolio Committee, 89, 101, 127, 202, 237
Partnership Against AIDS, 156, 164, 184, 269
party politics, 72–3, 101

Patent Act, 129
patent rights, 121, 122, 124, 126, 128, 130, 136, 141, 144, 145, 151, 193, 195, 209, 239, 244, 298
pattern I/II countries, 284
Paulus, Arrie, 36–7
Pauw, Jacques, 55
PCR count, 296–7
peer-reviewed scientific literature, 111, 113, 227
Pfizer, 238–9, 240, 316
Pharasi, Dr Bada, 129–30
pharmaceutical industry
    AIDS drugs strategy, 194
    and AZT, 107, 206, 256
    and Medicines and Related Substances Amendment Bill (No. 30 of 1997), 133
    and nevirapine, 260–1
    and Virodene trials, 131–2, 250
    approach of PhRMA, 124, 129, 141–2, 144
    argument with Eric Sawyer, 193
    Big Pharma appellation, 295
    brand-name and generic drugs and, 298
    Dr Manto Tshabalala-Msimang and, 216
    Dr Nkosasana Dlamini-Zuma and, 90–1, 106, 153, 158
    financial support of International AIDS Conference, 155
    fluconazole as first target of campaign against, 239
    Folb's rejection of Virodene and Medicines Bill, 127
    interdict, 138
    interpretation of Medicines and Related Substances Amendment Bill (No. 30 of 1997), 126
    mistrust of, 121–2
    opposition to competition, 123
    parallel importation, 293–4
    President Thabo Mbeki's accusation of TAC involvement in conspiracy with, 238
    President Thabo Mbeki's belief that CIA working covertly with American, 235
    regulation of, 125
    review of role of Medicines Control Council, 135, 136, 140
    Sarafina II controversy blamed on, 296
    social responsibility campaigns, 240
    South African Medicines Act lawsuit, 143, 145, 175, 192, 195, 241, 242, 243, 244–6, 247, 254
    TAC lawsuit, 271, 279
    US government's active support for, 196, 198, 200, 208–9
    Virodene research blocked by, 110
    world market, 128
Pharmaceutical Manufacturers' Association (PhRMA), 124, 128, 129, 144, 195, 196,

199, 203, 241, 334
Pharmaceutical Manufacturer's Association (PMA), 106, 122, 123, 127, 136, 203, 209, 240, 244, 245, 309, 334
physical abuse, 52, 53, 61, 82
physical symptoms of infection
  boils, 109
  coughing, 74
  diarrhoea, 110
  hepatitis, 186
  herpes sores, 109–10
  pigmentation changes, 216–17
  pneumonia, 16
  thrush, 160, 181–2, 238
  weight gain, 216–17
pilot projects, 151, 216, 254, 257, 259
Piot, Dr Peter, 174, 195, 333
Planned Parenthood Association, 165
plays, 10, 66–7
preventing mother–to–child transmission of HIV (PMTCT)
  advocacy of use of breast-milk substitutes, 208
  and AZT, 151–2, 157, 158, 181, 203, 207–8, 253–5
  and nevirapine, 205, 215–16, 240
  and TAC, 183–184, 208, 247, 248, 249, 259
  and Virodene, 251
  call for national programme, 182, 186, 188–189, 228
  controversy, 161, 164
  cost of, 156–8
  loss of child due to unavailability of, 237
  purchasing of unauthorised drugs for, 239
  research into, 257
  trials
    ACTG 076 trials (1994), 303–4
    Thai regimen (1998), 150, 152, 153, 304
    Petra trial (1999), 304
    HIVNET 012 (1999), 304, 309–10
    SAINT (South African Nevirapine) trial (2000), 304, 318
police, 54, 55, 57
political leaders, 71, 84, 167, 207, 212, 252
politics, 41, 57–8, 68–70, 71, 72–74, 75–76, 79, 99, 106, 138
population control measure, 41, 72, 232
portfolio committee, 128
Porton Down, 26
post-exposure prophylaxis, 234–5, 245, 266
poverty and AIDS, 13, 28, 30, 55, 72, 79, 106, 170, 173, 211, 225, 228, 247–8, 261, 265
pregnant women, 32, 76, 90, 94, 103–4, 141, 150
prescription drugs, 121–2
presidential priority programmes, 83
presidential task team, 266
presidential television address, 156–7

President's Advisory Panel on AIDS, 219–23, 254, 312–13, 314
pricing of medicines, 91, 123, 124, 128
primate origin of HIV, 19, 27, 29, 284
private health care sector, 91, 138, 154
productivity and AIDS, 272, 273
profits, 122, 137, 138, 139, 193, 195, 235, 239, 241, 243, 244, 260–1
promiscuity, 15, 20, 30, 40, 65, 66, 97–8, 170, 211
propaganda, 236, 242, 261
psychosocial factors, 23, 150, 170
Public Accounts Committee, 144
public health sector
  conflict between intellectual property rights and, 246
  funding of, 158
  medicines regulatory authority, 140
  primacy in pharmaceutical and health policies, 142, 143, 195–96
  provision of antiretroviral drugs, 91, 263, 269, 274
  provision of fluconazole, 182, 239
  provision of nevirapine, 248, 258
  provision of post-exposure prophylaxis, 234, 245
  TRIPS agreement and, 200
public hearings, 122
Public Protector, 102, 105, 122, 295

Q
Quirinale, 52

R
racism, 28–31, 39, 105–6, 186, 251, 263
Radio 702, 231
Ramaphosa, Cyril, 39
rape and HIV, 56–8, 60–1, 134, 167, 204, 234, 266, 290, 315
Rasnick, Dr David, 210, 212, 224, 226, 333
Rasool, Ebrahim, 255
Rath Foundation, 278–9
Reconstruction and Development Programme (RDP), 138, 162
redistribution of services and resources, 84
Rees, Dr Helen, 145, 205
regulations, 37, 198, 286
'Rethinking Core Concepts of AIDS' (seminar), 210
Reuters, 193, 240
review, 73, 135, 136, 140
Revised Drug Strategy, 142, 143, 195, 200, 241
right-wing strategies and agendas, 54, 74, 75, 291, 292
risk–benefit relationship, 132
risky behaviour, 42, 104, 120
Robbie, John, 203
Robbins, Dave, 171

Roberts, Dr Ian, 129–30, 196, 206, 212, 310, 333
Ross, Elisabeth Kübler, 16
Rupert, Anton, 90

S

SABC, 141, 260, 278, 314
Sachs, Justice Albie, 266–7
safer sex, 22, 33, 56, 164, 170
Saint trial, 207–8, 215, 253, 254, 310
sanctions, 196, 197, 198
sangoma, 23, 334
SAPA, 212
Sarafina, 95
Sarafina II (Mbongeni Ngema), 96–105, 107, 116–17, 144, 146, 156, 295
SARS, 30
Saturday Independent, 259
SA/US Bi-national trade commission, 196
Sawyer, Eric, 193, 196, 197, 308, 333
Scheepers, Caroline, 274–5
Schlebusch, Johan, 140, 301
Schoofs, Mark, 223, 225
schools, 70, 159, 164, 165–6, 203
Schoub, Prof. Barry, 224, 225–7, 333
scientific community, 27, 110, 116
scientific evidence, 29, 30, 44, 46, 117, 145, 206–7, 212, 223
Secure the Future, 194, 308
security forces, 31, 285
September Commission, 172
Serwadda, Prof. David, 26, 29, 333
Seventh International Global Network of People Living with AIDS (GAP+), 88
sex industry, 24, 27–8, 35, 38–9, 45, 51–5, 59, 77, 79, 168–9, 288
sexuality education, 70, 165
sexually transmitted infections (STIs), 36, 39, 41, 50, 54–5, 287
sexual networks, 66, 169–70, 287
Sexual Offences Act (Act 23 of 1957), 22
shebeens, 34, 35
Shell, Prof. Robert, 59, 289
Shenton, Joan, 31
Sher, Dr Reuben, 23, 24, 36, 37, 43, 176, 333
Shilowa, Premier Mbazima, 257
Shisana, Dr Olive, 96–7, 101, 102, 125–6, 140, 143–5, 295, 333
Sifris, Dr Denis, 21–2, 23, 24, 36, 44, 333
side effects, 112, 116, 117, 131, 151
Sidley, Pat, 242
signage, 24, 25, 50
Simelela, Dr Nono, 195, 254, 258, 308, 333
single-sex dormitory accommodation, 35, 37, 38, 40, 41, 72, 77–8
skin patch, 109, 117, 131
Slabber, Coen (Director-General of Health), 22
Smart, Rose, 67, 111, 162–3, 305, 308, 333
social responsibility campaigns, 240
socio-economic context, 72, 77–8, 106, 201, 211, 274
Sonn, Franklin, 123
South African Communist Party, 69, 233
South African Defence Force (SADF), 45–6
South African Institute for Medical Research (SAIMR), 20, 21, 24, 25, 36, 44
South African Medical Journal, 112
South African Medical Research Council, 61, 271–2
South African Medicines Act, 192, 193, 196, 198
South African Medicines and Medical Devices Regulatory Act (SAMMDRA), 198–9
South African Narcotics Bureau, 199
South African National AIDS Council (SANAC), 252
South African Rapists Association (SARA), 167
The Sowetan, 176, 186, 232–3
Special 301 Watch List, 142, 191–2, 195, 200
species barrier, 19, 27, 29, 284
The Star, 10, 145, 171
statistics, 12, 37, 43–4, 48, 61, 77, 225
stigmatisation, 12, 25, 28, 44, 50, 64, 66, 69, 86, 87, 97, 161, 162, 176, 179, 185, 201, 264, 277
strategic framework, 231
subtype B, 44
subtype C, 44, 46
Summit Club, 52–3
Sunday Argus, 96
Sunday Independent, 110, 131
Sunday Times, 31, 98, 112, 178, 282
Sunter, Clem, 273
support groups, 24, 63, 82, 87, 120, 134, 158, 216–17, 237
Supreme Court, 137
suspicion, 41, 111
Swart, Dr Kenau, 165
symbols, 70–1, 162
symposium on AIDS in Africa (first, 1986), 29
syphilis, 36, 41–2, 56

T

Tanzanian National Institute for Medical Research (NIMR), 249
task team, 129–30, 151
Taxol, 130
TB (tuberculosis), 10, 13, 16, 22, 30, 160, 211
technical advisory group on HIV and AIDS, 24
telephone advice line, 66, 162
television coverage, 88–9, 177, 197
third-force agents, 54, 55, 288–9
3TC, 152, 304, 310, 315

tiered pricing, 152–3
timeline, 324–6
Time magazine, 20, 230
Toms, Dr Ivan, 25, 69, 98, 333
Township AIDS project, 32–3
Township Fever (play), 100
toxicity, 115, 116, 118, 119, 131, 132, 204–7, 210, 215, 216, 226, 250
trade unions, 36–7, 235–6, 247
Trahar, Tony, 272
Treatment Action Campaign (TAC)
   and Dr Manto Tshabalala-Msimang, 212
   and nevirapine, 253
   and outcome of Saint trial, 215
   campaign for prevention of mother-to-child transmission, 183, 184, 208
   campaign in support of government, 242, 243, 244, 245–6, 247, 248
   court action against government, 255, 257, 258, 259, 260, 261, 263, 267–71, 278
   defiance campaign against drug company profiteering, 238–9
   Global March for Treatment, 227
   involvement of Busi Maqungo with, 237
   President Thabo Mbeki's accusation of conspiracy, 235–6
   response to legal letter, 251
   Revised Drug Strategy, 142
   rift between Napwa and, 185, 186, 188
treatment advocacy, 181, 182, 192
treatment programmes, 273, 277
triple therapy, 154, 206, 241
TRIPS (Trade-related Aspects of Intellectual Property Rights) agreement, 121, 126, 128–9, 142, 191, 192, 193, 195, 198, 200, 209, 240–1, 243, 245, 246, 298
TRIPS-Plus patent protection, 200
truck routes, 45, 55, 211, 287
Truth and Reconciliation Commission (TRC) amnesty hearings, 54, 57–8, 167
Tshabalala-Msimang, Dr Manto
   and antiretroviral therapy, 209, 223, 245–6
   and ARV, 217
   and AZT, 210, 212, 234
   and Big Pharma, 240, 245
   and fluconazole, 239
   and nevirapine, 215–16, 253, 254
   and TAC, 243, 247–8, 251, 257, 259–60, 270
   antagonism to AIDS fraternity, 214
   appointment as minister of health, 202–5
   as convenor of AIDS strategy group, 72
   attendance of Barcelona International AIDS Conference, 267
   berating of Anglo American, 272–3
   call on by ANC's health committee to reject denialists' views, 233
   chairing of parliamentary health portfolio committee, 101
   firing of deputy Nozizwe Madlada-Routledge, 281–2
   interview with *Radio 702* presenter John Robbie, 231–2
   involvement in NPPHC, 71
   liaison with advisory panel, 236
   outrage at Durban Declaration, 224
   overview of, 333
   parliamentary address (16 November 1999), 207
   ridiculed by medical doctors, 252
   SABC radio broadcast on World AIDS Day (1 December 2005), 278, 314

Tutu, Archbishop Desmond, 199

U
ubuntu, 14, 17
Ugandan government's AIDS control programme, 26, 29, 31, 70, 84, 203, 220, 260
UNAIDS (United Nations Programme on HIV/AIDS), 150, 156, 174, 195, 240, 255, 256, 260, 271, 274, 296
unemployment, 55, 77, 86, 167–8
United Democratic Front (UDF), 56, 57
United Nations, 36, 155, 200, 272, 286
university ethics committee, 116, 117
UN Security Council agenda, 199–200
urbanisation, 47, 49, 77, 167, 288
US-SA Bi-national Commission, 124
US National Institute for Allergies and Infectious Diseases, 30
US Secretary of Commerce, 123
US Trade Representative (USTR), 142

V
Van der Watt, Herman, 52, 54–5
Van Niekerk, Willie, 65
Van Vuuren, Paul, 55
Venter, Dr Rina, 70, 75, 333
vertical transmission (*see* preventing mother-to-child transmission of HIV)
vigils, 257–8
Viljoen, A.T., 75
The Village Voice, 223
viral load, 296–7
Virodene Pharmaceutical Holdings, 145
Virodene
   and Dr Nkosasana Dlamini-Zuma's support of, 124, 133, 135, 137, 138, 156
   mass media coverage of, 171
   President Thabo Mbeki's support of, 139, 147, 207
   Prof. Peter Folb's rejection of, 127, 132
   research into, 109–10, 115, 116, 117, 118–19, 121, 130–1, 136, 145, 146, 249,

250, 251, 262, 296–7
Visser, Olga, 109–15, 117, 130–1, 139, 145, 206, 251, 297, 310, 333
Visser, Zigi, 110–15, 131–2, 137–8, 139, 145, 206, 249, 250, 262, 297, 310
vitamins, 261, 278–9
voluntary counselling and testing (VCT), 264
Vulliamy, Ed, 108

W

walk-in HIV services, 49, 50
Washington Post, 194, 213
Webster, Prof. Eddie, 37, 39–40
Weg, Kenneth, 194
Whiteside, Prof. Alan, 222, 223, 273, 333
Witness to AIDS, 84
women
  empowerment of, 72, 182
  support groups, 63
  vulnerability of to AIDS, 51, 56, 73, 78–9, 167–8, 170, 179
working conditions, 37, 85, 264
workshops, 11, 12, 33, 159, 203, 280
World AIDS Day, 97, 133, 174, 200
World Bank projections, 13, 273
World Economic Forum (Davos, 1997), 161–2, 229
World Health Assembly (WHA), 142, 144, 191–2, 195, 200, 241, 247, 334

World Health Organisation (WHO)
  advice given by, 127, 128, 129
  AIDS prevention programme, 29
  and nevirapine, 215–16, 254, 260, 261
  antiretroviral treatment campaign, 246, 274
  approval of Revised Drug Strategy, 142
  endorsement of district health system, 89
  Global Programme on AIDS, 36, 76–7, 286, 296
  identification of extreme poverty, 228
  monitoring and analysis of implications of trade agreements for public health, 195–6
  rigorous testing of active ingredient of Virodene, 118
  South African representation to, 191
  standard treatment guidelines, 73, 91
  welcoming of Thai regimen, 150
World Trade Organisation (WTO), 121–2, 126, 147, 192, 208, 246, 298

Y

Young, Peter, 152
youth, 42, 68, 78, 104, 225, 226, 271–2, 321

Z

Zimmerman, Toni, 48, 333
Zuma, Dr Jacob, 61, 252, 269, 333
Zwane, Pule, 167